*The Person with
Alzheimer's Disease*

The Person with

Alzheimer's

Disease

PATHWAYS TO

UNDERSTANDING

THE EXPERIENCE

Edited by

PHYLLIS BRAUDY HARRIS, PH.D.

Professor and Director of the Aging Studies Program
Department of Sociology
John Carroll University
Cleveland, Ohio

THE JOHNS HOPKINS UNIVERSITY PRESS
Baltimore & London

© 2002 The Johns Hopkins University Press
All rights reserved. Published 2002
Printed in the United States of America on acid-free paper
9 8 7 6 5 4 3 2 1

The Johns Hopkins University Press
2715 North Charles Street
Baltimore, Maryland 21218-4363
www.press.jhu.edu

Library of Congress Cataloging-in-Publication Data
The person with Alzheimer's disease : pathways to understanding
the experience / edited by Phyllis Braudy Harris.
        p. cm.
Includes index.
    ISBN 0-8018-6873-4 (hbk. : alk. paper)—ISBN 0-8018-6877-7 (pbk. : alk. paper)
    1. Alzheimer's disease—Popular works.   2. Self-care, Health.
I. Harris, Phyllis Braudy.
    RC523.2 .P47 2002
    362.1'96831—dc21
2001002794

A catalog record for this book is available from the British Library.

To Gloria,

the inspiration for this book,

whose wit, wisdom, and friendship I will always cherish

Contents

List of Contributors   ix

Acknowledgments   xi

Introduction   xiii
   PHYLLIS BRAUDY HARRIS

Prologue: Notes from the Crying Room   xxxi
   GLORIA J. STERIN

Part 1 The Medical Experience

1. Testing Times: The Experience of Neuropsychological Assessment for People with Suspected Alzheimer's Disease   3
   JOHN KEADY AND JANE GILLIARD

2. Medical Experiences and Concerns of People with Alzheimer's Disease   29
   ROSALIE F. YOUNG

Part 2 The Impact of the Diagnosis on Everyday Life

3. Living with the Symptoms of Alzheimer's Disease   49
   ALISON PHINNEY

4. Making the Most of Every Day: Quality of Life   75
   REBECCA G. LOGSDON

5. Selfhood and Alzheimer's Disease   88
   STEVEN R. SABAT

6. *Social and Family Relationships: Establishing and Maintaining Connections* 112

LISA SNYDER

7. *Meaningful Communication throughout the Journey: Clinical Observations* 134

DOROTHY SEMAN

8. *Connecting to the Spirit* 150

JON C. STUCKEY

9. *Building Resilience through Coping and Adapting* 165

PHYLLIS BRAUDY HARRIS AND CASEY DURKIN

Part 3 Experiences with Formal Services

10. *The Experience of People with Dementia in Community Services* 187

CHARLIE MURPHY

11. *Volunteerism: Contributions by Persons with Alzheimer's Disease* 211

JANE STANSELL

12. *The Experience of Support Groups for Persons with Early-Stage Alzheimer's Disease and Their Families* 228

ROBYN YALE AND LISA SNYDER

13. *The Person with Dementia and Artwork: Art Therapy* 246

KATHLEEN KAHN-DENIS

14. *"I Can't Place This Place at All": The Nursing Home Experience* 270

JOHN KILLICK

Index 283

Contributors

Casey Durkin, M.S.S.A., clinical social worker and psychotherapist in private practice, Beachwood, Ohio

Jane Gilliard, B.A. (Admin), C.Q.S.W., director of Dementia Voice (Dementia Services Development Centre for the South West) and honorary special lecturer at the University of Bristol, Blackberry Hill Hospital, Bristol, United Kingdom

Phyllis Braudy Harris, Ph.D., professor and director of the Aging Studies Program, Department of Sociology, John Carroll University, Cleveland, Ohio

Kathleen Kahn-Denis, M.A., A.T.R.-BC, art therapist, Judson Retirement Community, Cleveland, Ohio

John Keady, R.M.N., Dip P.P., Cert.H.Ed., R.N.T., senior lecturer in nursing, School of Nursing and Midwifery, University of Bangor, Wales

John Killick, research fellow in communication through the arts, Dementia Services Development Centre, University of Stirling, Stirling, Scotland

Rebecca G. Logsdon, Ph.D., research associate professor, Department of Psychological and Community Health, Psychiatry and Behavioral Studies, School of Nursing, University of Washington, Seattle

Charlie Murphy, fieldworker for the voluntary sector, Dementia Services Development Centre, University of Stirling, Stirling, Scotland

Alison Phinney, R.N., Ph.D., assistant professor, School of Nursing, University of British Columbia, Vancouver

Steven R. Sabat, Ph.D., associate professor, Department of Psychology, Georgetown University, Washington, D.C.

Dorothy Seman, R.N., M.S., clinical coordinator, Alzheimer's Family Care Center, Chicago, Illinois

Lisa Snyder, M.S.W., L.C.S.W., clinical social worker, Alzheimer's Disease Research Center, University of California, San Diego

Jane Stansell, R.N., M.S.N., director, Alzheimer's Family Care Center, Chicago, Illinois

Gloria J. Sterin, Ph.D., retired, Shaker Heights, Ohio

Jon C. Stuckey, Ph.D., director, Office of Foundations and Grants, Messiah College, Grantham, Pennsylvania

Robyn Yale, M.S.W., L.C.S.W., clinical social worker and consultant to the Alzheimer's Association, San Francisco, California

Rosalie F. Young, Ph.D., associate professor of community medicine, Wayne State University School of Medicine, Detroit, Michigan

Acknowledgments

The quality of an edited volume is only as good as the efforts of its contributors. In this I have been extremely fortunate. I have had the opportunity to work closely with a dedicated group of scholars and practitioners who are truly committed to person-centered dementia care and research. I am indeed indebted to them.

I am very grateful to John Carroll University and the University Committee on Research and Service for continued support of my research in dementia studies. A university faculty research fellowship made it possible for me to be relieved of my regular academic responsibilities in order to finish the editing of this book.

I would also like to thank Wendy Harris, medical editor at the Johns Hopkins University Press, for her guidance and assistance, and Joanne Allen, whose skillful copyediting smoothed out the rough edges.

Last and certainly not least, I want to express my gratitude to the people with Alzheimer's disease and their families whose experiences appear in this book. They gave of their time and hearts to improve the quality of life of others who are struggling with this devastating disease.

Introduction

PHYLLIS BRAUDY HARRIS

> *You don't understand. They don't need to tell me I'm dying with Alzheimer's disease. I **know that**. . . . What they need to do—what **you** need to do—is help me figure out how to **live** with it.*

Mr. Spencer, a 56-year-old retired business executive diagnosed with early-onset Alzheimer's disease (AD), spoke these poignant words to me one summer evening. We were in the midst of a lengthy interview as part of a study aimed at gaining an understanding of AD from the perspectives of people in the early stages of the disease. As the ideas for this volume developed and the book began to take shape, I tried to keep his words in mind.

What Is the Purpose of This Book?

This book addresses the overall question, What is it like to live day to day with a dementing illness such as AD? With recent advances in neuropsychological testing and brain imaging, AD can now be diagnosed with 80–90 percent accuracy (NIA 2000). However, what does it really mean to receive such a diagnosis? How does it affect people's daily lives? How do they cope? And what lessons can be learned from their experiences in order to promote better-quality dementia care? The book seeks answers to these questions.

We have finally moved past the biomedicalization of this disease, and phrases such as *person-centered care*, *culture of dementia*, and *quality of life* are the new buzzwords in the field of dementia research and care. Yet the voices of the real experts—the people who have been diagnosed with a dementing illness—are still muted, and although they may sometimes be heard, often they are not truly listened to.

This book focuses on these people, persons with AD and related dementias. In the chapters that follow, the material is presented from the perspective of the person with AD, the lived experience of dementia. The terms *Alzheimer's disease* and *dementia* are often used interchangeably, and that is the case in this volume since it seeks to understand dementia as a social experience, not from a biomedical perspective. However, *dementia* is the all-encompassing term, describing a particular group of symptoms, with AD being the most common and well-known cause. Other common causes of progressive irreversible dementias are vascular dementia, frontal lobe dementia (including Pick's disease), and dementia with Lewy bodies. These dementias have common symptoms of memory deficits and other cognitive and functional impairments.

AD has metaphorically been described as a journey. Numerous books use that phrase in their titles, for example, *My Journey into Alzheimer's Disease*, by Robert Davis (1989); *Living in the Labyrinth: A Personal Journey through the Maze of Alzheimer's*, by Diana McGowin (1993); and *In a Tangled Wood: An Alzheimer's Journey*, by Joyce Dyer (1996). In this volume the metaphor is used to organize and try to make some sense out of the person's social experience with this disease. It starts at the time of neuropsychological assessment, often the first stop in the journey, and ends with the nursing home experience, often the last stop. This book is largely an exploration of the Western perspective of living with dementia; an examination of cultural differences between and within cultures is not included.

How Does This Book Add to Our Knowledge about the Experience of Alzheimer's Disease?

This volume presents for the first time an overview of the subjective experience of living with progressive memory loss, along with a compilation of some of the leading research in the United States and the United Kingdom. It delves further into the complexities and variability of a person's lived experience, an emerging area of research, examining the medical experiences, the impact of the diagnosis on everyday life, and experiences with formal services.

In the United States, the National Institutes of Health declared the 1990s the "Decade of the Brain," emphasizing the importance of the biochemical basis of behavior. As in the previous decade, the paradigm for viewing AD was the medical model, which sought to understand dementia as neurobiological or neuropsychological processes distinguishable from normal aging. This initiative led to major advances in biomedical research (NIA 2000), no doubt laying the groundwork for discovering the eventual medical treatment and causes of AD. The majority of social and behavioral research funded by the National Institute on Aging in the 1990s focused on the caregiver. Summarizing the research, Marcia Ory (2000) outlined eight major areas, including the prevalence of caregiving; the stressors, mediators, and effects of caregiver burden; and interventions to support family members. This research has produced seminal findings that will be indispensable in providing good-quality dementia care (Schulz 2000). However, out of the eight major research areas, only two included factors solely related to the person with AD.

Unfortunately, in the quest for valuable knowledge the person with the disease became somewhat lost. As some researchers noted, the prevailing medical model defined the condition primarily as a disease, neglecting the social and psychological factors involved in the definition and experience of the illness (Cotrell and Schulz 1993; Froggatt 1988; Lyman 1989). Herskovits (1995) pointed out in her critique of the AD movement that for the most part persons with AD, when seen, were stigmatized, objectified, and viewed as shells of their former selves, so that the attention focused on the needs of the caregivers, not the person with AD, who was deemed unworthy. Post (1995) was one of the first bioethicists to cause dementia researchers to rethink this stance.

A few researchers, such as Cohen (1991) and Sabat and Harre (1992), discussed the subjective experience of AD, but they were rarely heard or, if heard, largely disregarded. There were also a few firsthand narratives from individuals describing the experience of living with dementia (Davis 1989; McGowin 1993; Rose 1996), but these were viewed primarily as anecdotal.

In the United Kingdom, however, in addition to the parallel development in biomedical research and in research on the caregiver experience, there was also growing interest in the "person with dementia," emphasizing social-psychological care. Tom Kitwood and the Bradford Dementia

Group led this movement in dementia care (Woods 2001). They advocated a shift in emphasis from the biomedical paradigm to a paradigm that *recognized* and *valued* the subjective experiences of those with dementia. Such a shift places the concerns, needs, and interests of those individuals with dementia, as defined by them verbally and nonverbally, in the center of the dementia care arena (Kitwood 1990, 1993a, 1993b, 1997a, 1997b; Kitwood and Benson, 1995). Kitwood and Benson expounded on progressive ways of working with people with dementia, emphasizing the relationship aspects, guided by the principle, "Look at the person, not the diagnosis." Kitwood, in his last book before his death (1997a), summarized his work on personhood and person-centered dementia care over the preceding decade, emphasizing the importance of having an accurate understanding of a person's needs, wants, likes, values, interests, and abilities. He discussed the ethical, social-psychological, and neurological significance of dementia, a view that encompasses the whole person. Instead of defining a person experiencing dementia solely by his or her neurological impairment, Kitwood proposed a framework that emphasized the social-psychological experiences of the individual that interact with the neurological processes.

Previous to this shift most information about the experience of dementia had been secondhand, from interviews with and the observations and surveys of caregivers (see Aneshensel et al. 1995); Herskovits (1995, 148) observed that "very little was being asked of those with dementia, much was speculated and asserted about them." Now, because of the paradigm shift, writings of people with AD are being given more credibility. Works such as Henderson's *Partial View: An Alzheimer's Journal* (1998), with his insightful portrayal of the impact of the disease on himself and his family, are receiving attention.

Practitioners and researchers in both the United States and the United Kingdom have begun to shift their focus. Downs (1997) reviewed the literature on the emergence of the person in dementia research. She outlined three major areas of inquiry: the individual's sense of self, the person's rights, and the perspective of individuals with dementia. The last is the focus of this book. The emergence of this area is evidenced by the books of Malcolm Goldsmith (*Hearing the Voice of People with Dementia* [1996]), Robyn Yale (*Developing Support Groups for Individuals with Early Stage Alzheimer's Disease* [1995]), and more recently, Lisa Snyder (*Speaking Our*

Minds [1999]), Daniel Kuhn (*Alzheimer's Early Stages* [1999]), Sam Fazio, Dorothy Seman, and Jane Stansell (*Rethinking Alzheimer's Care* [1999]), and Steven Sabat (*The Experience of Alzheimer's Disease* [2001]). Goldsmith presents various accounts of people in the later stages of dementia, with the overriding goal of providing a more in-depth, diverse, and complex picture of individuals with this disease, underscoring the need to develop more flexible, person-centered services. Yale, through discussion of support groups for people with early-stage AD and their families, shares with us these persons' insights into their experiences with AD. Snyder describes, with a rich use of quotations, the lives of seven people in early-stage AD whom she met in her role as a social worker. Her goal is for us to see and hear them as people struggling with a disease rather than to simply view them, as they are most often viewed, in terms of the label "Alzheimer's victims." Kuhn was one of the first people to focus mainly on the needs and concerns of people and their families in early-stage AD, providing a guide for treatment and care. He included extensive quotations from persons with AD. Similar to Kitwood, Fazio, Seman, and Stansell urge us to rethink our notions about providing dementia care. They ask us to understand the necessity of including both the human element and relationships in our care, reminiscent of the I-thou relationship (Buber 1937), in order to assist the person with dementia to live as full and meaningful a life as possible. Sabat, through his case studies and analyses, assists us in reaching a deep psychological understanding of the impact of AD on the selfhood of a person.

Together, these writings help guide us to an understanding of the person's experience with dementia. This book represents another step on that path. The decade of the 1990s was a time of learning about the biomedical aspects of AD and caregiving; this next decade must also be a time of learning about the lived experience of AD.

What Methods Are Used?

The conceptual framework that undergirds the chapters in this volume is the unequivocal acceptance of the importance of the paradigm that recognizes and values the social and psychological experiences, the person's subjective experience of dementia. This does not negate the critical importance of obtaining an extensive medical understanding of the disease—its

symptoms, prognosis, progression, treatment and management, and biomedical ramifications. However, what the authors clearly state is, as Kitwood (1997a) advocated, "The person comes first."

As stated earlier, this paradigm shift started to occur only in the last
decade, so as much as one might intellectually agree with this premise, the
methodology for getting at the type of information that will broaden our
understanding of the perspective of a person with AD is still in its infancy.
Little is known about the subjective experience of living with a dementing
illness such as AD. Thus, the question then becomes, how best can we gain
access to the person's complex and variable world of dementia?

Quality-of-life (QOL) measures represent an attempt to quantify some
of that complexity, which would aid the clinicians who provide hands-on
care, as well as researchers. Some of the leading researchers have worked
on and written about designs for such measures for frail elderly people and
persons with AD (Albert and Logsdon 2000; Birren and Dieckmann 1991;
Brod, Stewart, and Sands 1999; Lawton 1991, 1997). In this volume, Logsdon (see chapter 4) clearly and concisely summarizes the research. QOL
measures for dementia are very useful global constructs to help us improve
the life of persons with AD, many of whom have lost the ability to communicate their needs and wants. It is one method of accessing and assessing the subjective experience of dementia. Yet, in trying to quantify the
subjective experience, we can lose the richness and the complexity of the
data before we really understand all the variables.

The quantitative approach to gathering information related to a social-
psychological phenomenon won't provide us with the in-depth knowledge
that is essential for our understanding of a person's experience. We are dealing with people who in the early stages of the disease are still able, if given
the opportunity, to rather eloquently give voice to their experiences, even
though their reading and writing skills may be impaired and their ability to
follow complex concepts may be limited. And in the later stages of the disease some meaningful communication is still possible (see Seman's and Killick's chapters, 7 and 14).

Therefore, multiple ways are needed to enter this "new culture of dementia care," as Kitwood and Benson (1995) called it, approaches that allow a close-up, more personal, in-depth view of dementia's impact. The
person's experience with dementia is, by its very nature, an ever-changing,
complex, confusing, all-encompassing, and life-altering experience that

affects self-identity, social relationships, physical, cognitive, and mental functioning, communication, spirituality, issues of autonomy, and above all his or her feeling of being accepted as fully human.

Alternative methodologies are needed to broaden our knowledge and generate different social realities. Leaders in the fields of social work and gerontology are beginning to recognize the importance of including such methods in their research (Witkin 2000; Branch 2000). Kitwood (1997a, 1997b) championed using more qualitative methods, such as analyzing accounts written by people with dementia, carefully listening to what people say in interviews or in a group context, and using poetry as a powerful and linguistic form to enter this uncharted territory. Qualitative research makes no claims to be representative of the population it is studying, but its purpose is to provide that in-depth examination.

This book advances this stance, using a multitude of methods, as well as QOL measures, for example, personal essays and memoirs, in-depth qualitative interviews, participant-observation, focus groups, community dialogues, case study analyses, clinical interviews and observations, dementia care mapping, checklists, poetry, artwork, and a review of writings by people with dementia. All are methods for trying to obtain a broader, richer view of dementia. Taken together, the chapters in this volume open a window of clarity onto the daily experiences of people living with AD. They assist us in accessing different pathways, all converging to increase our understanding of the person, a critical component in the provision of quality dementia care.

What Is the Structure of This Book?

This book traces the experiences of different persons with AD from the time of assessment through the nursing home experience. The authors present, based on their data, the perspectives of persons with AD in terms of one or more facets of that journey. Each chapter concludes with a discussion of lessons learned, specifically how the data presented might be used by health care professionals and family members to promote more person-centered dementia care.

Opening the book is a personal memoir of a researcher's experience of living with AD. In the prologue, "Notes from the Crying Room," Gloria Sterin's powerful writing style quickly pulls us into her world, beginning with the time when she began to suspect that she had AD. She discusses her experiences along this journey and honestly and openly shares her feelings and reactions to what has happened to her. Her poignant essay sets the stage for the rest of the book, introducing topics that are the focus of many of the chapters to follow.

The chapters are divided into three parts: "The Medical Experience," "The Impact of the Diagnosis on Everyday Life," and "Experiences with Formal Services." Part I, composed of two chapters, deals with the assessment and ultimately the diagnosis of probable AD or a related dementia. In a person's and family's struggle to ascertain what is happening to their lives a medical facility is often the first stop.

Chapter 1, "Testing Times: The Neuropsychological Assessment for People with Suspected Alzheimer's Disease," by John Keady and Jane Gilliard, introduces us to the assessment experience from the perspective of the person who suspects that he or she has AD. They guide us through three phases of the process of seeking help, which they have identified through in-depth qualitative interviews, allowing us to hear the voices of the men and women being assessed. Throughout the chapter, Keady and Gilliard argue that the assessment process need not be a poor early experience for people with dementia and their families. This experience can be dramatically altered by an effort by health care professionals to instill hope, by their being aware of the individual's unique biography, by their showing genuine respect for them as human beings, and by their treating persons with AD as partners in the diagnostic process rather than subjects.

Chapter 2, "Medical Experience and Concerns of People with Alzheimer's Disease," by Rosalie Young, takes us through the next stage of the journey, the disclosure of the diagnosis and the nature of the medical encounters. Through qualitative analysis of a series of focus groups involving people recently diagnosed with AD and some of their family members, their reactions and responses to this experience, as well as their coping abilities, emerge. Young also explores interactions and communications with physicians during this process and identifies a pattern of dyadic interaction, usually between a spouse and a physician, similar to the relationship between a parent and a physician in pediatric care. Recommendations for improving these interactions are provided.

Part II, the largest of the three parts, explores the impact of the diagnosis on people's everyday lives. Once the diagnosis has been confirmed, what does it mean to live with a dementing illness on a daily basis? The common symptoms of dementia—memory problems, getting lost, communication difficulties, diminishing insight, and difficulties using common everyday objects—are well known. In chapter 3, "Living with the Symptoms of Alzheimer's Disease," Alison Phinney through in-depth qualitative interviews shows what it is like to live with these symptoms. As Phinney explains, "To describe one's symptoms is to articulate something of the very meaning of the illness itself."

Chapter 4, "Making the Most of Every Day: Quality of Life," by Rebecca Logsdon, provides an overview of the concept of quality of life and its measurement. She demonstrates how the QOL-AD, a measure that she and her colleagues developed (Logsdon et al. 1999), can be helpful in dividing persons with AD into those with high QOL and low QOL. Using these categories, strategies to maximize QOL for people with AD can be developed and are suggested. QOL measurement provides a global perspective on the AD experience, and many of the chapters that follow delve further into the variability and complexity of the domains that the QOL measures identify.

A diagnosis of AD can have a devastating impact on one's psychological well-being, especially on one's concept of self and personal identity. Cohen and Eisdorfer (1986) have asserted that a loss of self accompanies AD. Yet Steven Sabat, in chapter 5, "Selfhood and Alzheimer's Disease," delves into the complexity of selfhood, revealing its components, and persuasively argues against the commonly held belief about the loss of self. He demonstrates through the analysis of case studies, clients he has seen in his clinical practice, that (1) the self of personal identity remains intact throughout many of the stages of this progressive disease, (2) there is a self composed of attributes that persists far into the course of the disease, and (3) the preservation of the social self is very much dependent on the quality of the social interactions experienced.

However, Alzheimer's is not a disease that affects just one person; it is a family disease on many different levels. Families are dramatically affected, as a whole caregiver literature attests. In chapter 6, "Social and Family Relationships: Establishing and Maintaining Connections," Lisa Snyder draws our attention to the person's perspective as the disease unravels his or her social roles, responsibilities, and relationships. Snyder's rich data are drawn from her clinical and group interviews analyzed for common themes, the writings of people with dementia, and a review of the literature and videos that document the perspective of the person with AD. Snyder emphasizes the importance of family and social relationships and advocates for evaluating the relational needs of the person with AD.

One of the major ways that dementia affects daily life is its impact on a person's communication skills. We have come to accept that as the disease progresses, significant communication becomes impossible for the person with AD. Yet in chapter 7, "Meaningful Communication throughout the Journey: Clinical Observations," Dorothy Seman calls this assumption into question. Her observations and clinical insights about people's interactions in a group context, an adult day care center, are keen. Seman demonstrates the enduring ability of people, even in the later stages of AD, to communicate with and relate to one another in meaningful, deep, and empathetic ways. The poignant vignettes that she shares allow us to broaden our perspective about the possibility of meaningful communication with persons with AD, a position she strongly advances throughout her chapter.

People often turn to religious and spiritual beliefs in times of crisis. Is this ability to connect to the social and sacred realm still possible for persons with AD? Jon Stuckey's premise in chapter 8, "Connecting to the Spirit," is that the human spirit has the capacity to emerge above the ravages of the disease and find its connection in a multitude of ways. Through a community dialogue on religion, spirituality, and AD we are introduced to people who openly reveal their spirituality, disclosing the meaning and peace it brings to their lives. Stuckey suggests guidelines for assisting persons with AD to maintain these connections.

On a daily basis persons with AD face the challenge of living and trying to maintain some control over lives that are constantly changing. How do they cope and adapt to the multiple onslaughts they experience? In the final chapter of part II, "Building Resilience through Coping and Adapting," Casey Durkin and I argue that the strengths of persons with AD are often overlooked in dementia care research. They are seen mainly as stressors or care recipients, yet many people are engaged in positive proactive coping strategies, such as using spirituality as Stuckey delineates. Through in-depth qualitative interviews, coping strategies are identified and the voices of the men and woman emerge to elucidate their experiences. Specific action steps for family members and health care professionals to promote positive coping are proposed.

The journey continues in part III, where the experiences of persons with AD in formal care settings are examined. Inevitably, as the disease progresses, persons with AD have some contact with formal dementia care services. Part III explores their experiences with community services, adult day care centers, early-stage support groups, and nursing homes.

In chapter 10, "The Experience of People with Dementia in Community Services," Charlie Murphy reveals through qualitative interviews, dementia care mapping, and a checklist for activities participants' evaluations of two community programs in Scotland: a drop-in center with a café-like environment for individuals with dementia and their family members and a befriending service (friendly visiting). Throughout the chapter Murphy's ethical concerns and sensitivity to the people that he is studying are apparent. He provides practical steps to consider when undertaking such a research evaluation of persons with AD and offers useful clinical insights about programming activities gained from the people's responses.

In contrast to Murphy, Jane Stansell, in chapter 11, "Volunteerism: Contributions by Persons with Alzheimer's Disease," urges us to view persons with AD not only as consumers of services but also as people still capable of providing services to others. She describes a volunteer program developed at an adult day care program in Chicago. Common themes of people's reactions to their volunteer work were gleaned from taped sessions of morning support groups and from staff notes on the volunteers' comments. Most important, Stansell's work shows that "persons with AD can be contributing members of society, not burdens."

Support groups for caregivers provide social emotional support, an opportunity to gather up-to-date information on AD-related issues, and a place to obtain helpful caregiving tips. These types of groups have been a mainstay of dementia care services. In the last decade, with the increased awareness of the social and psychological needs of persons with AD, early-stage support groups for them have been developed. In chapter 12, "The Experience of Support Groups for Participants with Early-Stage Alzheimer's Disease and Their Families," Robyn Yale and Lisa Snyder provides us with an overview of this movement, the different models, and steps to consider in developing such a program. From their evaluation research and clinical observations of early-stage support groups, which they have led for persons with AD and their families, they share with us the participants' reactions.

The last stop for some people in the Alzheimer's journey is the nursing home. When the care at home becomes too difficult and overwhelming for families, the services of nursing homes are sought, be it day care programs attached to a nursing home facility or institutional care itself. When people enter later stages of the disease and communication becomes more difficult, what pathways are available to access their feelings and thoughts about their condition? What are their experiences in nursing homes, their new and strange living environment? As Seman shows in chapter 7, meaningful communication is still possible.

The final two chapters speak to ways of continuing this communication in institutional settings, using alternative methods. In chapter 13, "The Person with Dementia and Artwork: Art Therapy," Kathleen Kahn-Denis introduces us to the medium of art, a nonverbal modality, as a way to reach persons with AD. She takes us through an analysis of three people's artwork, visually demonstrating how their personhood, humor, emotions, and insights resurface throughout the course of the disease. This process of creating subjective images not only can give people some control but is a way for them to still access and communicate their individual identities.

The volume closes with poems—powerful, poignant, eloquent words of people in the later stages of dementia fashioned together by John Killick in his chapter about the nursing home experience, aptly titled "I Can't Place This Place at All." Killick, through his ability to connect with people with dementia in nursing homes, allows us to interpret or understand their thoughts and learn about their losses and struggles to make sense out of the demands of the strange land in which they find themselves. Despite everything, their humor and humanity prevail and glimmer in their words. As Killick deftly demonstrates, the words the people speak are not gibberish but filled with meaning, words worthy of careful attention.

What Lessons Can Be Learned?

At the end of their chapters the authors discuss specific lessons learned related to their research or clinical findings. These are important lessons for students, health care professionals, researchers, and family members to digest and understand. There are, though, some lessons learned that are common to many of the chapters. These fall into three major categories: general insights learned about persons with AD, clinical implications, and lessons to consider when doing research with persons with AD.

General Insights

- Look at persons with AD as multifaceted human beings. Their diagnosis should not define the scope or terms of their relationships.
- Be cognizant that "Alzheimer's disease" is a powerful label that has a significant psychological impact on a person's self-concept and social relationships.
- Take the time to truly understand what the diagnosis of AD means for an individual and maintain a level of openness in that process.
- Individuals in the early and middle stages of AD can and often want to talk about their experiences of living with the disease.
- In order for persons with AD to deal with the disease, it is necessary for them to disclose their fears and concerns about the diagnosis to trusted persons.
- Persons with AD are capable of strong feelings and have the need for close human social interaction.
- Maintaining positive social relationships with significant others in their lives is of paramount importance to the quality of life of persons with AD.
- Persons with AD do not automatically lose the capacity to maintain meaningful connections to the social and spiritual realms upon being diagnosed with the disease AD.
- Persons with AD should be seen not as stressors but as people with strengths that can be used as resources.
- Relationships are the primary vehicle of care for persons with AD.

Clinical Implications

- The physician-person dyad is fraught with difficulties because persons with AD are not seen as partners in the process of assessment, diagnosis, and treatment. A person's report of symptoms must be listened to and taken seriously.
- The importance of instilling a realistic hope throughout the course of the assessment and treatment cannot be overestimated.

• It is important to be aware of the extent of depression that often accompanies a diagnosis of AD and the need to treat that illness.
• Referrals to support groups, activity programs, or counseling can be beneficial for some persons with AD and should be included as treatment options.
• It is necessary to understand each person's unique biography.
• A person with AD is capable of communication with meaning across the course of the disease, but clinicians need to modify their approach in order to give the person time to process and respond. Close attention should be paid to both verbal and nonverbal responses.
• Do not underestimate the significance of the environment, physical and social, in fostering or inhibiting relationships.
• Clinicians who think of persons with AD only in terms of loss and do not consider their abilities lose opportunities to promote the persons' independence and assist in maintaining their level of functioning.
• Many persons with AD describe their quality of life as good or excellent despite multiple losses.
• It is important to recognize the ability of persons with AD to adapt and use positive coping strategies to deal with the devastating losses.
• Persons with AD can face adversity, learn to cope, and build resilience.
• Most effective are multifaceted, multidisciplinary interventions that build on strengths, teach coping strategies, and provide assistance when necessary.

Recommendations for Doing Research with Persons with AD

• Interviewers must be knowledgeable and understanding about AD.
• Provide time to interview persons with AD and their family caregivers together and separately. Both need time to voice their concerns.
• It is of critical importance to take time and to gain the trust of persons with AD before the research is started.
• The true meaning of informed consent must be adhered to.
• Allow the person with AD to set the pace of the interview.
• It is possible to have meaningful and constructive interviews with people in the early and middle stages of AD. However, the researcher needs to be sensitive to any strain the interview may cause the person and adjust the length of the interview and questioning accordingly.

• The researcher needs to try to achieve a balance between intrusion and necessary data collection.

• Schedule interviews for the times during the day when the persons with AD are most productive.

As these recommendations suggest, much can be learned from the experts, the persons with AD.

Thus, by using multiple methods leading to a broadening of our understanding of the person's social reality of AD, we have opened various pathways to understanding the person and the lived experience of dementia. Also from this research come recommendations for providing quality person-centered dementia care. I hope that in the process we have at least partially fulfilled the plea expressed by Mr. Spencer in the quotation at the beginning of this introduction: to help him find ways to restructure a life with meaning, despite Alzheimer's disease.

REFERENCES

Albert, S. M., and R. G. Logsdon, eds. 2000. *Assessing quality of life in dementia*. New York: Springer.

Aneshensel, C. S., J. T. Mullan, L. I. Pearlin, C. J. Whitlatch, and S. H. Zarit. 1995. *Profiles in caregiving: The unexpected career*. San Diego, Calif.: Academic.

Birren, J. E., and L. Dieckmann. 1991. Concepts and quality of life in the later years: An overview. In *The concept and quality of life in the frail elderly*, ed. J. E. Birren, J. E. Lubben, J. C. Rowe, and D. E. Deutchman, 334–60. New York: Academic.

Branch, L. G. 2000. Editorial. *Gerontologist* 40 (4): 389.

Brod, M., A. L. Stewart, and C. Sands. 1999. Conceptualization of quality of life in dementia. *Journal of Mental Health and Aging* 5 (1): 7–19.

Buber, M. 1937. *I and thou*. Trans. R. Gregor Smith. Edinburgh: Clark.

Cohen, D. 1991. The subjective experience of Alzheimer's disease: The anatomy of an illness as perceived by patients and families. *American Journal of Alzheimer's Care and Related Disorders and Research*, May/June, 6–11.

Cohen, D., and C. Eisdorfer. 1986. *The loss of self*. New York: Norton.

Cotrell, V., and R. Schulz. 1993. The perspective of the patient with Alzheimer's disease: A neglected dimension of dementia research. *Gerontologist* 33 (2): 205–11.

Davis, R. 1989. *My journey into Alzheimer's disease*. Wheaton, Ill.: Tyndale.

Downs, M. 1997. The emergence of the person in dementia care research. *Aging and Society* 17:597–607.

Dyer, Joyce. 1996. *In a tangled wood: An Alzheimer's journey*. Dallas: Southern Methodist Univ. Press.

Fazio, S., D. Seman, and J. Stansell. 1999. *Rethinking Alzheimer's care*. Baltimore: Health Professions Press.

Froggatt, A. 1988. Self-awareness in early dementia in mental health problems in old age: A reader. In *Mental health problems in old age*, ed. B. Gearing, M. Johnson, and T. Heller, 131–36. Buckingham: Open Univ. Press.

Goldsmith, M. 1996. *Hearing the voice of people with dementia: Opportunities and obstacles*. Bristol, Pa.: Jessica Kingsley.

Henderson, C. S. 1998. *Partial view: An Alzheimer's journal*. Dallas: Southern Methodist Univ. Press.

Herskovits, E. 1995. Struggling out subjectivity: Debates about the "self" and Alzheimer's disease. *Medical Anthropology Quarterly* 9 (2): 146–64.

Kitwood, T. 1990. The dialectics of dementia: With particular reference to Alzheimer's disease. *Aging and Society* 10:177–96.

———. 1993a. Person and process in dementia. *International Journal of Geriatric Psychiatry* 8:541–45.

———. 1993b. Towards a theory of dementia care: The interpersonal process. *Aging and Society* 13:51–67.

———. 1997a. *Dementia reconsidered: The person comes first*. Buckingham: Open Univ. Press.

———. 1997b. The experience of dementia. *Aging and Mental Health* 1:13–22.

Kitwood, T., and S. Benson. 1995. *The new culture of dementia care*. London: Hawker.

Kuhn, D. 1999. *Alzheimer's early stages: First steps in caring and treatment*. Berkeley: Hunter House.

Lawton, M. P. 1991. A multidimensional view of quality of life in frail elder. In *The concept and quality of life in the frail elderly*, ed. J. E. Birren, J. E. Lubben, J. C. Rowe, and D. E. Deutchman, 4–27. New York: Academic.

———. 1997. Assessing quality of life in Alzheimer's disease research. *Alzheimer's Disease and Related Disorders* 11 (suppl. 6): 91–99.

Lawton, M. P., K. Van Haitsma, and M. Perkinson. 2000. Emotion in people with dementia: A way of comprehending their preferences and aversion. In *Interventions in dementia care: Toward improving quality of life*, ed. M. P. Lawton and R. L. Rubinstein, 95–119. New York: Springer.

Logsdon, R. G., L. E. Gibbons, S. M. McCurry, and L. Teri. 1999. Quality of life in Alzheimer's disease: Patient and caregiver reports. *Journal of Mental Health and Aging* 5 (1): 21–32.

Lyman, K. 1989. Bringing the social back in: A critique of the biomedicalization of dementia. *Gerontologist* 29 (5): 597–605.

McGowin, D. F. 1993. *Living in the labyrinth: A personal journey through the maze of Alzheimer's*. San Francisco: Elder.

National Institute on Aging (NIA). 2000. *Progress report on Alzheimer's disease*. Silver Spring, Md.: Alzheimer's Disease Education and Research Center.

Ory, M. G. 2000. Afterword: Dementia caregiving at the end of the twentieth century.

In *Interventions in dementia care: Toward improving quality of life*, ed. M. P. Lawton and R. L. Rubinstein, 173–79. New York: Springer.

Post, S. G. 1995. *The moral challenge of Alzheimer's disease*. Baltimore: Johns Hopkins Univ. Press.

Rose, L. 1996. *Show me the way to go home*. San Francisco: Elder.

Sabat, S. R. 2001. *The experience of Alzheimer's disease: Life through a tangled veil*. Oxford: Blackwell.

Sabat, S. R., and R. Harre. 1992. The construction and deconstruction of self in Alzheimer's disease. *Aging and Society* 12:443–61.

Schultz, R., ed. 2000. *Handbook on dementia caregiving*. New York: Springer.

Snyder, L. 1999. *Speaking our minds*. New York: W. H. Freeman.

Witkin, S. L. 2000. Editorial: Writing social work. *Social Work* 45 (5): 389–94.

Woods, R. T. 2001. Discovering the person with Alzheimer's disease: Cognitive, emotional, and behavioral aspects. *Aging and Mental Health* 5 (supplemental): S7–S16.

Yale, R. 1995. *Developing support groups for individuals with early stage Alzheimer's disease: Planning, implementation, and evaluation*. Baltimore: Health Professionals Press.

Prologue
Notes from the Crying Room

GLORIA J. STERIN

I had no idea when my husband had begun to notice signs in my behavior that made him suspect early-stage Alzheimer's disease (AD). However, I knew I was having inordinate difficulty preparing and presenting some of the lectures for a class I taught in a postdoctoral sociology program, not realizing then that only lectures based on new material caused trouble. Topics I had discussed frequently with former classes went smoothly. I lectured easily, stimulated lively discussion, and responded to questions without any problem. But when teaching new material, I found myself reading directly from notes. Or I'd become confused and lose my train of thought, forgetting where I was in the lecture and what I had planned to say.

I was puzzled and disturbed by the inexplicable unevenness of my performance. Concurrently, at home in the evening I struggled to compose a letter of condolence to a friend whose husband had died. I was having a dreadful time with that as well. Each time I paused to review what I had typed, I found segments repeated, often more than once, containing identical words and phrases. There were major problems with sequence, as I lost my train of thought and wandered into odd, illogical digressions. It was bizarre and becoming frightening.

To make matters worse, I began to notice a strange sensation I thought of as a fog in my head. At first infrequent and fleeting, it became progressively more intrusive and distracting, seeming to permeate my brain, making it hard to think clearly. Altogether, my world was becoming strangely unpredictable and unreal. The sense of unreality intensified as I constantly forgot what I was in the process of doing. I would go into a room to get something, but when I got there I had no idea what I wanted. I would have to return to where I had been before to find out. It was surreal.

Meantime, the letter to my friend had become a source of trauma approaching despair! This was incomprehensible; writing had always been my chief skill. At 14, in an essay contest I won a prize of $100 (a huge sum in 1938 Depression days) and a two-week trip to Toronto, Canada, from my home in Winnipeg. Now I could not compose a coherent letter to a friend. I spent so much time on that letter, it seemed to take on a life of its own! It was a long, difficult time before I faced the fact that something was seriously wrong.

Finally, in our car one day, I suddenly asked my husband (a physician) if he thought I had Alzheimer's disease. That idea had not consciously entered my head until I heard myself ask the question. Very gently and sadly, but without hesitation, he said, "Yes, I do." After that, I recall only a feeling of sick despair—for a long while I couldn't breathe—and asking a God I didn't believe in to let me die quickly. I could not imagine a future with such a disease.

For some time—I'm not sure how long—I lived apathetically, with little enthusiasm and recurrent depression, not sure what to do with the rest of my life. My husband was supportive and understanding, but we both were drained by the multiple consequences of our joint disaster. The major trauma for me has been the humiliation of dependency. The greater part of my life had been characterized by independence and confidence that I could meet any challenge. That was before I knew what kind of challenge I would finally face. My partner, lover, and best friend became transformed into my *caregiver*, a kind and loving word, but when applied to my husband, it summarized dramatically what had happened to my life. Because being cared about is one thing and conveys mutuality; being cared for is one-sided and not my cup of tea! I don't know how to live that role. Worse, I don't want to know! Imagine how difficult such an attitude has to make life for my unfortunate caregiver. I hate being the source of added difficulties for him, but I just don't know how to be gracefully dependent.

The timing and sequence of subsequent events is a blur now, but it must have been soon afterward that I first went to the Alzheimer Center. It was fortuitous timing. The newest drug for AD had just become available, and I was invited to participate in its testing.

There was a lift in morale when I began to participate in a research project on AD. I thought of it as making scrambled eggs (if you drop and break a carton of eggs, don't waste them; pick out the shells and scramble the eggs). To be of real use in life is a gift. We never realize, ordinarily, how critically important that is to self-esteem. Participation in the research was not always easy, often embarrassing, confronting me with the glaring deficits the tests revealed. But the staff was understanding and supportive, so respectful of a suddenly fragile dignity that I was never reluctant to participate in a testing.

There was a unique atmosphere there, unlike anything I had encountered before. Without exception, the staff were clearly dedicated to their work, seemed to like and respect their clients, and were exceptionally sensitive to the trauma and upheaval in the lives of the families they served. Everything was done to make visits there easy and pleasant. I once told my husband that I was sure everyone at the center had to be taking niceness pills, so uniformly kind, understanding, and sympathetic were they, so patiently genuine in their concern for us, "the demented ones."

Once I began regular visits as part of the study for evaluation of medication I was taking, I became less depressed and very much interested in the methods and mechanics of the assessment process. Before the onset of my unwelcome disease, I had obtained a Ph.D. in sociology and managed several fairly large research projects, some of which I had helped design. So naturally I was very interested in the way this piece of research was being carried out. From the first visit to the center, and throughout the study, I was impressed by the thoroughness of the testing procedures, the attention to detail I saw, but even more impressed by the kindness and professionalism of the staff.

Now about those tests: I was not trying to trick them—I am not sure that *trick* is exactly the right word. It just happened that after I had taken the same test at each evaluation, for I'm not sure how many visits, the words *apple, penny,* and *table* got into my memory and were just subsequently available. So when I heard the introduction to that particular set come up, I would answer the question before the tester had time to finish reading me the questions, surprising the testers.

However, my initial reaction to my neurologist was not as warm as my reaction to the rest of the staff. I'm not sure when it was, but it must have been after one of our first visits to the center. My husband was with me when my doctor came to see me, and before I had time to say anything to him, the two of them were having a virtual medical meeting on AD, while I listened, getting more and more frustrated because I was forgetting what I wanted to ask and they both seemed to have forgotten that I was there.

I felt as though I was being treated like a child, expected to sit quietly while the adults had their important discussion, which I could not be expected to understand. At a later session I got my act together, and when they started their conversation, I barged in and told the neurologist I had questions. He pushed back his chair, listened carefully, and answered very fully. In retrospect, it may or may not be true that he made some erroneous assumptions, but my failure to speak out sooner was just as much, if not more, to blame.

The center suggested that my husband and I join a support group for people with early-stage Alzheimer's and their spouses. This particular topic is harder for me to discuss than anything else I can think of. I went to one meeting of a support group. I was not sure I wanted to go in the first place. I did not go back. The support group seemed to be helping some people; however, I didn't want to be labeled. I didn't want my disease to be my defining characteristic. And in all of my former careers—nursing, social work, academic sociology, and sociological research, all related to the helping professions—I had been the helper.

After a while, I started writing down my feelings and reactions to my diagnosis in a file called "The Crying Room," where I "went" when feeling low. It was an offshoot of therapy sessions I had started soon after being diagnosed with AD to deal with a depression that threatened to be overwhelming. I had been in a turmoil of fluctuating emotions—fear, anger, shame, and suicidal thoughts. I hit bottom then, feeling that my life was effectively over. There seemed to be little in it for me anymore. One of my earlier careers had been social casework. I had done counseling in several settings, and I realized that now I myself needed some objective help. A therapist was recommended, and I went to see her. I liked her instantly.

The social worker was empathic, intelligent, and realistic. I felt that she understood where I was, and I left her office feeling better, more alive, than I had for some time. But driving home afterward, my husband asked how the session had gone, and with a sickening jolt I realized that I could recall nothing about what had transpired except the ambiance; the good feeling that I had had during the session had now evaporated. I had come to the car feeling lighter, relaxed, and energized. Now I felt like a pricked balloon—deflated! It's impossible to overstate the impact of that emotional nosedive after the buoyancy of the mood just moments before. As long ago as it was, I still recall vividly the sick feeling I had about that total memory wipeout.

My resourceful husband suggested I tape subsequent visits—an inspired idea, ultimately saving time and money. I taped and typed up all subsequent sessions. After several were done, I read through them at one sitting, curious to see what had changed over time. It was evident that talking out my feelings about the disease and my fears of the future had helped me to clarify my thinking and to recognize patterns in how I sometimes helped, but often hindered, myself in dealing with this new and weird phase of my life. It also made me realize that I had said most of what there was to say on the subject and had begun to repeat myself. Certainly I was far from resolving all the issues about how to play the hand I'd been dealt, but the tapes gave me an overview of where I was in my journey and a handle on what I still had to deal with. I lived one day at a time, not really unhappy but without much enthusiasm for a life that seemed to promise a downward spiral to a depressing end. I discontinued the sessions with the social worker, but at low moments I would reread one or more of the transcripts, which helped me focus on positives. The practical common sense of her approach helped me to switch from hopeless misery to action on my own behalf, to regain objectivity and remember that it really is better to light a candle than to curse the darkness. Objectivity favors mobilization of resources instead of drowning in misery.

Then. A colleague came back into my life to help me make a new career out of "scrambling eggs." We had taken a postdoctoral fellowship in sociology together but had not seen each other since. Though she was much younger than I, there was an empathy between us; we had similar perspectives about what matters in life. Now working in the area of AD, she had heard that I'd been diagnosed and called to see how I was. Our friendship expanded into collaboration. I could never have imagined that my last research project would be a study of my own disease! However, as an old saying goes, "If it works, don't knock it!" I am now on both sides of the fence at once, studying the disease I live with daily.

I have started to think in terms of reclaiming my life, to looking for ways to compensate for poor memory instead of giving in to depression. So, notes on my calendar, routines to create patterns for daily chores; not easy, often frustrating, and often I forget what I had planned to do. But I now tackle things that I'd been sure I could no longer do. It takes time for my new patterns to get safely into long-term memory and (I hope) stay there. It's also tricky; the rest of the world does not follow my routines. Unless I decide to be a hermit, I have to adapt to uncertainty a lot and let go of rigid routines when necessary.

I know now that I can take back some degree of control, retain some independence, which is good for morale. Patterns, once established, work pretty well, but if we travel or if routines are disrupted by visitors or spontaneous excursions, my shaky edifice of independence and efficiency crumbles, along with morale.

Thus, it is a very different world I live in now, and I am still trying to find my way in it. Strange. I forget so much these days. Events are randomly lost unless I'm reminded, and often even reminders fail to trigger recollection. What gets into long-term memory and stays, what disappears, is unpredictable now. I have noticed with fascination how trauma, especially blows to self-esteem, can trigger an indelible memory, when so much else is evanescent now.

Time is also strange now. Those events seem to me to have taken place a long time ago, but it has apparently been just a few years. Rarely these days am I surprised by time passing *more* quickly than I expected. In a way, I like that; it's nice to find that I have more time than I thought, to get ready to go out, for instance.

As I write, I can hear my husband's voice; feel the release of tension for both of us, the relief that I finally recognized reality, and feel the sadness for both of us at what must lie ahead. Yet I have learned much from this experience of living day to day with Alzheimer's. Let me emphasize two such lessons.

Lessons Learned

First, let us consider the impact of a word and reconsider *dementia*, the noun, and *demented*, the epithet. I have an axe to grind, and one that causes me serious discomfort. It is the name ascribed to this problem that I share unhappily with so many other senior citizens and not a few—deplorably— much younger persons who succumb, inexplicably, to the nightmare of AD.

Demented means literally deprived of mind, in my opinion a misnomer now that medication is available that vastly improves the ability to function, if not normally, at least with considerable awareness and, most wonderfully, restores the ability to think clearly, most of the time. I do not argue that even with medication memory is as good, as reliable, as it once was, but to a lesser degree that is true of many senior citizens who do not bear the brand of AD. But when names become labels, these have powerful psychological consequences, more powerful than we usually realize. The person is much more than only short-term memory, as critical as that faculty is to normal social interaction, even normal thought. Even so, there is a broad range of useful mental and social activities and abilities of which, aided by modern medicine, this person is capable.

Second, given the will, and supported by medication, one can learn to keep careful track of key things that must be remembered using paper and pencil to support and enhance short-term memory. Trouble arises from an inability to recall dependably, if at all, what has just happened, so what becomes crucial is the judicious selection of the things that should be remembered and written down on paper, kept always in the same place and consulted frequently. At best, this is not easy and takes practice. It cannot approach the efficiency of normal short-term memory, but it is much better than the haze of confusion and misery that attends just giving up.

If one has no legs, one must use crutches. In AD the crutches are routines, detailed and always followed with painstaking care and determination. This is clearly not for everyone, and not everyone with this disease needs or wants to do the hard work such control requires. But if one values autonomy highly, then it is worth everything to learn how to be independent to the maximum degree. There is a price to pay. Routines are antithetical to spontaneous events and pleasure. When those valuable familiar routines, lodged safely in old memory, are disrupted by fortuitous events, unexpected contingencies, or even just traveling away from home, confusion and loss of autonomy—and misery—can easily result. Perhaps, unless one is truly a control freak, as I am, the game is not worth the effort. For me, it is far more of an effort to let myself be looked after than to fall on my face in failure. Ultimately, I *can* do it myself, if I can keep working at it. I have relearned to do some things I thought I could no longer do. Such substitute mechanisms do not afford the flexibility of normal short-term memory but do offer alternative ways to maximize independence.

I tell myself that life is an adventure for all of us. We never know what lies ahead. We must learn to savor the moment and forgive the past; forgive, but not forget it, because in it lie the lessons learned for living as best we can and making the most of what will come next. The "crying room" is useful when things pile up and seem finally too much to bear. It doesn't hurt to cry a little, feel sorry for oneself a little, eat candy and be a child again. Then, finally, bored with self-indulgence, have a good laugh at your silly child, take a hot bath, and get on with living. There may well be another interesting experience around the next corner I won't want to miss.

Part I

The
Medical
Experience

1

Testing Times

The Experience of Neuropsychological Assessment

for People with Suspected Alzheimer's Disease

JOHN KEADY AND JANE GILLIARD

When objects are shown to her, she does not remember after a short time which objects have been shown. Asked to write "Auguste D," she tries to write "Mrs" and forgets the rest. It is necessary to repeat every word.
—Alois Alzheimer, 1901

This chapter is based on interviews conducted with fifteen people recently diagnosed with Alzheimer's disease (AD) who were willing to discuss its impact on their lives. This purposive sample was gained through a re-spected memory clinic in the United Kingdom, with all of the interviews undertaken individually by us over a two-year period. The primary focus of each interview was to explore the person's transitions, coping behavior, and subjective experience of living with AD. On all but one occasion the in-terviews included the perspectives of the family supporters,* reflecting the sense of "partnership" that characterized this study sample. A major area of concern arising from this study was the sense of insecurity and uncertainty that accompanied the experience of being psychologically assessed "for de-mentia," a sense that has only recently been acknowledged in the litera-

*We use *supporter* instead of *carer* or *caregiver* because those interviewed in the study did not identify with the implicit assumption of dependency contained in the latter terms.

ture (see, e.g., Cheston and Bender 1999; and Keady et al. 1999a, 1999b). Supporters in the sample also reported feeling "uncomfortable" about their role in the assessment process, particularly when they were asked to verify professional assessments of perceived areas of loss.

Using grounded theory and the constant comparative method as the main methodological vehicle (Glaser 1978; Glaser and Strauss 1967), this chapter constructs the meaning of assessment as it was experienced by those in the study sample, a process that was to lead to a medical diagnosis of "mild" AD using standard *DSM-IV* criteria (American Psychiatric Association 1994). Assessment is one of the first steps in the social process that we have termed "working together." Analysis of the study data indicated that the assessment had three temporal dimensions: (1) seeking help (assessment), (2) being told, and (3) moving on (see Fig. 1.1). Using the constant comparative method, each dimension was found to have supporting components. For the first dimension these emerged as (a) acknowledging the challenge, (b) playing the game, and (c) considering future options. The components supporting the second dimension involved (a) sharing understanding and (b) confirming doubts. The third dimension went beyond the early disclosure of the diagnosis and was employed once both partners in the process were ready to move forward together.

Only the first dimension and its supporting components are developed in this chapter; the remaining series of adjustments form substantial contributions to other areas of the book, and it is not our intention to replicate such discussion here. We shall commence with a brief review of the literature on the experience of assessment and its present status as a policy and practice imperative.

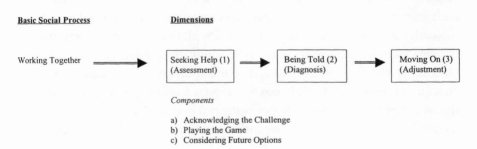

Fig. 1.1. Working together: linking the experience of dementia from assessment to adjustment

Assessment: Starting from a Level Playing Field?

The quotation at the start of this chapter is taken from Alois Alzheimer's handwritten case notes on Auguste D, a set of notes whose recent discovery has provided a fuller appraisal of Alzheimer's detailed observations and psychological assessments on his "unusual illness" (see Maurer, Volk, and Gerbaldo 1997, 1548). Indeed, as the quotation amply illustrates, the casenote entry reveals a process of psychological assessment and response that resonates through the years. On the other hand, following Auguste D's death in 1906, these entries were of limited interest compared with Alzheimer's anatomical observations of her "diseased" brain and the role and spread of neuritic plaques and neurofibrillary tangles within the higher and dominant areas of the brain structure, a spread that was to ultimately define the macroscopic hallmarks of "senile dementia" and map out the experience as medical territory for much of the twentieth century (for a more complete discussion, see Huppert, Brayne, and O'Connor 1994; and Lishman 1981).

However, as necessary as medical research remains, Alzheimer's written and anatomical observations contain both a paradox and a conundrum that continue to limit the efficacy of assessment practice in dementia care. To this day, a definitive diagnosis of AD is possible only on the death of the person suspected or assessed to have AD and subsequent anatomical observation of the diseased brain (Jacques 1992). The Alzheimer's Disease Society (ADS), now the Alzheimer's Society, suggested that assessment procedures leading to a clinical diagnosis of AD could be "about 80% accurate" (ADS 1995a; see also Piccini, Bracco, and Amaducci 1998; and Huppert and Wilcock 1997). This picture is complicated still further at the earlier stages of dementia, when other social, physical, and psychological conditions can conspire to "mask" its onset, thereby making a diagnosis more challenging (Burvill 1993), particularly when assessment is conducted exclusively in primary health care practice (Lepeleire and Heyrman 1999; Wright 1999).

On this latter issue, research has demonstrated consistently that the general practitioner (GP) is the first port of call for people concerned about their own health care needs (Pickard 1999), including poor memory performance (Briggs and Askham 1999). Steps that may eventually lead to a diagnosis of dementia presume that GPs in the primary health care team have the necessary skills, resources, and willingness to undertake such investigations. However, this may not always be the case. As an illustration, in the United Kingdom a recent extensive survey on GP diagnostic practice in twelve areas of England and Wales ($N = 1,000+$), conducted by the Audit Commission, found that only 54 percent believed that it was important to look actively for the early signs of dementia, while an underwhelming 52 percent considered it "beneficial to make an early diagnosis" (Audit Commission 2000, 22). Coupled with these alarming findings were the nihilistic attitudes displayed by GPs toward reaching a diagnosis of dementia, as typified in the report by the following example: "Dementia is untreatable, so why diagnose it?" (Audit Commission 2000, 21). Arguably, of even more concern is the finding in the report that fewer than half of the GPs questioned in the survey said that they used specific tests or protocols to "help them" diagnose dementia, a finding that raises an uncomfortable question about diagnostic standards in primary health care. These findings also need to be set against the recent policy backdrop that has emphasized the "vital importance" of early diagnosis and that such approaches should form an integral part of proactive mental health care practice (Department of Health 1996).

One way to clarify the confusion surrounding GP practice and an early diagnosis of dementia is to refer the person, as well as the supporter(s) as necessary, to specialist services (Wilcock, Bucks, and Rockwood 1999). To this end, the development of memory clinics in the United States and most European countries beginning in the late 1970s appears, prima facie, to be an ideal solution to this dilemma (Philpot and Levy 1987; Wright and Lindesay 1995). Indeed, studies have shown that in health districts where memory clinics exist, referral patterns and identification of dementia are increased in community samples (Audit Commission 2000; Thompson et al. 1997). This is due, in no small part, to the extensive range of tests that are available at such centers and the concentrated focus of professionals. For example, in memory clinic assessments of suspected dementia more extensive neuropsychological tests are usually triggered by a score of 18 or above on the Mini-Mental State Examination (MMSE) (Folstein, Folstein, and McHugh 1975). As Bucks and Loewenstein (1999) suggested in their informative guide, best practice indicates that such tests are conducted by members of a multidisciplinary team, which may comprise a neurologist, a psychiatrist, a social worker, a nurse, and a psychologist. Moreover, neuropsychological assessments are usually supported by results from a physical examination, laboratory tests, and anatomic or functional imaging as clinically indicated.

Writing about this intensive program as forming part of the practice of the Bristol Memory Disorders Clinic, in the United Kingdom, Bucks and Loewenstein (1999, 111) indicate that the battery of tests that may form part of the neuropsychological assessment includes the following:

- MMSE (Folstein, Folstein, and McHugh 1975)
- National Adult Reading Test (NART) (Nelson and Willison 1991)
- Digit Span (Wechsler Adult Intelligence Scale–Revised [WAIS-R]) (Wechsler 1981)
- Similarities (WAIS-R) (Wechsler 1981)
- Picture Completion (WAIS-R) (Wechsler 1981)
- Frenchay Aphasia Screening Test (FAST) (Enderby, Wood, and Wade 1975)
- Story Recall: Immediate and Delayed (Adult Memory and Information Processing Battery [AMIPB]) (Coughlan and Hollows 1985)
- Visual Recognition (Middlesex Elderly Assessment of Mental State [MEAMS]) (Golding 1989)
- Hopkins Verbal Learning Test—Recall and Recognition (HVLT) (Brandt 1991)
- FAS Benton verbal fluency (Lezak 1995)
- Wegl Colour Form Sorting (Grewal and Haward 1984)
- Cube Analysis (Visual Object Space Perception Battery [VOSP]) (Warrington and James 1991)
- Digit Copying (Kendrick 1985)
- Bristol Activities of Daily Living Scale (BADLS) (Bucks et al. 1996)

As Bucks and Loewenstein (1999) go on to explain, this extensive battery of tests usually takes about one hour to complete and is performed during one appointment at the memory clinic, with a second appointment necessary to explain the results or to conduct more tests. While the venue was different, this extensive assessment procedure was familiar to each participant in the reported study.

While memory clinics have been seen to play a major part in the "suc-

cess" of early diagnosis and medication trials (Wilcock, Bucks, and Rockwood 1999), they have been criticized for failing to provide people undergoing the diagnostic process with appropriate support and information
(Wright and Lindesay 1995), particularly upon their discharge from the facility (Bender 1996; Cheston and Bender 1999). Although this criticism
may highlight a number of competing concerns, it is arguably, unsurpris-
ing, particularly when people entering such services are seen more as "diagnostic subjects" than as full partners in the assessment process (Keady
and Bender 1998). In our opinion the most compelling reason centers on
the position of assessment as a cornerstone of professional practice (Jasper
1994; Nolan, Grant, and Keady 1996) and thus a part of the medical discourse in early dementia care. For instance, commenting on neuropsychological procedures in the assessment of suspected dementia, Wilcock and
Skoog (1999, 57) advised assessors that "a mental state examination should
also include an informal observation of the patient during the examination, assessing language, reasoning, memory, and also specifically apraxia,
aphasia, agnosia and left-right orientation."

This sense of professional "ownership" of diagnostic-testing procedures
may help to explain why there is such a paucity of literature on the social
context and subjective experience of the assessment process. However, a
study by Cheston and Bender (1999) provides some cause for optimism.
Supporting and developing an argument rehearsed earlier by Keady and
Bender (1998), Cheston and Bender suggested that the social context of
memory assessment needs to be a central feature of the assessment process
because without its integration into routine practice, neuropsychological
testing "accentuates into [their] fears of dependency and incompetence,
producing a sense of anxiety and threat" (1999, 200). Moreover, they contended that in their extensive experience as clinical psychologists, few people with suspected dementia were told why they were being assessed; thus
assessors often spun a complex web of deceit and euphemistic practice that
ended in uncertainty over how, and whether, to share a resulting diagnosis
(for a practice illustration in the memory clinic setting, see Gilliard and
Gwilliam 1996). Cheston and Bender (1999) argued that to compensate
for this imbalance in understanding, assessors need to implement a "person-focused" approach in which a philosophy of honesty, personal value,
and consent to treatment underpins professional practice. They acknowledged that this is not an easy solution, as it calls for much closer partner-

ships between assessors and those being assessed in which the assessment process is just one step. In this approach, assessment and the diagnosis of dementia are not ends but beginnings.

This reduction of the "power" held by the assessor was also noted by Genevay (1997, 17), who astutely observed, "To me assessment should include everything that happens in human interaction between me and my care providers that allows them to diagnose, treat and care for me." If practice is to improve, such subjective experiences must be valued and seen as integral to the assessment process; without this sense of value, the "person-focused" approach advocated by Cheston and Bender (1999) will not develop.

We shall turn to a theoretical exploration of this (subjective) experience of neuropsychological assessment after first providing some background information on the study design and approach to sample recruitment.

Study Design

Background

To operationalize the study aims, it appeared important to interview people who could openly discuss and reflect on their experience of "assessment" and how it felt to be on the receiving end of a neuropsychological screen for suspected dementia. This prestructuring of the sample was reinforced by Cotrell and Schulz (1993), who, while not wishing to discount the importance of the later experience of dementia (see Floyd 1988; Kitwood 1997), argued that "the most valuable insights regarding the psychological and experiential responses of persons with dementia are likely to be obtained during the mild to moderate levels of impairment when the individual is still able to verbalize an effective span of attention" (208).

In the reported study it was considered crucial that consent to participate be freely given and that the person having recently been through a diagnostic process was not in denial of his or her situation (Handron 1993), or unduly depressed (Verhey et al. 1993; Barker, Carter, and Jones 1994). In reaching an early diagnosis of dementia, most memory clinics adopt a longitudinal approach whereby the person being assessed initially undergoes a battery of psychological and physical tests (Philpot and Levy 1987). As indicated earlier, this was the practice at the memory clinic where the study reported here was conducted; at least one consultation was held before an opinion was offered on the efficacy of the test results. Even then, and as a matter of routine following an early diagnosis of dementia, the person being assessed (and the supporter if one existed) would be given an appointment to return to the memory clinic in six months to check on the reliability of the diagnostic procedure and explore personal coping responses. During this follow-up visit the person being assessed and the supporter were approached to be interviewed as part of the study.

Since it would have been inappropriate for either of us to "sit in" on the appointment, the decision whether to ask subjects to take part was left to the staff member responsible for providing the diagnosis and the follow-up visit. This was either the clinical neuropsychologist attached to the memory clinic or the doctor in charge of the case. This approach was thought to have two benefits. First an early, uniform diagnosis of dementia using *DSM-IV* criteria (American Psychiatric Association 1994) would have been reached. Second, a further clinical judgment would have been made to assess the person's (1) awareness of the procedure he or she had been through; (2) adjustment to and level of acceptance of the memory loss; (3) level of competence and ability to give informed consent to a procedure; and (4) retained verbal fluency and level of concentration.

It was considered essential that each of these four criteria be met before a person was approached for recruitment into the study. If the person did meet the criteria, the responsible clinical staff at the time of the follow-up visit would verbally introduce the aims of the study and then present the person (and the supporter if present) with a previously scripted letter of introduction and supporting information. Assuming participation, a prepaid envelope for return of the completed and signed documentation was also included, addressed to one of us. The letter also invited the participation of family supporters as part of the interview process. This was based on the experience of Pollitt and Anderson (1991) and the presumption that

- supporters acted as gatekeepers to the person with the early experience of dementia;
- protective strategies by supporters would be evident at this time (see also Bowers 1987); and
- the early adjustment to dementia could be seen as a system of personal and family adaptation, with both perspectives being important.

However, the introductory letter emphasized that the person living with the early experience of AD was to be the main focus of the interview. It was also decided to use a largely unstructured interview approach to help put the informant at ease. Lee (1993) suggested that conducting sensitive interviews requires an open and flexible approach in which the development of trust is essential: "Disclosure of sensitive or confidential information is usually only possible in these situations once trust has been established between the fieldworker and the people being studied" (103).

The timing of the interview therefore was designed to suit individual needs, with permission to tape-record the interview received from both the person with AD and the supporter(s). After some deliberation, it was decided that this request would be included in the initial pack sent before any visit to give the person with AD time to consider the request. The transcription also allowed the opportunity for a synopsis of the interview to be returned to the participants so that they could check it for accuracy; this was always returned to the person with AD and marked for his or her attention.

Sample Characteristics

The samples were gained via contact with a respected memory clinic in the United Kingdom, and as mentioned above, profile screening for the interviews was undertaken by members of the clinic's medical and neuropsychology staff. Further details of the sample composition and ethical considerations can be found elsewhere (see, in particular, Keady and Gilliard 1999, 238–40). Briefly, however, each interview was conducted and tape-recorded in the person's own home. Field notes were kept, and all tapes were transcribed and analyzed on the day of the interview. Ethical approval restricted the formal length of each interview to a maximum of forty-five minutes. To maintain qualitative rigor, all research participants had a diagnosis of mild AD. Further, on all but one occasion the family supporter of each person with AD wanted to be present during the interview. This resulted in a complete data set of fifteen people with AD (twelve women and three men aged 72–84 and 67–86 years, respectively) and, on fourteen occasions, their family supporters. A breakdown of the characteristics of each participant is displayed in Table 1.1.

Table 1.1. Interview Schedule

Interview	Person Interviewed	Age	Gender	Relationship (Person with dementia/Supporter)	Place of Interview	Length of Interview (minutes)
1	Person with dementia	67	Male	Husband/wife	Couple's home	45
	Supporter	—	Female			
2	Person with dementia	76	Female	Wife/husband	Couple's home	30
	Supporter	77	Male			
3	Person with dementia	72	Female	Wife/husband	Couple's home	25
	Supporter	72	Male			
4	Person with dementia	80	Female	Mother/daughter	Daughter's home	40
	Supporter	52	Female			
5	Person with dementia	86	Male	Husband/wife	Daughter's home	20
	Supporter	82	Female			
6	Person with dementia	73	Female	Wife/husband	Couple's home	45
	Supporter	76	Male			
7	Person with dementia[a]	78	Female	Wife	Person's home	30

		Age	Gender	Relationship	Location	
8	Person with dementia	84	Female	Wife/husband	Couple's home	40
	Supporter	87	Male			
9	Person with dementia	76	Female	Wife/husband	Couple's home	15
	Supporter	75	Male			
10	Person with dementia	74	Female	Wife/husband	Couple's home	25
	Supporter	77	Male			
11	Person with dementia	82	Male	Husband/wife	Couple's home	20
	Supporter	76	Female			
12	Person with dementia	79	Female	Wife/husband	Couple's home	35
	Supporter	82	Male			
13	Person with dementia	84	Female	Wife/husband	Couple's home	40
	Supporter	86	Male			
14	Person with dementia	81	Female	Wife/husband	Couple's home	30
	Supporter	81	Male			
15	Person with dementia	80	Female	Wife/husband	Couple's home	35
	Supporter	81	Male			

[a]No supporter present.

The study followed a grounded theory approach, with the data subject to constant comparative analysis (Glaser 1978; Glaser and Strauss 1967). As Glaser explained, in grounded theory, theory and theory development are grounded in empirical data and acts of everyday social life with the aim of generating a theory that "accounts for a pattern of behavior which is relevant and problematic for those involved and that this goal is not reached by voluminous description, but by clever verification" (1978, 39).

Findings

Seeking Help

The first dimension—seeking help—illustrates the early contact with professional service providers and the journey that led the person with (undiagnosed) AD (and the supporter) through numerous psychological assessments and screening procedures that varied in their level of sophistication and intensity. On each occasion this journey was initiated by the person's visit to his or her GP's office, followed by a relatively quick decision by the GP to refer the person to the memory clinic for further assessment. As it emerged through constant comparative analysis, seeking help contained three supporting components, identified as (a) acknowledging the challenge; (b) playing the game; and (c) considering future options.

Acknowledging the Challenge

For each person in the sample, the decision to seek help was initiated by a growing awareness that something quite serious was happening to him or her and that this experience could no longer be discounted. One participant in the study likened this process to "getting more and more frustrated" about his inability to "remember simple things," fearful that he was, in his words, "losing it big time" (interview 5). Significantly, in the sample this heightened level of awareness was shared with the person closest to him or her, who took these concerns seriously and saw them as a reason for concern, which led to a mutual decision to visit their GP to seek a medical opinion about the cause.

In acknowledging the challenge, the persons in the study recounted this first contact with the GP in a variety of ways, but the dominant expressions were of support and of being taken seriously. As one participant recounted,

"I felt she [the GP] listened to me and knew I had some sort of trouble. . . . She asked me some questions from a list and then spoke to us saying I had a memory problem. I was told I would need more help and that I should go to the centre [memory clinic] to find out more about it. So I went on from there" (interview 13).

At one level this first contact was a relief, as it validated the person's right to be concerned about himself or herself and his or her level of social or psychological functioning. However, at another level, after this first contact and mention of a referral "to the memory clinic" came the sudden realization that something really serious was happening and that further investigations would be necessary. This sudden realization resulted in a variety of responses, as the following slices of data attest:

- "After coming home [from the GP], I got worried that I would need more tests to find out what was wrong with me. I didn't know then if I would get any better." (interview 2)
- "I turned to my husband after we got back here [person's home] and we just held each other. Somehow we both knew that things had changed for good." (interview 10)
- "After hearing I needed to go to [names the memory clinic], I remember coming home and crying. I needed some time to think about things. Something was wrong with me and I had a problem, but I didn't know what." (interview 7)
- "I just got frightened." (interview 11)

The time gap between a GP referral and an appointment to the memory clinic was also seen as important, as it gave people with (undiagnosed) AD time to dwell on their anxieties and "figure out" a strategy for managing and, perhaps more important, reconstructing their experiences. Equally, this "time out" applied to other family members, giving them an opportunity to explore their own emotions and motivation for continuing with the referral. Interestingly, the location of the memory clinic within the health care setting proved an important issue, as this extract from the transcript of interview 1 suggests:

INTERVIEWER: Do you remember coming to [name of the hospital where the memory clinic was situated]?

PERSON WITH AD: Yeah, well, that's the latest one. We, er . . . to tell the truth I had the wind up me a bit there because being a local I knew what [the hospital] was and, er, it began to get on me a little bit, I think.

INTERVIEWER: What did it [name of hospital] mean to you?

PERSON WITH AD: Well, it was an asylum. That put the wind up me a bit [nervous laugh].

INTERVIEWER: So what did you think was happening to you, then?

PERSON WITH AD: Well, I thought that. . . . One picture comes to mind when anybody asks me this. A long time ago, we went to [name of area] by train and we used to pass [name of hospital] and, er, as you got far away you looked back and there was a whole row of windows and one of them, a small window, and in that window there used to be a lady sitting there quite a lot and, er. . . . Yeah, that used to get me a bit. It's getting me now actually [sniffs]. Yeah, that . . .

INTERVIEWER: Did you think that was what they were going to do to you, then?

PERSON WITH AD: No, not necessarily, but I suppose I thought of it, that lady up there. And we used to hear stories of her, the things she used to get up to. Only kid's talk, like. But, um . . . that preyed on my mind quite a bit [starts to cry and interview discontinued temporarily].

Here the location of the memory clinic resonated with the person's childhood images of mental illness, and to him, attendance at the clinic may well have confirmed that he was "going mad." It was therefore no surprise that he approached the neuropsychological assessment with a heightened degree of fear and anxiety, as well as a hesitancy to confirm the nature of his suspicions.

Over and above such anxieties, however, the referral to the memory clinic validated the person's right to be concerned about himself or herself, moving the process from an acknowledgment by the person being assessed that something quite serious was happening to a process that considered future attendance for "tests" and "more investigations." Propelled by GPs' concerns, this cognitive shift opened up the second component in seeking help, which we have labeled "playing the game."

Playing the Game

By calling the second component of assessment "playing the game," we are not suggesting that assessment is a game; the seriousness of the outcome confounds this notion. Rather, it would appear from the perspective of those being assessed that if the rules of participation are not made clear, then those taking part will place their own meaning and interpretation on the nature of events, including the relevance of the entire procedure to their own personal circumstances. For instance, during one interview the participant explained that during "the tests" he felt as if he were "in a trap" and that he knew, that the assessors knew, that they were "trying to catch me out" (interview 5). Observed through this lens, the purpose of assessment could be construed as predominantly controlling, with correct moves in the process symbolizing a game of chance and second-guessing. It is this movement that the name of the component attempts to capture.

This focus on chance extends to the design of the room where the neuropsychological assessment was conducted. One person with AD recalled it as being "unfriendly" and "cold," containing, as it did, a "large desk with lots of papers on it." The interviewee also recalled that there were "pictures of brains and things on the wall," which did little to settle her levels of anxiety. This interviewee went on to explain: "When I was there I wanted to look out of the window all the time to see something else, to take my mind off it, if you like, [pause] but he [her husband] kept telling me to give it my best go. My seat was against the wall too, and I've never liked sitting like that" (interview 6). Such experiences underscore the importance of integrating biographical information within an assessment process, teasing out the meaning it engenders for the person(s) concerned, however obtuse they may appear.

As already discussed, the delay in attending the memory clinic gave rise to feelings of uncertainty and anxiety, providing people with time out to consider—and in some cases plan—their response. Whereas the first encounter with the GP was relatively brief and served to confirm initial fears and suspicions, the next steps in the assessment were approached more cautiously. In discussing this next phase of the assessment process, participants spoke about the need to be "more prepared" and ready to anticipate "what might happen to me." Those in the sample certainly knew that their mental functioning would be probed and tested (a referral to a "memory clinic" simply reinforced this) and that therefore they needed to decide how to handle this turn of events. Moreover, while the environment of the memory clinic, the purpose of the visit, and the nature of his or her condition blended together to form a confused picture for the person concerned, it also raised anxiety for the supporter, particularly over his or her anticipated role in the process. As one supporter stated: "Before that first visit I had heard all sorts of things about the place. Mostly good, mind you, but I was more worried about [names her husband] and how he would cope if he had something bad. I must be honest and tell you that I was worried about that first visit there too. I didn't want to tell them too much about how he was getting on because it might have looked bad for him. I didn't want everyone to know our business" (interview 11).

For staff working at the clinic, such protective behavior meant that a delicate balance had to be struck between maintaining a person's sense of integrity and undertaking an assessment that aimed primarily to prove poor performance through the discourse and quantitative evidence of loss. While staff at the memory clinic undoubtedly did their best to allay such tensions in the opening part of the interaction, the start of the more formal testing procedures confirmed (to both partners) the seriousness of what was happening, as the following excerpts illustrate:

- "I was asked questions which I should have known but didn't. I knew they knew I wasn't doing so well, so I stopped giving out answers and said 'I don't know' to most things. It was easier then to get through it that way." (interview 4)
- "The first thing that happened was that they asked me questions on numbers and things. Adding up, I think. I have never been good at that type of thing, but I just did the best I could." (interview 8)
- "I thought it was important to do well, but I didn't know what I got right and what I didn't. That made it hard to know what was going on." (interview 12)
- "I could manage most of the questions but not all of them. I got scared as the time went on, as I wanted to do well and had trouble working out what was happening." (interview 13)
- "I had to draw a few shapes down and I had trouble doing it. I got a bit scared then." (interview 15)

This introduction of the more formal part of the assessment process was important, a point that was not lost on those taking part. Participants were asked to perform tasks about whose purpose and outcome they were given little information. Usually, the assessor's requests for responses were read from "charts" (interview 6), and one gentleman in the study likened the question-and-answer session to "being back at school," which, he explained, was "the last time anyone asked me to count out loud" (interview 11). Such perceived levels of threat evoked a number of coping responses, including

- taking time out during the assessment (interviews 1, 7, 9);
- being confrontational (4, 6, 8, 10);
- making excuses (9, 15);
- avoiding awkward questions (2, 4, 5, 7, 9, 12, 14, 15);
- relying on others for clarification (2, 6, 9, 12, 14); and
- strategic resistance (8, 10).

Such responses allowed participants to "step back" from the assessment process, giving them time to figure out the meaning (and rules) of what was happening and, perhaps more important, to reflect on the consequences of poor performance. Playing the game was a serious business. Of the coping strategies listed above, "strategic resistance" caused perhaps the most upset. The following exchange from interview 10 is illustrative:

INTERVIEWER: During the time of your assessment at the memory clinic were you aware of how you were doing?
PERSON WITH AD: Well, not really. I have always been forgetful and I thought it was just that.
INTERVIEWER: So you felt your memory loss was just a part of you?
PERSON WITH AD: Yes.
INTERVIEWER: Did you think all this interest in you was necessary?
PERSON WITH AD: No. I didn't need all those things they did.
SUPPORTER: Well, the thing about those tests is to help your memory. There is a chance that it could help. My view is to leave no stone unturned and try anything that is offered, even if there is only a glimmer of help. Don't you agree? [directed to person with AD]. I mean, there is nothing to lose and possibly something to gain.
PERSON WITH AD: I don't know, it just irritates me.
SUPPORTER: Well, they can tell from your memory if it is getting better or worse.
PERSON WITH AD: Well, I don't think so. It's just not worth it. All those things I had to do, they're so terribly childish. Add this, take away that, remem-

ber this, draw that. What's it all about? The tests are all very repetitive. I didn't bother in the end.

In this example of strategic resistance the person's performance and lack of engagement may well have helped to inform professional decision making on the diagnostic pathway, but a consequence was that the person being assessed was left with unresolved feelings of distress and anxiety over the performance. We do not mean to communicate the impression that professional workers were unfeeling and uncaring in their approach. Rather, the unresolved feelings appear synonymous with the diagnostic process, in which assessment procedures exist to probe for areas of loss with the true purpose of the tests, certainly during these early encounters, firmly embedded within a professional knowledge base.

Based on the study data, it appears that playing the game continues until the formal testing process comes to an end, a period of time short in its duration but vast in its implications. Closing the encounter left those engaged in the process with a further opportunity to interpret their experience and prepare for the follow-up visit. This period of reflection led to the third component in the dimension, considering future options.

Considering Future Options

After completion of the battery of neuropsychological tests, a second appointment for people attending the memory clinic was scheduled for about a month later. During the interval both those being assessed and their supporters had time to reflect on their performance and motivation for attending the clinic. For family supporters the feeling was generally positive, as the diagnostic process served to "sort things out" and to help clarify future options. However, those undergoing the diagnostic process undoubtedly experienced increased levels of anxiety during and after this time as the seriousness of what they had been through began to sink in.

In the phase of considering future options, couples whose interpersonal relationships were close were more likely to construct some sense of value and meaning out of their experience, building a partnership whereby "they faced the future together" (interview 2), forming a barrier against external threats. This dynamic was exhibited most clearly in the following exchange (interview 6):

INTERVIEWER: When you returned to the clinic for your next appointment, what sort of things were going through your mind?

PERSON WITH AD: Well, I wanted to get it over with. I had a letter saying the time I should be there.

INTERVIEWER: Were you worried about what would happen to you?

PERSON WITH AD: Yes. The first time the tests just went on and on and I got tired. So I just wanted to go there and get it over with.

SUPPORTER: That's right. After that time, we decided to face things together. Mind you, that probably says more about us than anything else. I wasn't too happy when they asked me questions in front of her, especially when she hadn't got things quite right. But I wanted to know what was happening and at least they could help us with that.

For the person with (undiagnosed) AD, this sense of partnership appears to have been crucial in fostering a positive attitude toward the assessment process and gaining some meaning from it. However, this finding should not be accepted at face value. Based on further analysis of the data, it appears that a continuation of "strategic resistance" (to the assessment process or to the experience of memory loss) from the time of engaging in the battery of neuropsychological tests had a crucial impact on shaping future transitions and decision making. Indeed, instead of bringing people closer together, "strategic resistance" acted to drive the couple further apart. In many ways, this dynamic added an extra layer of stress on an already stressful situation, with the external assessment procedure confirming the seriousness of the situation for one partner (the supporter) in the process, while for the other, the person with dementia, it was simply an irrelevance. Thus in relationships involving persons with AD for whom "strategic resistance" was the overriding coping style, the seeds were sown for a culture of recrimination to grow and germinate. Undoubtedly, this experience was not helped by the limited explanatory information provided by assessors at the time of the neuropsychological testing.

In considering future options, therefore, different outcomes were available to each participant in the study, including, of course, an option not to return to the memory clinic and proceed with further tests and/or to receive the results. Indeed, to varying degrees, all of the participants in the study shared a reluctance to return to the memory clinic, although such an outcome was necessary if the results of the tests were to be shared and acted on and the implications understood.

Lessons Learned

From our data we gleaned important conditions that needed to be present in the assessment process to assist the person with (undiagnosed) AD and the supporter to move forward, namely:

- a good prior relationship between the person with (undiagnosed) AD and the supporter;
- a willingness by the person with (undiagnosed) AD to openly disclose fears, concerns, and coping behaviors with a trusted person;
- a willingness by the trusted person (supporter) to hear, validate, and act on these concerns;
- a mutual decision to do something about their concerns, with the two parties recognizing and agreeing that "this is (or might be) serious";
- a reasonably quick decision to seek a medical opinion about the cause of the serious signs;
- primary health care teams' taking the reported signs and symptoms seriously and having the necessary knowledge and skills to facilitate an early diagnosis of dementia. Alternatively, the primary health care team's response may be to refer the person being assessed or the couple to more specialized support services, such as a memory clinic;
- an absence of strategic resistance during neuropsychological assessment; and
- an early diagnosis and that diagnosis, as well as the prognosis, being made known to the person with dementia and the supporter.

These conditions need to be tested further, but their occurrence seems important if support and a diagnosis of AD are to occur at an earlier point. Moreover, these conditions incorporate the underlying assumptions about the provision of quality dementia care reported by the King's Fund Centre (1986). This project paper detailed the principles of "good service practice," and by astutely avoiding such exemplars, the report's authors were able to set out a challenge to service providers and policymakers. This was achieved by citing five key principles that outlined philosophical beliefs about personal empowerment, calling for an acknowledgment that (1) people with dementia have the same human value as anyone else irrespective of their degree of disability or dependence; (2) people with dementia have the same varied human needs as anyone else; (3) people with dementia have the same rights as other citizens; (4) every person with dementia is an individual; and (5) people with dementia have the right to forms of support that do not exploit family and friends (King's Fund Centre 1986, 7–8).

Future Recommendations for the Assessment Process

Although the last decade witnessed a move toward sharing an early diagnosis (ADS 1995b; Heal and Husband 1998; Husband 1999; Pitt 1997), little thought has been given to developing appropriate professional support (Kuhn 1999; Moniz-Cook et al. 1998) to how to handle the disclosure of the diagnosis to the person with dementia (Gilliard and Gwilliam 1996; Rice and Warner 1994). Indeed, given the current climate of professional nihilism, it is not surprising that those involved were often bewildered about the meaning and purpose of the "assessment process" and the battery of cognitive tests that they completed. The interview data indicate that the assessment process only tended to lead to a poor early experience with professional interventions. Moreover, the very term *memory clinic* suggests a more passive activity than what was actually taking place.

Unfortunately, such experiences do not appear to be an isolated phenomenon, as the anxiety and misunderstandings over "being assessed for dementia" were later shared in a separate, larger survey of people experiencing the first stages of dementia ($N = 62$) (Keady et al. 1999a, 1999b). To improve the situation, two aspects of assessment might usefully be developed. First, assessment could be improved by a greater awareness of the person's unique biography. The Gloucester project (Johnson et al. 1989) described the input of services to older adults using such a framework and found that the approach worked well. As Johnson explained in an earlier text (1986, 10), the biographical approach to assessment is centered on three key principles: (1) to establish a clear interest in the person; (2) to avoid a focus on "problems" and "needs"; and (3) to express a genuine interest in the person's life and what he or she sees as major themes and life events.

By looking for the meaning of social events, the assessor, in this approach, is more concerned with meeting individual needs than with dispensing the resources that services have to offer. This shift in the role of the assessor from one of "expert" to one of "enabler" was warmly received by recipients in the reported project (Johnson et al. 1989), although in today's cost-conscious climate, with its push for speedy assessments (ADS 1997; Department of Health 1990), there may be little opportunity for such initiatives to develop.

Second, biographical approaches to assessment suggest that the role of psychometric tests might be more limited than is currently the case (Cheston and Bender 1999). A model that places people with (undiagnosed) dementia in a position of greater control, so that their anxieties are lessened and a fuller picture of their circumstances emerges, might be more helpful. Although formal testing still has a role, especially if there is a need to investigate subareas of cognitive performance, the person with (undiagnosed) dementia must be seen to appreciate its purpose. One way to move in this direction would be to provide participants with more detailed information about the purpose of assessment and the interpretation of the results. Arguably, this would help to reduce the perception of threat, and those with (undiagnosed) dementia would be treated as partners in the diagnostic process rather than as subjects. However, while this would appear to be central to moving practice forward, such openness demands a more inclusive and transparent agenda to dementia whereby the element of fear surrounding a diagnosis is minimized.

Finally, instilling hope in both people undergoing or having an early diagnosis of dementia and those who care about them is of the utmost importance to the assessment process. This instillation of hope might be crucial in helping to shift public attitudes about the nature of the condition. Conceivably, this hope might be conveyed through the prescribing of the "new drugs" for dementia, although much still needs to be understood, particularly around the social construction of quality of life for people living with dementia (see, e.g., Cohen 1991; Hutchinson, Leger-Krall, and Wilson 1997; Parse 1996; Tappen et al. 1999; Whitehouse et al. 1997; Woods 1999; and Logsdon's chapter [4] in this book). Also, hope and some control can be encouraged through including discussion of strategies for memory enhancement as part of the assessment process. While such interventions are presently in their infancy, as Moniz-Cook et al. (1998) reported

in their pilot study, psychosocial support appears crucial in helping to improve the well-being and adjustment processes for both persons living with
the early experience of AD and their supporters.

This chapter only scratches the surface regarding what it is like to be on
the receiving end of a neuropsychological assessment for (suspected and
eventually diagnosed) AD, and we must consider ourselves to be at the beginning of a knowledge base. However, we hope that by outlining some of
the experiences, processes, components, and conditions, we have taken
one small step along this particular road of understanding.

REFERENCES

Alzheimer's Disease Society (ADS). 1995a. *Dementia in the community: Management strategies for general practice*. London.
———. 1995b. *Right from the start: Primary health care and dementia*. London.
———. 1997. *No accounting for health: Health commissioning for dementia*. London.
American Psychiatric Association. 1994. *DSM-IV: Diagnostic and statistical manual of mental disorders*. 4th ed. Washington, D.C.
Audit Commission. 2000. *Forget me not: Mental health services for older people*. London.
Barker, A., C. Carter, and R. Jones. 1994. Memory performance, self-reported memory loss, and depressive symptoms in attenders at a GP-referral and a self-referral memory clinic. *International Journal of Geriatric Psychiatry* 9:305–11.
Bender, M. 1996. Memory clinics: Locked doors on the gravy train? *Psychology Special Interest Group for the Elderly Newsletter* 58 (October): 30–33.
Bowers, B. J. 1987. Inter-generational caregiving: Adult caregivers and their ageing parents. *Advances in Nursing Science* 9 (2): 20–31.
Brandt, J. 1991. The Hopkins Verbal Learning Test: Development of a new memory test with six equivalent forms. *Clinical Neuropsychologist* 5:125–42.
Briggs, K., and J. Askham. 1999. *The needs of people with dementia and those who care for them: A review of the literature*. London: Alzheimer's Society.
Bucks, R. S., D. L. Ashworth, G. K. Wilcock, and K. Siegfried. 1996. Assessment of ac-
tivities of daily living in dementia: Development of the Bristol Activities of Daily Living Scale. *Age and Ageing* 25:113–20.
Bucks, R. S., and D. A. Loewenstein. 1999. Neuropsychological assessment. In *Diagnosis and management of dementia: A manual for memory disorders teams*, ed. G. K. Wilcock, R. S. Bucks, and K. Rockwood, 102–23. Oxford: Oxford Univ. Press.
Burvill, P. W. 1993. A critique of current criteria for early dementia in epidemiological studies. *International Journal of Geriatric Psychiatry* 8:553–59.
Cheston, R., and M. Bender. 1999. *Understanding dementia: The man with the worried eyes*. London: Jessica Kingsley.
Cohen, D. 1991. The subjective experience of Alzheimer's disease: The anatomy of an

illness as perceived by patients and families. *American Journal of Alzheimer's Care and Related Disorders and Research* 10 (2): 6–11.

Cotrell, V., and R. Schulz. 1993. The perspective of the patient with Alzheimer's disease: A neglected dimension of dementia research. *Gerontologist* 33 (2): 205–11.

Coughlan, A. K., and S. E. Hollows. 1985. *The Adult Memory and Information Processing Battery (AMIPB)*. Leeds: St. James's University.

Department of Health. 1990. *NHS and Community Care Act*. London: HMSO.

————. 1996. *Assessing older people with dementia in the community: Practice issues for social and health services*. Wetherby: HMSO.

Enderby, P., V. Wood, and D. Wade. 1975. *Frenchay Aphasia Screening Test (FAST): Test manual*. Windsor, England: NFER-NELSON.

Floyd, J. 1988. Research and informed consent: The dilemma of the cognitively impaired client. *Journal of Psychosocial Nursing* 26 (3): 13–18.

Folstein, M. F., S. E. Folstein, and P. R. McHugh. 1975. Mini-mental state: A practical guide for grading the cognitive state of patients for the clinician. *Journal of Psychiatric Research* 12:189–98.

Genevay, B. 1997. See me! Hear me! I know who I am! An experience of being assessed. *Generations: Bulletin of the British Society of Gerontology* 21 (1): 16–18.

Gilliard, J., and C. Gwilliam. 1996. Sharing the diagnosis: A survey of memory disorders clinics, their policies on informing people with dementia and their families, and the support they offer. *International Journal of Geriatric Psychiatry* 11:1001–3.

Glaser, B. G. 1978. *Theoretical sensitivity*. Mill Valley, Calif.: Sociology Press.

Glaser, B. G., and A. L. Strauss. 1967. *The discovery of grounded theory: Strategies for qualitative research*. Chicago: Aldine.

Golding, E. 1989. *The Middlesex Elderly Assessment of Mental State*. Bury St. Edmunds: Thames Valley Test Company.

Grewal, B., and L. Haward. 1984. Validation of a new Weigl scoring system in neurological diagnosis. *Medical Science Research* 12:602–3.

Handron, D. S. 1993. Denial and serious chronic illness: A personal perspective. *Perspectives in Psychiatric Care* 29 (1): 29–33.

Heal, H. C., and H. J. Husband. 1998. Disclosing a diagnosis of dementia: Is age a factor? *Aging and Mental Health* 2 (2): 144–50.

Huppert, F., C. Brayne, and D. W. O'Connor, eds. 1994. *Dementia and normal aging*. Cambridge: Cambridge Univ. Press.

Huppert, F., and G. Wilcock. 1997. Ageing, cognition, and dementia. *Age and Ageing* 26 (suppl. 4): 20–23.

Husband, H. J. 1999. The psychological consequences of learning a diagnosis of dementia: Three case examples. *Aging and Mental Health* 3 (2): 179–83.

Hutchinson, S. A., S. Leger-Krall, and H. S. Wilson. 1997. Early probable Alzheimer's disease and awareness context theory. *Social Science and Medicine* 45 (9): 1399–1409.

Jacques, A. 1992. *Understanding dementia*. 2nd ed. Edinburgh: Churchill Livingstone.

Jasper, M. A. 1994. Expert: A discussion on the implications of the concept as used in nursing. *Journal of Advanced Nursing* 20:769–76.

Johnson, M. 1986. The meaning of old age. In *Nursing elderly people*, ed. S. J. Redfern, 3–17. Edinburgh: Churchill Livingstone.

Johnson, M., B. Gearing, T. Dant, and M. Carley. 1989. *Care for elderly people at home: Final report*. Buckinghamshire: Open Univ. Press.

Keady, J., and M. Bender. 1998. Changing faces: The purpose and practice of assessing older adults with cognitive impairment. *Health Care in Later Life: An International Research Journal* 3 (2): 129–44.

Keady, J., and J. Gilliard. 1999. The early experience of Alzheimer's disease: Implications for partnership and practice. In *Dementia care: Developing a partnership in practice*, ed. T. Adams and C. Clark, 227–56. Edinburgh: Churchill Livingstone.

Keady, J., J. Gilliard, C. Evers, and S. Milton. 1999a. The DIAL-log study 1: Profiling the experience of people with dementia. *British Journal of Nursing* 8 (6): 387–93.

———. 1999b. The DIAL-log study 2: Support in the early stages of dementia. *British Journal of Nursing* 8 (7): 432–36.

Kendrick, D. 1985. *Kendrick cognitive tests for the elderly*. Windsor, England: NFER-NELSON.

King's Fund Centre. 1986. *Living well into old age: Applying principles of good practice to services for people with dementia*. Report No. 63. London: King's Fund Publishing Office.

Kitwood, T. 1997. *Dementia reconsidered: The person comes first*. Buckinghamshire: Open Univ. Press.

Kuhn, D. 1999. *Alzheimer's early stages: First steps in caring and treatment*. Salt Lake City: Publishers Press.

Lee, R. M. 1993. *Doing research on sensitive topics*. London: Sage.

Lepeleire, J. D., and J. Heyrman. 1999. Diagnosis and management of dementia in primary care at an early stage: The need for a new concept and an adapted procedure. *Theoretical Medicine and Bioethics* 20:215–28.

Lezak, M. D. 1995. *Neuropsychological assessment*. 3rd ed. New York: Oxford Univ. Press.

Lishman, W. A. 1981. *Organic psychiatry*. 2nd ed. Oxford: Blackwell Scientific.

Maurer, K., S. Volk, and H. Gerbaldo. 1997. Auguste D and Alzheimer's disease. *Lancet* 349:1546–49.

Moniz-Cook, E., S. Agar, G. Gibson, T. Win, and M. Wang. 1998. A preliminary study of the effects of early intervention with people with dementia and their families in a memory clinic. *Aging and Mental Health* 2 (3): 199–211.

Nelson, H. E., and J. Willison. 1991. *National Adult Reading Test (NART): Test manual including new data supplement*. Windsor, England: NFER-NELSON.

Nolan, M., G. Grant, and J. Keady. 1996. *Understanding family care: A multidimensional model of caring and coping*. Buckinghamshire: Open Univ. Press.

Parse, R. R. 1996. Quality of life for persons living with Alzheimer's disease: The human becoming perspective. *Nursing Science Quarterly* 9 (3): 126–33.

Philpot, M. P., and R. Levy. 1987. A memory clinic for the early diagnosis of dementia. *International Journal of Geriatric Psychiatry* 2:195–200.

Piccini, C., L. Bracco, and L. Amaducci. 1998. Treatable and reversible dementias: An update. *Journal of the Neurological Sciences* 153:172–81.

Pickard, S. 1999. Co-ordinated care for older people with dementia. *Journal of Interprofessional Care* 13 (4): 345–54.

Pitt, B. 1997. "You've got Alzheimer's disease": Telling the patient. *Current Opinions in Psychiatry* 10:307–8.

Pollitt, P. A., and I. Anderson. 1991. Research methods in the study of carers of dementing elderly people: Some problems encountered in the Hughes Hall Project for later life. *Generations: Bulletin of the British Society of Gerontology* 16 (summer): 29–32.

Rice, K., and N. Warner. 1994. Breaking the bad news: What do psychiatrists tell patients with dementia about their illness? *International Journal of Geriatric Psychiatry* 9:467–71.

Tappen, R. M., C. Williams, S. Fishman, and T. Touhy. 1999. Persistence of self in advanced Alzheimer's disease. *Image: Journal of Nursing Scholarship* 31 (2): 121–25.

Thompson, P., F. Inglis, D. Findlay, J. Gilchrist, and M. E. T. McMurdo. 1997. Memory clinic attenders: A review of 150 consecutive patients. *Aging and Mental Health* 1 (2): 181–83.

Verhey, F. R. J., N. Rozendaal, R. W. H. M. Ponds, and J. Jolles. 1993. Dementia, awareness and depression. *International Journal of Geriatric Psychiatry* 8:851–56.

Warrington, E. K., and M. James. 1991. *The Visual Object Space Perception Battery*. Bury St. Edmunds: Thames Valley Test Company.

Wechsler, D. 1981. *The Wechsler Adult Intelligence Scale—Revised*. New York: Psychological Corporation.

Whitehouse, P. J., J.-M. Orgogozo, R. E. Becker, S. Gauthier, M. Pontecorvo, H. Erzigkeit, S. Rogers, R. C. Mohs, N. Bodick, G. Bruno, and P. Dal-Bianco. 1997. Quality-of-life assessment in dementia drug development: Position paper from the international working group on harmonization of dementia drug guidelines. *Alzheimer Disease and Associated Disorders* 11 (3): 56–60.

Wilcock, G. K., R. S. Bucks, and K. Rockwood, eds. 1999. *Diagnosis and management of dementia: A manual for memory disorders teams*. Oxford: Oxford Univ. Press.

Wilcock, G. K., and I. Skoog. 1999. Medical assessment. In *Diagnosis and management of dementia: A manual for memory disorders teams*, ed. G. K. Wilcock, R. S. Bucks, and K. Rockwood, 48–61. Oxford: Oxford Univ. Press.

Woods, B. 1999. The person in dementia care. *Generations: Bulletin of the British Society of Gerontology* 23 (3): 35–39.

Wright, G. 1999. Dementia: Early diagnosis and the primary healthcare team. *General Medical* 8:17–19.

Wright, N., and N. Lindesay. 1995. A survey of memory clinics in the British Isles. *International Journal of Geriatric Psychiatry* 10:379–85.

2

Medical Experiences and Concerns
of People with Alzheimer's Disease

ROSALIE F. YOUNG

I was devastated. The bottom fell out.
—Man in AD support group

We have little knowledge of the concerns of people with Alzheimer's disease. Also lacking are first-person reports about how they react to the diagnosis, the way they interpret their present state, and even whether they perceive future loss of independence, memory, and life itself as catastrophic (Cotrell and Lein 1993). Contributing to the lack of information is the nature of their medical experiences, especially as they concern medical encounters between individuals with AD and physicians. Although there is increasing interest in the personal world of people with this disease (Cohen 1991), attention is seldom paid to their subjective experiences. Persons with AD are often relegated to the status of inanimate objects (Cotrell and Schulz 1993). Whether this occurs because investigators believe that the individual is unable to understand or is incompetent is not known, but this situation prevails despite the person's abilities, health status, or level of impairment.

This investigation of the medical experiences and concerns of persons with early-stage AD was prompted by the need to have firsthand information about personal reactions and responses to the diagnosis. It sought to find out exactly what these individuals were saying, the problems they were experiencing, and the nature of the Alzheimer's experience as they perceived it.

The words of the individuals who participated in this investigation reveal that becoming depressed after receiving the diagnosis was common. Yet they adjusted to the disastrous news and began to face the situation. They learned to cope with the inevitable. At the present time, all of the study participants are in the process of reconstructing their lives based on the unfortunate reality they have to face. Most are hopeful, especially for drugs that promise to arrest the progression of this deadly disease.

This chapter presents first-person reports of the subjective world of persons with AD. The words and phrases they spoke, which were both simple and elegant, can guide us toward understanding. The same words can also help us identify ways to improve the medical encounters of persons with AD and family caregivers.

How Issues and Concerns Were Identified

Focus group meetings were convened for individuals diagnosed with AD and family caregivers. All were members of early-stage AD support groups. The groups met twice monthly under the auspices of the local chapter of the Alzheimer's Association. I was invited to attend four meetings held over a six-week period. The meetings lasted one and a half to two hours each. They were held in a community center, where participants sat around a large table. At the end of each meeting the group mingled over refreshments.

Participants in three focus groups included twenty-four persons with AD and three caregivers that accompanied them. An additional ten caregivers participated in a fourth focus group, for family members. Most were spouses, but two were adult children of women with AD. Men and women were represented almost equally. They ranged in age from late sixties to mid-eighties. All were Caucasians of European ancestry. Each focus group comprised five to eleven persons.

Each meeting was conducted as follows:

I was introduced by the group facilitator, and then the members of the focus group introduced themselves. The purpose of the my visit was discussed, and group members were advised that the main agenda item would be talking about AD-related topics.

I gave a brief presentation mentioning that participants would be asked directly about the meaning of AD, their feelings after being informed of the diagnosis, how they were coping, and whether there had been adverse effects on their families. Participants were asked to be candid. They were encouraged to (a) provide first-person reports of their lives after diagnosis and (b) listen to accounts of and offer comments about the personal experiences of others attending the meeting.

Comments were elicited about participants' willingness to discuss personal feelings and to disclose their emotional reactions.

I asked participants to respond to four questions. All of the questions were original to the study, but two were derived from questions used to determine the meaning of disabling illness (Luborsky 1995). These questions were formulated according to principles for focus group interviews (Stewart and Shamdasani 1990). The questions were: (1) "What does it mean to you to have AD?" (2) "What kinds of things have you or your family done to prepare for the future?" (3) "What would you like to say to others who were recently told that they have this disease?" and (4) "Tell me about your doctors and the experiences you have had with health care providers." This last question was based on comments made during the first meeting that reflected the need for a specific question.

Participants were asked to fill out an original instrument that indicated mood state (Fig. 2.1). The form included four faces, each reflecting a different mood. Individuals checked the face that best reflected their mood at the times. Next, they completed a second copy of the form to best indicate their mood upon receiving the diagnosis. Including standardized test batteries to measure affect was not considered to be in the best interests of this investigation. Such batteries (e.g., the CES-D Depression Scale) include a series of items that require choosing among four or five response categories. Not only do individuals have to ponder the meaning of eleven to twenty or more questions but they must indicate whether the behavior or state occurred "very often," "often," "sometimes," or "rarely," and for some depression indexes they must indicate how often during the past week. It was believed that providing paper-and-pencil tests about the frequency of mood states would neither provide the information sought (e.g., the type of emotional response that followed diagnosis of AD) nor fit the focus group format since participants would be likely to concentrate on answering formal questions, thus disrupting the conversational flow.

Please check the face that shows your mood when you found out you had
Alzheimer's Disease.

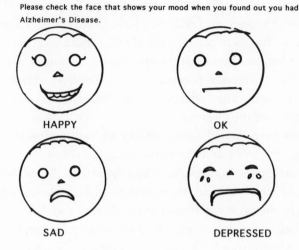

Fig. 2.1. Mood states

CONVERSATION FLOWED EASILY during the four meetings. The focus
group setting seemed to foster friendly exchanges, as well as disagreements,
even among persons who were initially reluctant to express their concerns.
However, among persons accompanied by spouses responses were less spontaneous. A husband, for example, might first look at his wife before answering. While in some cases these nonverbal exchanges were for confirmation of what was being said, in other cases the person appeared to be
asking forgiveness for disclosing feelings or impressions.

   Notes were taken on all responses and conversations. Direct quotes were
written out completely. After each meeting the investigator's field notes
were fully written up. Audiotape or videotape recorders were not used.

   After all four focus group sessions were completed, the full notes were
analyzed. Themes were identified, and categories were developed. The procedures used represented the qualitative analysis methodology of thematic
analysis. Several response themes emerged. They involved the individuals'
emotional reaction, the meaning they ascribed to the disease, modes of
coping, family effects, and medical encounters. These themes fell within
the domains of (1) receiving and reacting to the diagnosis; (2) depression,
anger, and coping; and (3) medical encounters, communication, and frustrations.

Themes

Receiving and Reacting to the Diagnosis

Several participants reported fearing that they had AD before they received the formal diagnosis. They had experienced the phenomenon of *anticipatory dementia* (Cutler and Hodgson 1994) and worried that they might be afflicted. Thus, the diagnosis was actually a confirmation of their worst suspicions.

Meaning ascribed to disabling illness can involve three domains: self-concept; the continuity of personal meaning; and generalized worry (Luborsky 1995). Whether individuals with AD share these frames of meaning has not yet been discovered. Nor is it known whether they view the potential loss of role functioning as worse than death, as has been observed for other diseases (Ditto et al. 1996).

Thus, once they had been formally diagnosed, the individuals had to determine the personal meaning of the disease. Therefore, in response to the question, "What does it mean to you to have AD?" most of the respondents discussed their initial reaction.

They reported great difficulty in dealing with the diagnosis. Clearly, they feared future mental and physical disability. They interpreted the diagnosis as a catastrophic event that would affect every aspect of their lives, and the personal meaning of the disease was focused on loss. Multiple losses were identified: loss of functional ability, loss of independence, loss of self-image.

Essentially, meaning was framed as the threat to life and self. As one man stated, "When I heard, I wanted to go out the window—but I live on the first floor." Another respondent sadly reported, "I can't even think of what the disease does to a person."

One man stated, and others concurred, "I was just devastated. The bottom fell out." But another man remarked, "As bad as it was, I think I would have been more devastated if I found out I had lung cancer—at least I have some time and don't need surgery."

Some individuals refused to speculate on the meaning of functional loss but reported that they had been very upset about being told of the disease. "There are times you are discouraged; you just don't see any future and the future you can imagine is terrible."

On being asked to describe their initial reactions, they responded that they had had great difficulty accepting the diagnosis. Shock and disbelief had been common. A woman in her eighties said, "I couldn't believe it when I found out. I didn't feel any different. Now I'm waiting for the Lord to take me. But I have learned to live each day." "It took me two years to get used to the idea," said one man, sadly shaking his head. And in a regretful tone a man in his sixties said, "I might have to stop driving if my doctor has his way. This will be a big blow."

In several remarks made by individuals with AD and their family companions the family context of the disease was confirmed. Not surprisingly, people revealed that the family unit was severely impacted. While the individuals were upset and shocked, the family unit also was strained.

"Considering what the future would hold I have given durable power of attorney to my family," one woman stated sadly. Some individuals nodded in agreement, while others felt that she was just giving up. These different responses illustrate one of the two ways that families were affected. The first was by creating a sense of divisiveness between the person with AD and his or her spouse or child. Indeed, several family caregivers revealed that they felt the need to conceal their feelings from the person for whom they were caring. Spouses, in particular, seldom shared their thoughts and fears and sometimes withheld information in an attempt to protect their husband or wife. However, some families faced the disease together, discussed the future, and became more cohesive. This second type of family response was indicated in several ways. For example, some families acted to make their lives richer. Other tried to face the threat together, sharing their concerns and also their feelings. Some tried joint coping mechanisms, such as going to the library together to research the newest articles or jointly fulfilling leisure pursuits. Many families tried to maximize the quality of their family life during this period of intact functioning. "We try to ski, swim, play golf, or tennis almost every day, so as not to let this beat us down," said one woman with AD. Another reported: "We moved to be closer to our daughter. We want to see her as much as we can."

Depression, Anger, and Coping

Participants often found it difficult to adjust to the situation. Many had fallen into a sad, depressed state and found little that was positive in life.

Several adverse emotional responses were mentioned that were consistent with published reports of intense psychological aftereffects (Pearson et al. 1989; Reisberg and Ferris 1985; Teri and Uomoto 1991). The affective responses included depression and, to a less extent, anxiety. Some participants reported simultaneous depression and anger.

Clearly, a depressive response accompanies most chronic disease, and certainly life-threatening illnesses. Yet, for persons with AD, depression is one of the most prevalent affective responses. It is estimated to occur in at least 30 percent of the cases (Teri and Wagner 1992). The rate of depression may be as high as 50 percent at earlier stages of the disease (Pearson et al. 1989). Perhaps those who become depressed after the diagnosis may have greater insight and therefore are more aware of their own bodily functioning than those with less insight (Seltzer, Vasterling, and Bussell 1995). For these people, depression may be a response to their knowledge of their own bodily decline. For some, however, it may be a bereavement function, giving them the opportunity to mourn their future loss (Reifler and Larson 1989).

The method used to find out if people were, or had been, depressed was to ask all individuals that attended the four meetings to complete forms indicating their mood state (see Fig. 2.1). As noted above, on one form participants were to indicate what their mood state had been at the time they received the diagnosis. They were instructed to try to remember how they had felt when they returned home from the doctor's office.

Review of the first set of mood forms indicated that more than half (55%) had been depressed when they received the diagnosis. Another 22 percent circled the "sad" face. Together, these two groups represented more than three-fourths of the participants. The remaining 23 percent circled the face labeled "OK." These figures are higher than those reported in the literature, which indicates the rate of depression in early-stage AD to be approximately 50 percent. This difference may reflect the particular population that participated in the study, or it may relate to the type of instrument was used to measure depressive affect.

Since the literature also indicates that emotional devastation may lessen over time, the individuals were asked to move to the present time and indicate their general mood state during the week this meeting was held. As expected, for some persons with AD the depression had lessened and apparently run its course. Just 22 percent were depressed, none were sad, 77 percent were "OK," and 22 percent even circled the happy face. While the reduction in the rate of depression was expected, the drop from 77 percent to 22 percent for the depressed and sad mood states was not. In this case, the figures were lower than those reported in the literature for early-stage AD.

After completing the mood form, participants were encouraged to discuss depression. They were first asked to talk about their initial depressive response. Next they were asked why they believed this had occurred. "I suspected I had Alzheimer's because I knew something was wrong, but once I found out I was very down," said one man, who indicated that he had found it very hard to deal with the diagnosis, as did another: "I had a very tough time." One woman described the length of time that she had been very depressed: "I was in a complete fog for almost three months."

None of the participants reported receiving medication to treat the depression. One man stated, "I got started on Cognex; my mood improved." However, physicians prescribe this medication to help stabilize cognitive impairment, not for treatment of depression. Accordingly, not a single person reported being referred to a mental health professional for consultation or therapy. Despite the lack of pharmacological or professional intervention, most of the individuals reported that their depression had subsided.

When asked whether they felt that they had adjusted, most nodded their heads "yes." "You adjust to things you never thought you could—not driving, losing your independence," said one, and another said, "I'm not as pessimistic as I was four months ago." However, for one man the loss of driving privileges and other losses, including giving up his business, had perpetuated the depression: "It's been three years since I found out, but in the meantime they took away my car, my business, and everything that was important to me. I knew it was coming and I know I should move to some positive action, but I'm so down."

Family members were also depressed. However, they tried to prevent their husbands, wives, or parents from discovering this. They shared their feelings during the meeting of the family support group. Several reported that they always tried to keep their own spirits up in order to avoid upsetting or discouraging their loved ones.

Depression was not the only affective response. Many felt angry or cheated. As one man stated, "I was so angry when I found out. Now I'm not so angry, because there's really nothing I can do about it."

Generalized anger often gave way to specific targets. Participants were angry with medical providers for not finding a better way to treat the disease, and they were angry that science had not been able to find a cure. One person asked, "How come I have to look up information in the library? Why doesn't my doctor know what the new medical treatments are?" Another asked angrily, while others nodded their heads in agreement: "Why can't they find a cure? Why are they spending all of the money on cancer research?"

During the meeting of the family members' support group one wife stated: "He gets so upset sometimes." As repeatedly reported by these persons with AD, there was great difficulty accepting the diagnosis, and they often became depressed or angry. Yet, without medical help they somehow had developed ways of dealing with the situation that diminished their depressive response, if not their anger. Indeed, most of the persons with AD reported that they had developed positive ways of coping.

The literature shows that persons with AD have a wide range of coping behaviors (Cohen 1991). Some of the participants reported that they tried to avoid thinking about the disease, which may have helped them escape from reality. This coping behavior, which has been observed in other types of situations (Kahana, Kahana, and Young 1987), probably is a denial technique that enables persons with AD to avoid acknowledging the illness and eventual loss of physical, cognitive, and social functioning (Reisberg et al. 1989). Therefore, it may serve a protective function. Other individuals deal with the threat of future losses by cognitive restructuring, which casts the event in a different context. It may make the situation more manageable (Cohen 1991). Often persons with chronic disease seek information, which is an instrumental type of coping (Felton, Reverson, and Henrichsen 1984). Our participants sought information from others during the early-stage support group meetings and also welcomed informational talks from health and social service personnel. A few were more diligent and personally searched the literature for news of new pharmacological agents to help avert functional decline. Others sought out alternative medical providers or tried herbal remedies. Some behaviors typically associated with AD may actually be coping strategies (Cotrell and Lein 1993). Individuals may show repetitive actions of speech as they try to master the situation; alternatively, they may withdraw and retreat to defend themselves against fears of dependency (Verwoerdt 1981).

The range of coping strategies was quite wide. An energetic, youthful-looking man reported that he engaged in instrumental coping of the information-seeking type: "I try to find out about all the clinical trials and read all the books I can. I visit libraries and have become somewhat able to decipher medical journals. Often I have questions but try to find someone who can answer them."

One woman took advantage of the opportunity to learn new skills: "I started taking piano lessons; I always wanted to." Musical expression was also the method of choice of one man who continued his part-time job: "I dress in my tuxedo and play music at the mall; I will continue as long as I remember the songs people like to hear, because it really makes me feel good to do this." "I tap dance," said another man. "I'll never be Fred Astaire, but who cares?"

An older woman calmly reported her cognitive-restructuring behavior: "Everyone dies of something, and with this disease I have lots of notice. I'll be around for a while and can live my life pretty much as I want." One man stated matter-of-factly, "My father and grandfather had the disease so I expected it. When it came, I accepted it because I knew I had many years until I would lose everything." And in an almost preaching tone another man stated: "Tell [others] to do everything they can as soon as they can, enjoy all they can, realize attitude is important; if you can't drive and someone else can, go for it!"

Medical Encounters, Communication, and Frustration

Most of the individuals in the study were under the care of primary care physicians. Some had visited neurologists for confirmation of the diagnosis and then switched back to their regular physicians. As the group conversations progressed, they revealed that they had little confidence in, or good interaction with, their physicians. Almost universally, persons with AD reported their medical encounters to be very unsatisfactory and frustrating. Many remarked that medical professionals disappointed them. Spouses or other family members shared some of the dissatisfaction and frustration.

In general, there were two types of frustrating or unsatisfactory encounters. First, both persons with AD and their families were very disappointed by the medical care received, and second, they were very dissatisfied with communication and interaction patterns. Regarding the first, they were concerned about physicians' failure to pursue medical interventions. Doctors were portrayed as unknowledgeable, and frustration with medical man-

agement was common. Medical personnel were also criticized for not offering serious treatment. Doctors appeared to be letting the disease take its
course and not trying to arrest or even manage it. With regard to the second complaint, both persons with the disease and their family members felt
that only a paucity of information was being provided, especially about possible treatment options. They were particularly bothered about this information gap. They also believed that the office visits provided nothing but
an assessment of physical or mental limitations, with doctors advising them
that drugs might eventually hold some promise. This is consistent with the
attempt to medicalize AD (Lyman 1991). Accordingly, the interaction patterns were strictly disease-oriented, not person-oriented.

A sense of anger resulted from the strictly medical nature of the visit.
One spouse stated, in very strong terms: "Will you tell doctors what's going
on with us? These people are so ill informed." Regarding the paucity of information physicians provided, a person with the disease asked: "Why should
I have to do my own research? I'm constantly calling the Alzheimer's Association
or talking to people here in the group. That's where I get my information, not
from my doctor." Frustration with the nature of the medical care they received was a commonly expressed theme. Family members and persons
with the disease alike found the medical care system in general and their
own physician in particular to be unresponsive to their health needs.

The second type of medical dissatisfaction arose from the nature of the
medical encounter, especially as it involved communication and interaction. Almost every person with the disease expressed unhappiness with
communication patterns. The major complaint was that doctors seldom
communicated with them; rather, the communication was directed toward
spouses or family caregivers. Throughout the medical encounters the caregiver was asked to be the source of information, and the person with AD
was seldom asked direct questions. Persons with AD were not even told directly of the diagnosis. "My doctor told me nothing," said one man. "He told
my wife and she had to break it to me."

Other men concurred that only their spouse was directly informed of the
diagnosis and that physicians made determinations of health and functioning by querying the accompanying family member. The literature
shows that it is quite common to expect family members to be proxy reporters about health status and functional decline of persons with AD
(Green et al. 1993; Kiyak, Teri, and Borson 1994). Seeking information

about whether the person can remember certain things or is able to use public transportation, the physician asks the family member. Physicians often encourage caregivers to preempt the person with dementia and directly answer their questions (Teri et al. 1989). One man told us angrily, "Any answers you want, ask my wife, just as the doctor does."

Clearly, such an interaction pattern ignores the patient's own concerns and facilitates the caregiver's gatekeeper role (George 1989). This person provides information and screens or inhibits the diseased person's conversation. Perhaps this is done lovingly, in an attempt to protect the latter, but it may not be beneficial. It may actually increase the anxiety level of the person with AD (Young 1998).

An analysis of these remarks about medical encounters reveals a clear pattern of dyadic interaction. The medical encounter predominantly involves a spouse-physician dyad. Traditional medical interaction models proposed a patient-physician dyad, but this was found wanting, so the models were expanded to include a triadic interaction pattern (Bloom 1965). In this model the physician, patient, and family member are included in disease presentation, medical management decisions, and overall communication.

There is no model of physician-patient interaction that circumvents the patient, except for pediatric care. Very young children and infants do not interact directly with physicians, and communication is with their parents. That these focus group participants reported the typical form of the medical encounter to be a physician-caregiver dyad suggests that persons with AD are being infantilized by the medical profession. Persons with AD were particularly offended by being ignored or treated like children. "Tell me why I need to be treated like a child by my doctor. Why should I put up with it?" asked one participant. "Why don't they listen to us? Why do they avoid us, or ignore us?" asked another.

Individuals complained bitterly about other aspects of their interaction and communication with physicians. They were very concerned that they were not respected, that they were not being treated as competent adults, and that their decision-making powers were being taken away. Said one man:

My doctor asks me how I am, nods when I tell him, and then asks me to step outside. He and my wife discuss me and then call me back and tell me what to do.

That's how I lost use of my car and was forced to give up my business. The doctor told her I would deteriorate and not be able to take care of the business, so to sell it while she could still get a pretty penny for it.

This man was very resentful and expressed relief that his wife was attending the family-support group meeting and thus could not hear his comments. However, his remarks generated several nods of agreement. One man advised this individual to stay in the room at the next visit to the physician and not comply with the request to step out. Another frustrated man stated: "He tells [my wife] how to deal with the disease, not me."

Other frustrations with physicians were that they lacked understanding. The persons with AD also complained that they had received little help, support, or interest from the medical care system. Physicians were reported as cold and distant. Two men that had lost their driving privileges perceived their physicians as punitive for initiating this action.

Perhaps due to the dyadic nature of the medical encounter, some individuals believed that their physician and family caregiver were colluding to take away their independence and relegate them to the role of an "object," as one stated. As the result of these experiences, many people with the disease felt anger not only toward their physician but toward their spouse as well.

Lessons Learned

Several lessons were learned from directly asking persons with AD to talk about what the disease means to them and to identify ways that they are dealing with the situation. First, this means of eliciting information provides knowledge of the subjective world of these individuals that would not be forthcoming in other ways. We gain essential knowledge of what these people are going through now, what they previously experienced, and how they are managing and adjusting. We can use this information to better understand the people involved and their experiences. Such knowledge and understanding put health care or social service personnel in a better position to help persons with AD and their families.

The results of this inquiry can provide valuable guidance for the medical care system as well. One extremely important lesson is how both persons with AD and their family members can be better served by health professionals. These firsthand reports showed that there is much room for improvement in interaction and communication patterns. It was quite obvious that a triadic interaction pattern involving the patient, the physician, and the family member was not being implemented for delivery of the diagnosis, medical management decisions, or psychosocial need assessments. Nor was there evidence of the classic medical dyad (patient and physician) in either conversation or general communication. Therefore, health professionals can greatly benefit the person with AD and or her family by improved interaction strategies. There are several ways to accomplish this. First, the patient should be present when the diagnosis is delivered so that the spouse or family caregiver will not have to decide if and when to tell the person with AD the "bad news." Communication that excludes the individual with the disease lessens the likelihood of a positive medical encounter. Second, the diagnosis, and especially the prognosis, should be presented in hopeful terms. After all, medical research has identified many promising treatments for this disease. The new field of gene therapy is specifically addressing genetic determinants of AD and seeking to find ways to modify a person's genetic profile. Physicians can provide information about new and potentially useful medical treatments and might also suggest enrollment in clinical trials. Any of these could make the person's medical encounter more helpful.

A third approach would be to recommend social services. After all, persons with AD and their family caregivers have many needs. Often they do not know about services to aid either or both of them. Many families think that outside of nursing home care or home care aides, there are no appropriate formal services. Although more agencies and programs that offer services are needed, many service agencies are in place in major urban communities. Respite care for caregivers, adult day care for persons with AD, and support groups for both are appropriate recommendations for physicians to make. Fourth, physicians should also become aware of the extent of the depression brought on by an AD diagnosis. Once they have this knowledge, they might try to ameliorate depressive symptomatology through medication. They could talk directly to persons who have been diagnosed with AD about their feelings, fears, mood states, and similar matters. If appropriate, they might also refer the individuals to a mental health provider. The physician should be involved in the psychological, social, and service needs of the entire person with AD and his or her family. Finally, the physician should treat the person with AD with respect. Even when cognitive loss is severe, many persons with AD listen when questions are posed, acknowledge that they have been spoken to, and are able to respond to a smile or friendly greeting.

Another lesson learned from direct questioning of people at early stages of the disease is that asking persons with AD to answer questions and talk about their situation can enhance their self-esteem. It shows them that they are valued and respected and that others wish to hear their opinions. It reinforces the fact that they are not incompetent. Indeed, the participants in this study showed, and reported, that they were quite pleased that their views were being sought and that they were being asked about their problems. Some talked about matters that they had never discussed with their loved ones.

Conclusion

When people are encouraged to report their feelings, talk about problems, and share the ways they deal with anticipated loss, valuable information can be gathered. It was clear to me that twenty-four persons with AD and ten family members wanted to tell their stories. Rather than being reluctant reporters, individuals with the disease appreciated the opportunity to be treated as adults rather than as children or as incompetent, to be pitied or ignored. They were not hesitant to reveal their fears, emotional responses, or depressed state or to express their anger and frustration. Their personal statements revealed complex but fairly predictable subjective responses to both the diagnosis and the prognosis of functional loss.

The initial reaction was one of shock and emotional devastation. However, this gave way over time to a second stage, in which there was less emotional devastation and a gradual adjustment to the situation. By the second stage, most people had stopped denying that they had a fatal disease that would cause them to lose everything they valued; they had begun the long process of dealing with the situation. The strategies they used to adjust included active coping, especially information gathering attempts, enrollment in clinical trials, and participation in support group meetings.

The medical encounters of these individuals were extremely frustrating. Often corroborated by spouses were reports of medical professionals ignoring the person with the disease and failing to offer medical alternatives or suggestions or even to provide basic understanding and support. Persons with AD were being infantilized, and spouses were encouraged to humor them while watching for signs that the persons with AD might need to stop working, driving, or caring for themselves. The basic dignity of these people was being denied by the medical profession.

Whether one's interest in the situations of individuals with early-stage AD is that of a researcher, a social service provider, or a provider of medical care, it should be recognized that they are real people and thus should be taken seriously. They should not be ignored, overlooked, or considered to be unreliable reporters. Firsthand reports of their situations and experiences should be encouraged, and the information they provide should be heeded. Furthermore, they should be respected. Health professionals, in particular, may better serve persons with AD and also their family members by treating the former respectfully, as adults, and encouraging them to express themselves.

REFERENCES

Bloom, S. W. 1965. *The doctor and his patient*. New York: Free Press.

Cohen, D. 1991. The subjective experience of Alzheimer's disease: The anatomy of an illness as perceived by patient and families. *American Journal of Alzheimer's Care and Related Disorders and Research*, May/June, 6–11.

Cotrell, V., and L. Lein. 1993. Awareness and denial in the Alzheimer's disease victim. *Journal of Gerontological Social Work* 19:115–32.

Cotrell, V., and R. Schulz. 1993. The perspective of the patient with Alzheimer's disease: A neglected dimension of dementia research. *Gerontologist* 33 (2): 205–11.

Cutler, S. J., and L. G. Hodgson. 1994. Anticipatory dementia: A continuum of concern about developing Alzheimer's disease. Paper presented at the annual meeting of the Gerontological Society of America, Atlanta, November.

Ditto, P. H., J. A. Druley, K. A. Moore, J. H. Danks, and W. D. Smucker. 1996. Fates worse than death: The role of valued life activities in health-state evaluations. *Health Psychology* 15 (5): 332–43.

Felton, B. J., T. A. Reverson, and G. A. Henrichsen. 1984. Stress and coping in the explanation of psychological adjustment among chronically ill adults. *Social Science and Medicine* 18 (10): 889–98.

George, L. K. 1989. Services research: Research problems and possibilities. In *Alzheimer's disease treatment and family stress: Directions for research*, ed. E. Light and B. Lebowitz, 401–31. Rockville, Md.: NIMH.

Green, J., F. C. Goldstein, B. E. Sirockman, and R. C. Green. 1993. Variable awareness of deficits in Alzheimer's disease. *Neuropsychiatry, Neuropsychology, and Behavioral Neurology* 6 (3): 159–65.

Kahana, E. F., B. M. Kahana, and R. Young. 1987. Strategies of coping and post-institutional outcomes. *Research on Aging* 9:182–99.

Kiyak, H. A., L. Teri, and S. Borson. 1994. Physical and functional health assessment in normal aging and in Alzheimer's disease: Self-reports vs family reports. *Gerontological Society of America* 34 (3): 324–30.

Luborsky, M. R. 1995. The process of self-report of impairment in clinical research. *Social Science and Medicine* 40 (11): 1447–59.

Luborsky, M. R., and E. M. Riley. 1996. Understanding the meaning, expression, and experience of depression in later life: Anthropological perspectives. In *Aging and depression in long term and residential care*, ed. R. Rubinstein and M. P. Lawton. New York: Springer.

Lyman, K. 1991. Bringing the social back in: A critique of biomedicine and dementia. *Gerontologist* 29:597–605.

Pearson, J. L., L. Teri, B. V. Reifler, and M. A. Raskind. 1989. Functional status and cognitive impairment in Alzheimer's patients with and without depression. *Journal of American Geriatric Society* 37:1117–21.

Reifler, B., and E. Larson. 1989. Excess disability in dementia of the Alzheimer's type. In *Alzheimer's disease treatment and family stress: Directions for research*, ed. E. Light and B. Lebowitz, 363–82. Rockville, Md.: NIMH.

Reisberg, B., and S. Ferris. 1985. A clinical rating scale for symptoms of psychosis in AD. *Psychopharmacol Bulletin* 21:101–4.

Reisberg, B., S. Ferris, A. Kluger, E. Franssen, M. deLeon, J. Mittleman, J. Borenstein, K. Rameshwar, and R. Alda. 1989. Symptomatic changes in CNS aging and dementia of the Alzheimer's type: Cross-sectional, temporal, and remediable concomitants. In *Diagnosis and treatment of senile dementia*, ed. M. Bergener and B. Reisberg, 193–223. Berlin: Springer-Verlag.

Seltzer, B., J. J. Vasterling, and A. Bussell. 1995. Awareness of the deficit in Alzheimer's disease: Association with psychiatric symptoms and other disease variables. *Journal of Clinical Geropsychology* 1 (1): 79–87.

Stewart, D. W., and P. N. Shamdasani. 1990. Recruiting focus group participants and designing the interview guide. In *Focus groups: Theory and practice*, ed. D. W. Stewart and P. N. Shamdasani, 51–68. Newbury Park, Calif.: Sage.

Teri, L., S. Borson, A. Kiyak, and M. Yamagishi. 1989. Behavioral disturbance, cognitive dysfunction, and functional skill. *Journal of the American Geriatrics Society* 37:109–16.

Teri, L., and J. Uomoto. 1991. Reducing excess disability in dementia patients: Training caregivers to manage patient depression. *Clinical Gerontologist* 10:49–63.

Teri, L., and A. Wagner. 1992. Alzheimer's disease and depression. *Journal of Consulting and Clinical Psychology* 3:379–91.

Verwoerdt, A. 1981. Individual psychotherapy in senile dementia. In *Clinical aspects of Alzheimer's disease and senile dementia*, ed. N. E. Miller and G. D. Cohen, 187–209. New York: Raven.

Young, R. F. 1998. The subjective experience of Alzheimer's disease. *Gerontologist* 38 (1): 297–99.

Part 2

The Impact
of the Diagnosis
on Everyday Life

Living with the Symptoms of Alzheimer's Disease

ALISON PHINNEY

It's scary. Yeah, it's scary. . . . I suppose in a way it's like being in a fog, and you can't find your way out of it. . . . I mean, not knowing is frightening.
—Sandra, a 78-year-old retired professor of nursing

It is vitally important to understand how people with early Alzheimer's disease experience symptoms. Symptoms are an important dimension of any illness. They may serve as signals of underlying disease, and descriptions of symptoms help us to understand what it is like to live with an illness. Therefore, we listen carefully as our patients, our family members, and our friends tell us about their physical symptoms—pain in the left shoulder or dizziness upon first getting up in the morning. We pay attention when they describe their mental or emotional symptoms—hearing voices or feeling sadness and despair. However, persons with AD are often ignored or discounted when they try to explain the symptoms they live with. We tend to assume that their reports are not accurate or reliable, telling ourselves that perhaps they do not recognize their symptoms or that they have forgotten them (Geldmacher and Whitehouse 1996). Clinical research in this area is replete with studies of Alzheimer's symptoms as they have been observed by others, but very little is known about what the symptoms are like for the person with the illness.

Recent research has tried to look at how persons with AD perceive their symptoms, but the question has been posed in terms of how aware they are of their symptoms (DeBettignies, Mahurin, and Pirozzolo 1990; Derouesne et al. 1999; Vasterling et al. 1997; Weinstein, Friedland, and Wagner 1994). Asking how aware they are presumes that as outside observers we can accurately perceive the person's symptoms and that our interest in the person's perspective is limited to the question of how impaired that perspective is. This question reflects the way in which we have traditionally viewed AD as a disease of cognition in which the ability to self-reflect breaks down. Symptom experience, regarded as an issue of (self-)awareness, becomes yet another indicator of decline rather than an expression of the richness and complexity of the person's illness experience.

The purpose of this chapter is to direct the focus to persons with AD and their perception and interpretation of their own symptoms in order to better capture some of this richness and complexity. The view in this chapter is that symptoms are an expression of lived experience, that to describe one's symptoms is to articulate something of the very meaning of the illness itself (Benner and Wrubel 1989; Kleinmann 1988).

Study Methods

Data Collection

The following discussion is based on findings from two studies that consisted in interviewing and observing a total of thirteen persons with early AD and their family caregivers. The in-depth, semistructured interviews (tape-recorded and transcribed) lasted from 45 to 100 minutes. Depending on the study, persons with AD were interviewed two or three times, and family members were interviewed one or three times. Both studies also included an observation component; persons with AD and their families were observed for several hours as they went about their usual daily activities. The research questions focused on how the person with AD experienced symptoms, the meaning the illness had for them, and how they coped with and adapted to the changes in their lives. Family caregivers were asked to talk, not about their own experiences, but about what they thought it was like for the person with AD to live with the disease. Thus, data were obtained from three sources to help provide a more complete picture of how persons with AD experience the symptoms of the disease.

The participants were eight women and five men who ranged in age from

TABLE 3.1. Characteristics of People with Alzheimer's Disease

Person with AD	Age	Years since Diagnosis	MMSE Score[a]	Previous Work	Living Situation
Maggie	71	1	16	Medical transcriptionist	With spouse
Bebe	88	3	18	Office receptionist	With daughter
Christina	68	0.5	18	Gallery sales agent	With spouse
Bob	81	1	23	Professor of music	With spouse
Mary	70	2	17	Homemaker	Assisted living
Jim	76	4	22	Public-utility foreman	With spouse
Tom	64	2	23	High-school teacher	With spouse
Sandra	78	4	19	Professor of nursing	With friend
Roy	86	2	18	Office manager	With spouse
Edith	89	4	17	Music teacher	Assisted living
Joyce	73	2.5	20	Homemaker	With spouse
Harold	81	1	24	Office manager	With spouse
Laura Mae	82	3	18	Homemaker	With spouse

[a]Mini-Mental State Examination.

64 to 89 (Table 3.1). All but four lived in their own homes with their spouses (two women lived in assisted living facilities, one woman lived at home with her daughter, and one lived at home with a longtime friend). The length of time since persons had been diagnosed with AD ranged from six months to four years, or an average of 2.3 years, and the levels of dementia ranged from mild to moderate (16–24 on the Mini-Mental State Examination, or MMSE). All the participants either had participated in previous AD research or were members of early-diagnosis support groups. It was through these connections that they had heard of this research and volunteered to take part. All of the participants were Caucasians who lived in comfortable middle-class rural, suburban, and urban communities. Everyone had at least a high-school education, and eight of the participants had attended college for two or more years. Four participants had a graduate-level degree.

Data Analysis

The findings are based on the results of a thematic analysis whose emphasis was on revealing the patterns and meanings of lived experience (van
Manen 1990). Interviews and field notes were read in their entirety several
times, and notes were made in the margins about issues and concerns raised
by the participants. The issues and concerns were formulated into more
general themes, which were compared across the cases for similarities and
differences. In addition to looking for themes across the entire text, I summarized each set of interviews and notes to capture some of the important
meanings in each person's experience. The analysis was thus a process of
going back and forth between the specific and the general, of understanding the "particular" in the light of the "universal" (van Manen 1990, 79).
To make the process more rigorous, I had colleagues review portions of the
raw data and the analyzed text.

Findings

Analysis of data from the thirteen participants involving the experience of
symptoms revealed five themes: (1) "I can't remember"; (2) "I worry about
getting lost"; (3) "Everything is more difficult"; (4) "Conversations don't
always fall into place"; and (5) "I'm sort of oblivious." I discuss each of these
in turn, using extensive illustrations from the interview texts. In all cases,
pseudonyms are used to protect people's identity.

"I can't remember"

Everyone spoke of being unable to remember things that they thought they
should know, such as names of people or recent occurrences. This kind of
forgetfulness involves an inability to call to mind certain factual knowledge. People spoke of trying to recall a recent event and not being able to
do so. It is not as if it never happened. Rather, while they may know intellectually that they were involved in the event (i.e., they know *of* it), they
no longer know *about* it. They are losing knowledge of what is happening
in their world. They realize that they no longer know something they knew
at one time and that they cannot retrieve that information.

Maggie is able to describe what this is like. Laughing with embarrassment, she explains: "It's almost like I'm a blank all the time. I mean really. [little laugh] It's kind of weird. I can't remember what I do from one next to the, from one day to the next. What did I do you know?" Being a "blank" is a realization that comes to Maggie when she steps out of her usual routine and tries to remember something.

MAGGIE: Well, this morning I enjoyed [my walk].
INTERVIEWER: Yeah. Can you remember where you went?
MAGGIE: Yeah, I uh . . . It's funny, I say "Yeah" and then I look over there [indicating the window by the table] and I forget what. [little laugh] But anyway . . .
INTERVIEWER: Is that what you meant, when a minute ago you said everything becomes a blank?
MAGGIE: Yeah, . . . yeah, something like that.

In other words, the blankness of forgetting is a feeling that comes when she steps back to adopt a reflective stance. The sad irony is that Maggie is finding that she has to take this stance more and more, being always attentive and mindful in order to prevent complete confusion and disorientation. For example, she watches her surroundings carefully when she is out for a walk so that she does not get lost. She no longer takes going for a walk for granted. So it is possible that Maggie's efforts to cope make her more aware of this blankness. Later on she describes this blankness as being without thoughts or words. "Well, it's kind of like just being a zombie . . . not using your brain. You're maybe just looking at what's around. Don't think about, . . . don't think about it. Don't . . . I don't talk to yourself about it."

Several of the participants, Maggie included, describe their problem as one of "short-term memory." Bob feels that his problem is that it is difficult for him to get information into "permanent storage." He explains: "What I find difficult though, is remembering . . . uh . . . remembering things. Maybe peoples' names, or what I did or what I went to the store and didn't get, or things like that, that are not planted back there." He and his wife, Ashley, explain that he can only remember one thing at a time.

ASHLEY: We both know that if we are talking together and I ask you to do something, or just talking about a subject, it has to be just one thing. It can't be . . . if it's something like "Please take out the garbage," that's OK, but it can't be "Please take out the garbage and on the way back in please bring in the six-pack of Coke from the garage and then would you get the newspapers together." I mean it has to be one item. Hmm?

BOB: Yeah, I think it . . .

INTERVIEWER: Would you agree with that?

BOB: I tend to find it difficult, yeah. Cause I can't remember, it seems to get erased by the second idea.

INTERVIEWER: The first one gets erased by the second?

BOB: Yeah. So I try to . . . stay with the first part of it.

Bob describes what it is like to forget: "[It's like] having a goal that you're not going for. You can't reach it because you don't remember what it is. Sometimes I guess I get angry or upset just at the fact that I have troubles, and uh . . . then it makes it worse of course." He gets angry when he is having difficulties, and then his concentration slips and his memory fails him further.

Maggie certainly finds this to be the case. As she struggled to tell me a story, she became increasingly frustrated by her inability to remember. She stumbled over her words to tell me how it gets worse as she becomes more frustrated.

MAGGIE: Well, when I left [my job] we had these little . . . [laughs uncomfortably] How can I tell you if I can't . . . ? We . . . uh . . . it gets worse when I . . .

INTERVIEWER: Get frustrated?

MAGGIE: [Nodding, speaking at the same time as the interviewer] Get frustrated. Maybe I can wait.

INTERVIEWER: It'll come back.

MAGGIE: Anyway . . . I gave the guy some . . . this other fellow who worked there. . . . No, I can't do it, I can't.

When talking about what it feels like when she forgets something, Maggie responds quickly.

INTERVIEWER: When you have a problem with your memory now, what is that like for you?

MAGGIE: Frustration. Uh huh. Yeah.

INTERVIEWER: What does that feel like?

MAGGIE: It feels like shit, if you want to know.

This frustration and anger were echoed by several of the participants. Some said that they felt angry at themselves. Christina often chastises herself in the hope that it will help her find the motivation to fight back against the illness. "I scold myself because 'You are trying so hard Christina to understand this disease and try to . . . uh . . . conquer it and there you are. You haven't conquered it, and maybe you won't conquer it.' And I talk to myself like that. I'm trying to make the best of it, if possible to conquer it."

Sandra claims that being forgetful is her main problem. She is especially distressed at not being able to remember things that have happened recently or are going to happen soon. Her response is not one of anger but one of fear. "It's scary. Yeah, it's scary. Um . . . I suppose in a way it's like being in a fog, and you can't find your way out of it. . . . I mean, not knowing is frightening."

Sandra does not say anything more about how and why "not knowing" is frightening, but there are a number of possibilities. In part it may be frightening because being unable to remember leaves her feeling adrift, unable to grasp what is happening around her. It may also be frightening when Sandra's memory failure causes her to lose trust and confidence in herself. Her fear may come in part from this feeling of profound vulnerability.

In summary, participants felt that they were often unable to get hold of information that they thought they should know. This feeling of being a blank was frustrating, embarrassing, and also frightening. But it is worth pointing out that not all of the participants were upset by their forgetfulness. Some feel that it is to be expected because they are getting old. Bebe says that for her, being forgetful is as natural as being unable to run quickly. It happens because her brain, like the rest of her body, is slowing down. It is sometimes consternating, but it is nothing to really be worried about. "Well, I think everybody does [have memory problems]," she explained. However, when I asked her more about it, she was unable to describe this experience. "No. Don't, can't even remember it. . . . I'm not concerned about it. I think I'm just doing what nature does to you as you get older."

"I worry about getting lost"

Being lost was a major concern of most of the participants. Many had a story to tell about finding themselves in an unfamiliar place or not knowing how to find their way from one place to another.

Jim is someone who worries a great deal about getting lost when he is out walking the dog in his neighborhood. He feels unsure of himself and is only comfortable if there is someone to accompany him or if he follows the same route each time. Even though he has lived in the same house for almost forty years, his surroundings are strangely unfamiliar to him now. In contrast, the neighborhood where he grew up, in a nearby city, seems much closer and familiar in his mind.

> Just the other day I was going to go down and get something that, uh . . . see if I can remember what it was. [The supermarket], I think it was. Yeah, it was at [the supermarket]. And, uh, I couldn't remember the names of any of the streets on the way down there. . . . In a residential area where there is nothing but houses . . . when you get out walking and the streets are going zig and zag . . . I just if it was in [the city], I, in [my old neighborhood] or something, I know them backwards and forwards, but here I'm not that familiar with the streets. When I get down the street a ways I get lost.

Jim can no longer be in the world in a completely unreflective way when he is out walking. As he himself explains later on, he has lost the capacity to just go without giving it a second thought: "And, uh, it's just everything is taken for granted until this happens and then all of a s-sudden you think, 'Oh, I got to think now, how do I get back to where I'm came from?'" Jim attributes the unfamiliarity of his surroundings to forgetfulness since he does not remember the names of the streets. But it is more than that. As he describes his experience, it is almost as if the fabric of the world itself has changed.

Feeling lost was experienced by many as a sense of being in unfamiliar terrain, feeling that the world around them did not make any sense. Joyce explained this most clearly when she said that her world seemed to be constantly changing. "I try to go out every day, just to see if things have changed that much. But they do . . . I can see the same things I've seen for years, and they're different. Everything is different. I can't explain it."

The way Tom describes it, there are times when he is not able to make sense of the world around him. For a brief moment his world loses meaning.

> [You] just don't know where you are for a moment. Now, um, . . . that's happening a little more frequently and a little more strong—once in a while I'll get to a place that I don't know, and I've been there a hundred times and I don't know, I

don't know where I am. And then it just snaps right in. . . . Suddenly I am where I am supposed to be. This happens very fast. Even before you know it and there is any significant action. Just a feeling that I am not here. Now I am here.

Tom continues to walk comfortably around his local community, and he still drives to other towns and cities to run errands for the family. As far as he can recall, and as far as his family is aware, he has never become truly lost, unable to find his way around a place. But he has these uncomfortable moments of feeling lost in the world, moments that are becoming more frequent and more intense.

Others have had actual experiences of losing their way, not knowing where they were or being unable to find their way home. Maggie loves to go out walking every day, but it is always with some trepidation, given her concern about getting lost. This happened to her once when she was shopping at a large mall about twenty blocks from her house. It was before she knew she had AD.

MAGGIE: [Little laugh] I don't want to get lost.
INTERVIEWER: Has that ever happened to you?
MAGGIE: Uh, yeah, once . . . uh, before I even knew about this several years ago . . . uh, yeah, several years ago. I went to, uh . . . let's see now. Oh, . . . [little laugh] I went to a store, not downtown, but Rockline? What is it?
INTERVIEWER: Rockhurst.
MAGGIE: Rockhurst. And it was very crowded. People were pushing. Everyone was pushing. You know, in there, and I got very confused. This was the first thing. And I, um [clears throat], I kind of lost my memory there, and I went and I saw a lady and I asked her if she would help me. Which she was very nice. I didn't even know about Alzheimer's. And, uh, . . . I said, "Can you help me find how to get home?" [little laugh, clears throat] And she told me where to go, and I got on the bus or the train or whatever it is, and I made it home. But I'll never, haven't done that again.

Maggie makes a point of describing the circumstances, implying that the environment of the crowded mall caused her to become confused. Perhaps she was unable to see clearly where she was because the crowds were making it hard for her to find the signs she needed to find her way to the bus. Or maybe once she realized that she couldn't find her way, she needed to really concentrate but could not because of the distractions.

Others spoke of feeling uncomfortable in new places. Bob travels frequently with his wife, although it is becoming increasingly difficult for him.
He has trouble finding the bathroom in a strange place at night. He has uri-
nary urgency and is anxious to avoid being incontinent.

BOB: Well, I'm reluctant about [traveling]. I wish I didn't. . . . We'll be the
guests in a lot of homes, and, uh, this has a twist to it. . . . If I feel the urgency
to urinate, I get out of bed and get in the bathroom as quick as I can. That's an-
noying, and we had one experience with . . . Andrew is, uh, Ashley's oldest
son—tall, big fellow, down in the southern part of this state. And we were down
there, and he has a sprawling big home, and I found myself needing to urinate
very badly. I couldn't find the bathroom. It was really, really rough, but I did find
it. But there were about three of them, and you had to go down this hallway and
that . . . just terrible. And, uh, I'm worrying about that [for our next trip back
East] because we're going to be in one home that I know is very big and similar
to the one down south. . . .
INTERVIEWER: It's hard to find your way around a new place.
BOB: Yeah, especially if you get the feeling like being in a hurry.

This story reveals that Bob's difficulty finding his way around a new place
is not necessarily a problem in and of itself. Rather, it is an obstacle that he
has to surmount in order to cope with the immediate problem of making it
to the bathroom in time. Finding his way is more difficult when he is in a
hurry and thus perhaps less able to pay careful attention to his surroundings. Finding his way does not present any difficulties in his own home, but
it is something that he is unable to do in an unfamiliar place.

In summary, participants often felt as if their surroundings were unfamiliar, even places they thought they knew well. Their surroundings sometimes seemed strange and hard to make sense of, and people found themselves having to pay careful attention to cues in their environment. But
even with this extra effort, sometimes they could not find their way.

"Everything is more difficult"

People describe becoming less able to engage in meaningful activity; more
specifically, they find it difficult to use objects or devices. They often lose
things that they need in order to get along during the day and spend con-

siderable time searching for them. Some report that their activities are slowed down and that they often have to stop and think about what to do next. Sometimes they cannot make sense of the objects that are at their disposal and do not know how to use them. People find that they have to work much harder at simple tasks. As Tom puts it, "Everything is more difficult now."

Losing Things

People complain of having trouble finding things around the house. They spend a lot of time looking, which often keeps them from engaging in a desired activity. Maggie says that she is always asking herself, "Now what did I do with that?" She explains that she has trouble keeping track of her belongings and that she has to stop and think when she is looking for something in the house. Each morning when she gets ready to go for her regular walk, she cannot just automatically pick up her purse and head for the door. Rather, she has to stop and think about where her purse might be, and then she starts looking. Her husband points out that she may see the purse but not recognize it as being what she is looking for and continue her search. He often has to help her look. He has suggested that she leave her purse in the same place every time but met with limited success.

Jim's experience is much the same. His medications are kept in a small box near the fireplace so they will be in easy view. Even so, he can never find them. Unlike Maggie, he doesn't spend much time looking for the box. Instead, once he realizes that he doesn't know where it is, if he doesn't immediately see it when he glances around the room, he asks his wife for help. Without her there to tell him, he would be unable to find the pills.

Losing things is something that happens often to Christina, although she rarely complains about it. One example involves the box that contains her notes from her master's exam, which she and I were speaking of one day. She had told me several times in previous interviews of her plan to review these notes to help her remember what she had learned when she was in school so many years before. On this particular day I had seen the box on the kitchen stove an hour earlier, but Christina apparently did not remember that it was there. But this did not seem to bother her. She expressed no frustration or concern, nor did she seem in the least upset or bothered. "Yeah. Right. The box is out. It might be right in here [looking on the adjacent table but unable to find it]. I've hidden it for a while, and that's my next project. [pause] I think it's upstairs in my bedroom, it's somewhere."

Christina's present equanimity stands in contrast to the early days of the disease, when she would become extremely anxious and fearful when she could not find something. She saw it as a sign that things were getting worse, and since she knew what lay ahead (given her strong family history of AD), she experienced what she now calls "extreme suffering." She was entirely focused on her feelings, which she says made it even more difficult to find things.

> INTERVIEWER: You used the term *extreme suffering*.
> CHRISTINA: Yeah.
> INTERVIEWER: Is that what that was like?
> CHRISTINA: It was. Because I knew what I was facing, and . . . uh . . . it was in the early stages when it was hitting and I couldn't find . . . because of the worry I think that I couldn't find anything. And . . . and . . .
> INTERVIEWER: So it was making it worse.
> CHRISTINA: It was making it worse, and the fe- . . . fear of the . . . of the whole thing just was rising every minute, and oh gosh, here it is I can't find, and I'd get so frustrated and so upset, and I would cry and I would look and look, and then I wouldn't find it because I was not really concentrating on what I was looking at. I was more concerned about my feelings and . . . and you know what was happening to me—I'm declining! I'm declining!

Eventually she was able to overcome this by changing her attitude— telling herself, "Either you find it or you don't." She does not say that she has overcome the problem of not finding things, but it is no longer an issue in her life. It doesn't bother her anymore because she doesn't let it. On the other hand, her inability to find these notes is one of the things that is keeping her from following through on her plan to review this material.

Feeling Confused

People admit that there are occasions when they do not know what to do next, when they do not understand what is happening around them and do not know what is expected of them. Maggie, for example, recalled going to a busy Laundromat by herself and becoming confused. She couldn't remember how to use the machines and had to ask for help.

MAGGIE: Oh, I'll tell you something that happened. I went to go . . . to the . . . I was going to say to church [little laugh]. To the . . . to the linder . . . to the Laundromat. . . . I went to the Laundromat and it was crowded, and that really threw me off. I couldn't remember what I was supposed to do. And I was putting in . . . the money in a place, and I was just all mixed up. And people were looking at me and giving me dirty looks [little laugh] and . . . I even lost some of my clothes—people had to come and help me. There was a lady there, and I said, "I'm sorry, I've got Alzheimer's." And she was very, very nice. It was horrible. And I didn't want to say anything. [clears throat] . . . And I put a lot more money in there than I needed, and people were looking at me. It was awful. . . . But there were nice people there, but it's just so crowded. When I went in I started putting my clothes in the wrong place. [little laugh] . . . Well anyway . . . Cause I was, I put the clothes . . . where it was supposed to be already done.

INTERVIEWER: In the dryer?

MAGGIE: Yeah, in the dryer. Yeah, and I was putting too much money . . . I don't know how I didn't even run out of money. So I don't know what I was doing. [little laugh] I don't think I will do that . . . go again myself—I was so humiliated.

This is an example of the breakdown of meaningful activity. Maggie found herself completely unable to make sense of the situation, and there is a great deal at stake in her being able to do so. One concern is her capacity to do a simple chore like the laundry on her own. She worries about losing her independence and eventually ending up in a nursing home. But more immediate is her concern about how she must have looked. Her confusion was visible for all to see, and she was ashamed and humiliated that she had appeared incompetent in front of others.

Tom described how he feels when he has directions to follow and cannot keep track of what he is supposed to do.

TOM: Well, you got family around you, you can get mixed up and confused. [laughs]

INTERVIEWER: [Laughing] How so?

TOM: Yeah!

INTERVIEWER: What do you mean?

TOM: Ooh, too much noise. Uh, somebody asking me or telling me to do something. I don't get the directions for that in time to do what I have to do next. And then I . . . will be told to do A, and then before I can really think out A I've got B to do. And then I go back to A and I can't remember what A was.

Both Tom's and Maggie's accounts of confusion suggest that their environment seems chaotic. Tom refers to his family around him, saying there is "too much noise" and suggesting that too much is being demanded of him. Maggie describes the Laundromat as busy and crowded and says that this "threw her off." Both suggest that they need to concentrate more these days in order to do the simplest activities. As Tom explains it, everything takes more time and conscious effort.

TOM: It's just everything works more slowly, that's it.

INTERVIEWER: What is it like being slower?

TOM: Um, I have to scan everything in my car when I drive it. I have to look at everything and make sure I've got everything ready to start the car. Otherwise I'll forget something.

Tom is more cautious now. For example, he no longer just jumps in the car and goes. He has to consciously take account of the task at hand and think carefully about what he has to do. What used to be automatic has become deliberate and mindful.

In summary, participants felt that their everyday activities were becoming more difficult to accomplish. They often lost track of things around the house and needed help to find them. They found themselves becoming confused when faced with equipment that once posed no problem. Every step in a task takes careful attention and conscious effort, and sometimes they are not sure what to do next. The simplest of activities can no longer be taken for granted. For some people this was devastating, especially when they felt that others were watching and judging them. But others seemed accepting of this change in their lives and were resigned to having to work harder at simple tasks.

"Conversations don't always fall into place"

People with AD describe their trouble using language or participating in conversations. They often have trouble finding the right word or expressing a thought. They have to pay careful attention in order to follow along in a conversation.

Difficulty Expressing Oneself

Tom was always one whose thoughts and words came quickly. It was important to him as a schoolteacher to be able to express himself clearly, quickly, and easily. He finds that he has slowed down mentally since the onset of AD. He has to think and speak slowly in order to be understood by those around him. "I speak in an impaired fashion. I speak slowly, to get my words right." But he is still misunderstood sometimes. "I'll be speaking to somebody, I'll get the wrong words, say the wrong thing. . . . When I'm speaking gibberish sometimes the words don't come out right." Later on he explains that sentences "don't work very well."

When asked about the most significant changes that have occurred as a result of AD, Maggie describes her difficulty in expressing herself. "Not being able to say things that I want to say, you know. Forgetting what I was going to say." She characterizes this as a problem of forgetting and thinks of it as "getting in trouble" with herself. She has the sense that it happens often, and it was the only problem that stood out when she was asked to think about changes resulting from AD.

There were several occasions during the three interviews when Maggie's ability to express herself completely broke down. The following excerpt from the beginning of the third interview is a good example.

INTERVIEWER: You were saying [earlier] that you have problems with spelling more than you used to.

MAGGIE: Yeah! Yeah. It's amazing. And the . . . the . . . I don't recognize some of the things now, you know, like, uh, what was I going to say? Maybe I'll think of it. [clears throat] It's harder for me to, uh, understand, uh, oh . . . [little laugh] oh, how to put it? I don't even know if that is what I'm supposed to . . . hmm . . . I dun-. . . . I'm confused right now. But I knew that [clears throat] I do have some trouble with . . . [little laugh] what am I talking about?

INTERVIEWER: You were talking about writing. Writing things.

MAGGIE: Yeah. Yeah . . . yeah, I can't read my own writing, you know. I guess that's part of it or something.

INTERVIEWER: You have trouble recognizing the words?
MAGGIE: Hmm, uh-huh. [little laugh] Something like that.
INTERVIEWER: It's hard to describe?
MAGGIE: It is. It's hard to describe. Exactly.

Here Maggie was having trouble expressing herself. It is not clear whether she had the thought and could not find the words or the thought itself was elusive. Whatever the case, eventually she lost what it was she was even talking or thinking about, and the communication broke down completely.

Difficulty Participating in Conversations

Sandra admits that she was never a great conversationalist, but now it takes special effort to stay involved in a conversation.

SANDRA: So, uh, I think I also probably try harder, really try to stay more alert, more active in conversations, and it's an effort, but I do, I do make the effort, and I think, I think I succeed. Most of the time.
INTERVIEWER: But does it tire you out?
SANDRA: Somewhat, yeah, yeah. . . . Yes, because you're making an extra effort to be alert and to remember. I can't drift off anytime.

Sandra's understanding of the sense of a conversation may be unaffected, but being actively involved in a conversation is no longer a skill that she can take for granted.

Roy describes this same thing. He feels slower; he needs more time to think about what he wants to say, and sometimes he can't follow a conversation. He speaks slowly and ponderously as he explains:

Well, I . . . I . . . I . . . things don't come to me that fast, and it takes me a little time to think about what I want to say, so . . . so it isn't like you carry on a conversation and everything falls into place all the time. Sometimes it doesn't . . . you recognize that . . . your reaction, uh, to conversations that you may, that you look at a little different, you really notice that, uh, maybe you're not following like you used to be able to follow a conversation.

Jim says that he is less active in conversations now because he worries that he may not understand or follow what the others are talking about. He stays quiet because he doesn't want to embarrass himself or others.

INTERVIEWER: Do you find that you converse less with people now than you did?

JIM: Yes. I just stand back and listen.

INTERVIEWER: What has made that change?

JIM: Well, the part of it is, the point you were just trying to make is I don't . . . I was just thinking the other day I can't really join in here because I go to . . . ha . . . what's the subject and may-, may-, maybe they've been talking a lot about it and I haven't heard all that they have been saying. So I would sound kind of foolish if I say something that's . . . that has no relation to what they have been talking about.

INTERVIEWER: So you would be worried that you would embarrass yourself?

JIM: Yeah. Or embarrass them too. They're friends, and they are . . . So I am a little leery.

Even though he is quiet, he is very much present in the experience. Behind his listening, Jim is actively engaged in the discussion around him. He describes the work this involves.

JIM: Yeah, I just sort of . . . I have to concentrate and everything, and I used to sort of sit back and let it go, you know, but now I have to concentrate. They may ask me a question, so I better listen and see what they are talking about. This just occurred to me, you know, that they are talking to him and him. They are going to ask me and I wouldn't even know what the subject is that they were discussing would be.

INTERVIEWER: So it's a lot more hard work, it sounds like.

JIM: Yes. Yes, yes. And you really don't accomplish a lot in spite of it.

INTERVIEWER: What do you mean?

JIM: Well, if you can't remember, you can't remember. You just have to keep churning it over in your mind, but then you get hung up on one thing and you've forgot all these other things.

INTERVIEWER: Right. Right. Or you get hung up on one thing and their conversation has continued on.

JIM: Yeah, right.

Jim has to pay careful attention in a conversation. He cannot just "sit back and let it go" as he once did. He concentrates very hard to remember what is being said in case he is asked to comment. But despite all this hard work, he still gets lost in the flurry of words. The conversation moves on, leaving him behind trying to keep fresh in his mind what has already been discussed. It is as if he is no longer a native speaker, as if English has become for him a foreign tongue.

In summary, participants often had trouble finding the words to easily express themselves. They realized that it took longer for them to formulate and articulate their thoughts and also that it was difficult for them to keep up with a conversation. The result of this is that people are often quieter than before since they do not want to risk embarrassing themselves in front of others.

"I'm sort of oblivious"

Persons with AD have the most difficulty describing the times when they are only vaguely aware that something is amiss.

Sandra admits that she is forgetful, but she is not always aware of its being an issue. Her forgetfulness is not always obvious to her. "I think I . . . you know, I think there . . . sometimes I see it in myself, I mean it's **glaringly** apparent . . . hmm . . . but sometimes I don't."

Often she will only realize that she has forgotten something if someone else mentions it. She is also conscious enough of her forgetfulness that she increasingly relies on her datebook. In a certain sense the symptoms are invisible to her. She knows she has AD and therefore expects to have certain problems, but she only becomes aware of these problems when she notices how much she relies on her coping strategies.

SANDRA: I feel certainly that I have [deteriorated somewhat]. Over time I'm sure, I mean it's going to happen.

INTERVIEWER: There's nothing specific that's making you say that, or just the sense that it must be?

SANDRA: I have so many props. [laughs]

INTERVIEWER: What do you mean?

SANDRA: I mean I write everything down [laughing], and I keep notes for myself on my calendar . . . hmm . . . that, uh . . .

INTERVIEWER: Are you doing that more than you used to, do you think?

SANDRA: I think I **rely** on it more. I think I have, you know . . . I have been pretty faithful in keeping the calendar, you know, for some time, but I do rely on it more, I do go to look at it to see what am I supposed to be doing today. And, uh . . . so, in that respect I would say yes.

Being unaware of her symptoms is a curious experience that Sandra seeks to explain by suggesting that in part she is "in denial," not wanting the symptoms to exist since they might indicate that the disease was getting worse. Also, she points out that it is possible that she simply forgets the symptoms; that is, that she is aware at the time but cannot remember enough to describe her symptoms later on.

Sometimes persons with AD base their knowledge of their own symptoms solely on what other people tell them they have observed. Otherwise they seem to be unaware that anything is wrong. Mary, for example, only recognizes that something is amiss when her daughters tell her about it. But even then she does not experience the changes herself; she simply accepts that what her daughters tell her is true. In telling me how she came to know that she had AD, she explained that her daughters came for a visit and found her dirty and unable to take care of herself.

MARY: You know, I think I was just sort of oblivious to all that was going on. I mean, it sounds strange even to me.

INTERVIEWER: Did you believe them when they told you this?

MARY: I couldn't believe it. I mean, I knew it must be true because they're my kids and they wouldn't lie to me, but at the same time it was difficult for me to really grasp that.

INTERVIEWER: You didn't see it yourself?

MARY: No, I didn't see it myself.

Mary admitted only that it seemed "strange" that she could be having these experiences and not be aware of them, but her daughter Meg revealed more about what this experience must be like for Mary. In the excerpt below she describes the almost crazed look in her mother's eyes when she realized for a brief moment that she was really lost and that she had not known it before.

MEG: She stayed with us for three nights, and by the third night she was very agitated. She could not go to sleep. It's 10:30 at night, and my husband and I are watching television, and she keeps coming out and she'd say, "Oh, I heard the television and I didn't know what it was. Oh you're staying overnight!" She really thought that we were at her house. And then it's like, "No Mom, we're in *our* house." [pause] "Oh." [pause] And then she realized for a moment, and you could tell that this *really* freaked her out. There's a sound in her voice. It gets tight. And there's, her face kind of sets, you know, so, and there's just a way that she gets that's really worked up. And there's also a look in the eye that is . . . it's crazy. It's not rational anymore. I don't know how to describe it.

INTERVIEWER: Is this a fleeting thing? What happened after you told her that?

MEG: Okay, that was fleeting. But then she went, she kind of flipped back over to, "Okay, we're in this house," and then two seconds later she is back at her place. And she would keep coming out, and she . . . she . . . she wears lots of bracelets, and rings, and she fidgets with them. The more she gets agitated, she plays with them and she turns her rings, and she rubs her thighs, like she is petting the dogs.

Meg's description of her mother's reaction gives us a sense of the fear and panic that Mary must have felt when she realized that she was not where she thought she was. But her recognition of being lost disappeared almost as quickly as it came. As Meg tells it, Mary reverted immediately to believing that she was in her own home again, although she continued to seem unsettled. It is impossible to know whether Mary simply forgot what Meg had told her or whether not knowing where she was was just too terrifying a prospect to face.

Mary's experience reveals that it can be painful to have others point out problems of which you are otherwise unaware. Several participants said that they preferred to spend time alone because then they could remain oblivious to their symptoms. This was a major concern for Christina. Her daughter explained: "Mom reiterated that she really feels fine alone and it's good for her to be alone part of the time because she feels she is in charge. She feels she is competent when she's alone because she isn't reminded of being otherwise because of [her husband's] presence as a competent person."

Of course, the conflicting claim here is that Christina is increasingly reliant on her husband for help. She wants to maintain her close relationships with family and friends, but at the same time these relationships are uncomfortable because in the presence of others she is increasingly self-conscious and aware of her symptoms. Most of the time she feels that she is fully in command of herself. It is only when a moment of failure is pointed out by someone else that she realizes that she is not always aware of what is happening to her. "[My daughter] reminds me . . . she makes me aware of it."

To be made aware of one's symptoms can be painful in part because it forces people to recognize the possibility that the disease is real and may be progressing. It is more comfortable to remain oblivious to the symptoms and believe that nothing has changed. This helps people maintain the hope that the disease will stabilize or that the diagnosis was wrong after all. On the other hand, being unaware of one's symptoms may cause people to feel uneasy. Laura Mae's husband explained that after an evening spent socializing with friends she would invariably turn to him to ask whether she had been alright, whether she had said anything she should not have said. Laura Mae suspects that symptoms may reveal themselves without her being aware, and she is concerned that she may have embarrassed herself or others by her behavior. She told me that what was most difficult about AD was "not feeling sure of myself." For Laura Mae it is most disquieting to realize that there might be a difference between her own experience of symptoms and what others observe. It is increasingly difficult for her to trust herself in her everyday dealings in the world.

In summary, participants often realized that their symptoms were largely invisible to them. This was hard for them to understand, and they wondered whether they were denying the extent of their impairment or simply forgetting the symptoms. Whatever the reason, it was difficult for most participants to accept that others might see symptoms that they themselves were unaware of, which in turn often made it difficult for them to accept help. This sense of being oblivious left people feeling uncomfortable, in some circumstances even panicked.

Lessons Learned

Symptoms Have a Depth of Meanings

The findings discussed above are important in that they point toward a richer understanding of dementia symptoms than currently exists, an understanding that takes into consideration symptoms as they are *lived* and *articulated* by people who actually have the illness. Certainly a great deal of valuable work has been done by researchers and clinicians alike to identify and describe symptoms of memory loss, disorientation, aphasia, and so on. But these technological accounts of illness remain abstracted from the meaningful context of lived experience. Therefore, while we know a considerable amount of what these symptoms look like as raw behaviors, we know very little indeed about what it means to live with them. And as long as we exclude from our accounts the lived experience of people with dementia, the language for understanding such experiences will remain meager and impoverished.

So it is that we must heed the voice of those with dementia in order to create the possibility of a richer language of dementia symptoms, one that allows us to speak of *symptoms as meaning*. Understanding what it is to live with symptoms of dementia means seeing the symptoms as situated in the context of people's current and past life experiences and understanding the concerns that people bring to the situation. It means being open to the emotional significance of the symptoms and understanding why the symptoms matter to people. And not least, it means understanding how people make sense of symptom experiences, which can be very elusive and difficult to grasp.

Of course, this is not to say that the person with the illness can necessarily provide the complete story of what it is like to live with symptoms. Undoubtedly, it is often difficult for those with dementia to recognize and remember what has happened to them. Therefore, in order to obtain a more complete picture of symptom experience in AD, it is necessary to include information obtained from other sources (e.g., direct observation and interviews with reliable informants). But this does not justify excluding the person's lived understanding of symptoms from accounts of AD. As difficult as it might be for people with the illness to describe their symptoms, findings from these two studies reveal how much they have to say about the matter when given the opportunity and time.

Interventions Strategies

By listening carefully to these stories, clinicians, caregivers, and family members might devise more appropriate and effective ways to help persons with AD cope with their symptoms. The most obvious intervention may not be the best if it does not take into account the person's lived experience. For example, writing directions and street names on a slip of paper may not help someone like Jim, whose experience of being lost is not so much that he forgets the way but rather that he feels that the world itself is strange and unfamiliar. As Jim pointed out, he only feels comfortable if there is someone to accompany him or he is in the neighborhood where he grew up, a place that still feels very familiar. He has tried writing down street names, but it does not really help.

Findings from this research show that people in the early stages of AD may fall silent in conversations, not because they are distracted or disinterested but because they have trouble keeping up with the pace of the conversation; they do not want to risk embarrassing themselves or others by saying something inappropriate. Knowing this, the conversational partner might try to slow down, making extra effort to repeat or rephrase previous comments and making sure that the person with AD is following along. Simply allowing persons with AD sufficient time to think about what they want to say and to find the words to express their thoughts might go a long way toward promoting their continued involvement in conversations.

As people with dementia find it more difficult to accomplish simple tasks, we need to consider what this experience is like for them. For example, if they are constantly losing things, it may not be simply because they have forgotten where to look. If the person is actually unable to recognize the item in question, it will not be sufficient to simply leave it in the same place each time. Family members in these two studies found that they typically needed to help the person more directly by telling them where to look or pointing to the item itself. Likewise, when people find it difficult to use familiar equipment, depending on the extent of their confusion it may be helpful to simply allow them more time, or they may need gentle assistance that does not expose their confusion and compound their embarrassment.

Some people may find such assistance reassuring to the extent that they feel safe and protected, but what stood out in these interviews was how difficult and painful it can be to receive help when it makes someone so acutely aware of his or her embarrassing symptoms. For example, Maggie feels humiliated by her symptoms because she worries that people will think she is stupid or foolish. At the same time that reminders may help her remember a recent event, they may also remind her of her profound impairment and cause her further shame. It is important for clinicians, caregivers, and family members to be sensitive to the terrible dilemma faced by someone like Maggie. She needs help, but in accepting it she is forced to face the terrible fact of her own decline.

But there may be kinder, less obvious ways to offer assistance. Maggie's husband, Ted, has found ways to gently remind her of things without making the forgetfulness so visible and intrusive: "In saying, 'Do you remember?' I don't, I don't try to start sentences with that anymore. Cause, uh, . . . I'll just say, I'll just word it differently, so that if, if she doesn't remember it, it's not, it doesn't come out as being critical or she's failed a test or something like that—I'll say things more like, 'It, wasn't it fun when we, when we took a trip to Colorado?' and she'll think about it and say, 'Yeah, I remember that. It was fun.' And, uh, rather than saying, 'Remember when we were in Colorado, we did such and such?' Well, she might not remember it, and that would then kind of end the conversation." Ted helps Maggie remember recent events without challenging her so that if she does not remember, she is not forced to admit her failure. Embarrassment is avoided, and their conversation continues.

It is important to recognize that there may be subtle yet important differences in how individuals experience symptoms. These differences make it essential to listen carefully to people's stories about their symptoms and then tailor interventions to address each person's experiences.

Bearing Witness to Suffering

As well as informing interventions to help persons with AD cope with their symptoms, findings from these two studies remind us that it is important to take the time to listen when they tell us about the pain and despair of breakdown. It is important to bear witness to the failures, the confusion, and the chaos that people experience when they are forgetful, lost, or unable to express themselves easily. Dementia is a frightening disease for all of us, and it can be difficult to hear these stories and be reminded of our own vulnerabilities. But in opening ourselves to this suffering, we create possibilities for relationships with people who are struggling with multiple losses and who feel that they are being ignored, discarded, or left behind by the world around them.

Several participants told me that their doctors did not listen to them and that their illness tended not to come up in their everyday conversations with family and friends. It was only in the context of their support groups or in research interviews that they had the opportunity to talk about what it was like to be forgetful, slow, or unaware and what this meant to them. The participants emphasized that it was important that others understand what they were going through. The symptoms mattered deeply to them in ways that were not easy to articulate. Above all, they wanted others to listen when they struggled to describe these difficult experiences. Clinicians, caregivers, and family members would do well to heed this message.

Conclusion

The findings discussed in this chapter show that people with early AD are indeed able to describe their experience of symptoms, sometimes haltingly, at other times with startling clarity. They speak of being forgetful and feeling lost in a world that seems strange and unfamiliar. Their activities are slowed down as the most simple of tasks come to require careful attention and consideration. They find it increasingly difficult to express themselves through words, and conversations become a challenge. And finally, many realize that they are often not completely aware of the changes they are experiencing. It is as if their symptoms are often invisible to them.

These findings speak to the importance of listening to people's symptom stories as they struggle to tell us what is wrong. These stories are difficult, but they inform our understanding of what it means to people in the early stages of AD to be forgetful and slow, to feel lost and confused. This deeper and clearer understanding will guide us in developing appropriate and effective interventions to help people better cope with their symptoms.

REFERENCES

Benner, P., and J. Wrubel. 1989. *The primacy of caring: Stress and coping in health and illness.* Menlo Park, Calif.: Addison-Wesley.

DeBettignies, B. H., R. K. Mahurin, and F. J. Pirozzolo. 1990. Insight for impairment in independent living skills in Alzheimer's disease and multi-infarct dementia. *Journal of Clinical and Experimental Neuropsychology* 12:355–63.

Derouesne, C., S. Thibault, V. Baudouin-Madec, D. Ancri, and L. Lacomblez. 1999.

Decreased awareness of cognitive deficits in patients with mild dementia of the Alzheimer type. *International Journal of Geriatric Psychiatry* 14 (12): 1019–30.

Geldmacher, D. S., and P. J. Whitehouse. 1996. Evaluation of dementia. *New England Journal of Medicine* 335:330–36.

Kleinmann, A. 1988. *The illness narratives: Suffering, healing, and the human condition.* New York: Basic Books.

van Manen, M. 1990. *Researching lived experience: Human science for an action sensitive pedagogy.* London, Ont.: Althouse.

Vasterling, J. J., B. Seltzer, B. D. Carpenter, and K. A. Thompson. 1997. Unawareness of social interaction and emotional control deficits in Alzheimer's disease. *Aging, Neuropsychology, and Cognition* 4 (4): 280–89.

Weinstein, E. A., R. P. Friedland, and E. E. Wagner. 1994. Denial/unawareness of impairment and symbolic behavior in Alzheimer's disease. *Neuropsychiatry, Neuropsychology, and Behavioral Neurology* 7 (3): 176–84.

Making the Most of Every Day

Quality of Life

REBECCA G. LOGSDON

From the first suspicion that something is wrong through the progression of cognitive, behavioral, and social changes that occur following a diagnosis, Alzheimer's disease affects individuals' lives in profound ways. Cognitive and functional abilities decline, and individuals become less able to engage in meaningful, pleasurable activities (Logsdon and Teri 1997; Teri and Logsdon 1991). Communication and social skills may deteriorate, precipitating interpersonal conflicts (Pearson et al. 1989; Reisberg et al. 1987). These losses have an impact on the emotional state of both the diagnosed individual (Teri et al. 1994) and their loved ones (Drinka, Smith, and Drinka 1987). Thus, dementia sets into motion a set of events that can have an impact on all aspects of the individual's quality of life (QOL).

Despite these losses, it is evident that some individuals with AD maintain a high QOL throughout the progression of the disease (Volicer and Bloom-Charette 1999; Volicer, Hurley, and Camberg 1999; Whitehouse and Rabins 1992). As we explore individuals' perceptions of their own QOL, we can identify characteristics of individuals who report a good QOL and use this information to develop interventions aimed at maintaining or improving QOL with AD. This chapter discusses QOL with AD, its assessment, factors associated with self-reported QOL, and strategies for maximizing QOL for individuals with dementia.

Quality of Life and Alzheimer's Disease

QOL is an elusive concept that has been defined in a variety of ways depending on the context and on the conceptual orientation of the investigator (cf. McSweeney and Creer 1995). From a bioethical standpoint, QOL has been defined as the essential conditions beyond mere survival that are needed for individuals to have experiences that provide meaning and joy (Post and Whitehouse 1995; Roy 1992). From a medical standpoint, QOL includes appropriate physical, social, and role functioning, mental heath, and perception of health (Cella 1992; Wilson and Cleary 1995). In a review of the state of research on the QOL of frail older adults, Birren and Dieckmann (1991) recommended that QOL be considered a multidimensional construct including social, environmental, health, spiritual, and emotional states. Lawton (1991) provided a theoretical framework for QOL in older adults that includes four areas of importance: behavioral competence, objective environment, psychological well-being, and subjective perception of and satisfaction with one's overall QOL. A report of the Institute of Medicine (1986) echoed these views of QOL specifically for older adults with chronic illness, describing QOL as a sense of well-being, satisfaction with life, and self-esteem that is achieved through good care, the accomplishment of desired goals, and the ability to exercise a satisfactory degree of control over one's life. Despite their differences, all these definitions share common themes. The importance of the individual's personal sense of satisfaction with various areas of his or her life is recognized by all, as are the contributions of physical comfort, emotional well-being, and interpersonal connections.

QOL is an important concern for individuals with AD, as new treatments are being developed to improve cognitive function, delay decline, or treat behavior problems. Assessment of QOL provides a subjective evaluation of treatment that takes into account important areas that are not assessed by traditional cognitive tests or behavioral checklists. It provides an avenue for the person with AD to participate directly and meaningfully in evaluating treatment outcomes. QOL assessment also provides a framework that enables persons with AD and their families to weigh the costs and benefits of treatment and to evaluate the "clinical significance" of any improvement to their lives. Finally, QOL assessment provides important information about the specific areas of improvement associated with different types of treatment, thus guiding both future research and clinical care.

Assessment of QOL with AD

QOL is a highly personal and subjective construct that can best be assessed by the person whose life is being evaluated (Patrick et al. 1988; Pearlman and Uhlmann 1991). However, assessing QOL in individuals with AD is not a simple task because cognitive or other difficulties may impair an individual's ability to comprehend complex questions and communicate responses in ways that are easily understood and measured (Lawton 1994; Rabins et al. 1999). Eventually we must rely on proxy reports (Albert et al. 1999; Rabins et al. 1999) or direct observations (Lawton et al. 1999; Volicer, Hurley, and Camberg 1999) of QOL for individuals in advanced stages of AD. However, it is important to assess self-reports of QOL whenever possible, especially since QOL ratings are increasingly being used to influence decisions regarding care and treatment of individuals with AD (Logsdon and Albert 1999; Whitehouse et al. 1997; Winblad et al. 1997). Recent investigations indicate that individuals with mild to moderate AD can reliably and validly describe their own QOL when questions are structured and presented in an understandable and supportive interview-based format (Brod et al. 1999; Logsdon et al. 1999; Selai et al. 2000). For a more detailed discussion of research on assessing QOL at different stages of AD, the reader is referred elsewhere (e.g., Albert and Logsdon 2000; Salek, Walker, and Bayer 1998; Volicer and Bloom-Charette 1999; Walker, Salek, and Bayer 1998). The remainder of this chapter focuses on self-report assessments of QOL among individuals with early- to middle-stage AD using the Quality of Life-AD (QOL-AD), a measure developed by Logsdon et al. (1999).

Development and Description of the QOL-AD

Any assessment of QOL must meet certain requirements. An assessment must possess adequate psychometric qualities, including reliability, validity, and sensitivity. It must possess face validity, make sense to the respondent, and include questions that reflect the respondent's own beliefs about what is important to QOL. It must not be excessively burdensome for the respondent in terms of time required or intrusiveness (Walker, Salek, and Bayer 1998). For individuals with AD, additional requirements must be considered. It is particularly important that the language be clear and straightforward so that individuals with mild to moderate language impairment can understand and respond to questions. It must focus on present feelings rather than requiring memory for past events or feelings. It is helpful for the measure to be administered as a structured interview in order to avoid the requirement for reading and remembering instructions and so that the respondent may ask questions if there is an item that he or she does not understand. Response options should be simple, concrete, and consistent across items. Finally, it is important that the measure be brief in order to minimize fatigue and burden on the respondent.

The QOL-AD was designed to meet all these requirements. It consists of thirteen items rated on a four-point scale, with 1 being poor and 4 being excellent. Original items were reviewed by individuals with AD and their families, as well as experts in the field of geriatrics and gerontology, in order to maximize the construct validity and to ensure that it focused on QOL domains thought to be important in AD. The QOL-AD includes assessments of the person's relationships with friends and family, concerns about finances, physical condition, and mood, as well as an overall assessment of life quality. It is administered as a structured interview using standardized instructions. The interview requires about ten minutes, and individuals with AD find the process interesting and easy to complete. The QOL-AD has been successfully completed by individuals who scored as low as 4 on the Mini-Mental State Exam, or MMSE (Folstein, Folstein, and McHugh 1975). In a sample of 180 subjects no one with an MMSE score greater than 10 was unable or unwilling to complete the QOL-AD (Logsdon, in press). The measure has been demonstrated to have good internal reliability (α = .88). The test-retest reliability after a one-week interval is also excellent, with an intraclass correlation of .76. The construct validity of the QOL-AD has been demonstrated by its correlation with measures of activities of daily living (R = .37), depression (R = −.53), and engagement in pleasant activities (R = .40) (Logsdon et al. 1999).

Table 4.1. Demographic Characteristics of Whole Group and Low- and High-QOL
Subgroups

Characteristic*	Whole Group (N = 155)	Low QOL (N = 32)	High QOL (N = 28)
Age mean (SD)	77.2 (6.8)	76.7 (6.2)	76.9 (6.7)
Education mean (SD)	13.5 (3.5)	12.7 (3.2)	14.0 (3.2)
Years-since-onset mean (SD)	4.5 (3.0)	4.4 (3.0)	4.1 (2.1)
Sex	88 male (57%)	20 male (56%)	16 male (44%)
Marital status	128 married (83%)	25 married (78%)	24 married (86%)
Ethnicity	141 Caucasian (91%)	28 Caucasian (87%)	23 Caucasian (82%)

*SD = standard deviation.

Quality of Life in Community-Residing Individuals with AD

The QOL-AD is currently being used in a longitudinal investigation of community-residing individuals with AD. Before examining how individuals describe their QOL, I shall describe the entire group of 155 subjects who have completed their baseline assessment, then compare two subgroups of individuals: those who report exceptionally high QOL (score 1 standard deviation or higher above the mean score, $N = 28$) and those who report exceptionally low QOL (score 1 standard deviation or lower below the mean score, $N = 32$). Demographic information about the whole group, as well as the high- and low-QOL subgroups, is provided in Table 4.1. Although the high-QOL subgroup appears to have a slightly higher level of education than the low-QOL group, there are no significant differences between the groups on any demographic variables.

Table 4.2 shows mean scores for each of the thirteen QOL-AD items (possible range, 1 to 4) and the total score (possible range, 13 to 52) for the entire group and for the low- and high-QOL subgroups. For each of the three groups memory was rated lowest, as expected. The items on which there was the greatest difference between the high- and low-QOL groups were energy (1.5-point difference) and ability to do chores (1.4-point dif-

Table 4.2. Mean and Standard Deviation of Item Scores for Whole Group
and Low- and High-QOL Subgroups

Item	Whole Group (N = 155)	Low QOL (N = 32)	High QOL (N = 28)
Physical health	2.9 (.74)	2.2 (.74)	3.5 (.51)
Energy	2.8 (.73)	2.0 (.57)	3.5 (.51)
Mood	2.8 (.73)	2.2 (.67)	3.5 (.51)
Living situation	3.4 (.59)	2.8 (.49)	3.9 (.34)
Memory	2.2 (.76)	1.8 (.61)	2.9 (.73)
Family	3.4 (.59)	3.1 (.62)	3.8 (.50)
Marriage or closest significant relationship	3.6 (.60)	3.1 (.69)	3.9 (.28)
Friends	3.1 (.69)	2.6 (.61)	3.6 (.49)
Self as a whole	2.8 (.65)	2.3 (.54)	3.3 (.72)
Ability to do chores	2.8 (.74)	2.1 (.62)	3.5 (.58)
Ability to do things for fun	3.1 (.69)	2.4 (.72)	3.7 (.53)
Money	2.9 (.72)	2.3 (.78)	3.4 (.69)
Life as a whole	3.1 (.68)	2.6 (.70)	3.9 (.45)
Total	38.6 (5.3)	31.3 (2.7)	46.3 (2.3)

ference); the groups differed the least on relationship with family, and marriage or closest significant relationship (less than 1-point difference).

Table 4.3 shows differences between the low- and high-QOL groups on a variety of characteristics. Although it appears that the high-QOL group scored slightly higher on the MMSE, this difference is not significant, nor are there any differences in level of impairment on instrumental activities of daily living. The groups differ significantly on activities of daily living, physical function/mobility, depression, and frequency of pleasant events; these differences indicate greater impairment to activities of daily living and mobility, more depression, and fewer pleasant events in the low QOL group.

Table 4.3. Differences in Characteristics of Low- and High-QOL Subgroups

Characteristic	Low QOL (N = 32)	High QOL (N = 28)
MMSE score[a]	17.5 (5.6)	19.4 (4.7)
Activities of daily living[b]	10.2 (4.3)	7.9 (2.4)*
Instrumental activities of daily living[b]	21.8 (5.9)	21.4 (6.0)
Physical function/mobility[c]	55.5 (28.7)	71.6 (22.2)*
Physical function/role[c]	56.2 (38.1)	67.0 (34.7)
Caregiver burden[d]	19.6 (17.1)	13.5 (9.1)
Depressive behavior problems[e]	1.0 (.86)	0.5 (.56)*
Disruptive behavior problems[e]	0.7 (.63)	0.4 (.36)
Memory-related behavior problems[e]	2.5 (.84)	2.6 (.99)
Depression[f]	10.2 (5.0)	3.5 (3.3)**
Pleasant events[g]	24.1 (6.1)	29.9 (5.2)**

[a]Mini-Mental State Exam (Folstein, Folstein, and McHugh 1975).
[b]Lawton-Brody Physical and Instrumental Self Maintenance Scale (Lawton and Brody 1969).
[c]Medical Outcomes Studies (Stewart, Hays, and Ware 1988).
[d]Screen for Caregiver Burden (Vitaliano et al. 1991).
[e]Revised Memory and Behavior Problems Checklist (Teri et al. 1992).
[f]Geriatric Depression Scale (Yesavage et al. 1983).
[g]Pleasant Events Schedule—AD (Logsdon and Teri 1997; Teri and Logsdon 1991).
$*p < .05; ** p < .001.$

Thus, the use of the QOL-AD in a structured interview format provides a vehicle for individuals with mild to moderate AD to talk about how they perceive their own QOL.

Case Examples

Communication, particularly spontaneous verbal expression, often becomes impaired early in the course of AD. Because of this, most participants in the longitudinal investigation found it easier to express themselves in response to specific questions asked as part of the QOL-AD interview than to spontaneously talk about their QOL. However, some subjects with more intact verbal abilities commented on their experiences in more detail. These spontaneous comments reinforce some common "themes" from the structured interview. Individuals with high QOL tended to focus on their abilities, whereas those who reported low QOL tended to focus on the loss of abilities. For example, two individuals who had recently given up driving were mildly cognitively impaired and relatively independent in activities of daily living. One stated, "I still do my quilting, and I fix dinner every night," while the other reported, "I had to give up driving, and that just about did me in. I feel pretty worthless." Individuals with high QOL reported positive relationships with others ("My husband and I have always had a lot of friends, we go out to dinner with a group of five couples once a month"), while those with low QOL expressed dissatisfaction ("My daughters live a couple of blocks away, but I hardly ever see them. They only come over when they need something"). Finally, individuals with high QOL tended to maintain prior interests ("I read the sports pages every day"), while those with low QOL had given up many interests ("I used to have the most beautiful yard on the block, but now I don't have the energy to even plant flowers in the front beds").

Although these are only a few brief samples of what individuals say about their QOL, they suggest subtle differences that are difficult to quantify yet may influence how individuals view their lives. The significance of support from others, whether family, friends, or formal care providers, is apparent, as is the importance of pleasant and meaningful activities.

Lessons Learned

Individuals in the early to middle stages of AD can and often want to talk about their experiences with the disease. The QOL-AD interview provides a framework for a discussion of the individual's own perception of how he or she is doing in a variety of areas and allows a balanced focus on what is retained as well as on what is lost with the disease. Most individuals in this study rated their overall QOL as good or excellent, despite losses that many of us would consider devastating. In working with individuals with AD it is important to recognize the importance and the adaptive nature of focusing on strengths, identifying activities that are meaningful and pleasant, maintaining positive relationships with significant others, and making the most of every day.

These findings suggest targets for clinical interventions focused on improving QOL. A multifaceted, multidisciplinary approach to care is likely to be most effective in enhancing QOL as the disease progresses. Interventions that focus on maximizing functioning and teach caregivers strategies for supporting the abilities of the person with AD while providing needed assistance can be helpful in maximizing QOL. Well-intentioned caregivers often "take over" tasks from the person with AD, especially when the individual is struggling or frustrated by a task. These caregivers can learn alternative approaches, such as providing step-by-step instructions or "hands-on" assistance to allow the individual to continue to engage in activities of daily living.

For individuals who have mobility limitations that negatively impact QOL, structured exercise programs may be helpful to build strength and endurance and to keep the individual mobile. Being able to walk up and down steps, get in and out of a car, and get out of a chair or bed are all QOL-enhancing activities that can be preserved into the late stages of AD for most individuals.

Identifying and treating both major depression and subclinical depressive symptoms are important aspects of care for individuals with AD. Some depressive symptoms, such as lack of activity, irritability, lack of response to pleasant stimuli, and isolation are often dismissed as "part of the disease." There is considerable evidence, however, that these symptoms are responsive to treatment and that addressing them enhances QOL for both the person with AD and his or her caregivers. Support groups and activity programs for persons with AD can provide social relationships, a network of peers, and appropriate pleasant events for individuals at all stages of the disease, as well as provide needed respite for caregivers. Finally, maintaining a positive focus on what the person can do, rather than constantly dwelling on what has been lost, appears to be a key to preventing depression and maintaining a high QOL.

Conclusion

Although Alzheimer's disease is a devastating illness, many individuals are able to find meaning and quality in their lives despite the progression of cognitive and functional deficits. By identifying and providing appropriate services, health care providers, family members, professional caregivers, and others can make a difference in the lives of those with Alzheimer's disease.

ACKNOWLEDGMENTS

This ongoing research is supported by grants from the National Institute on Aging (AG-13757, AG-10845, and AG-05136) and from the Alzheimer's Association (FSA-95-009). I gratefully acknowledge the contributions of my colleagues Linda Teri, Ph.D., Laura Gibbons, Ph.D., and Susan McCurry, Ph.D., who provide valuable insight and advice, Amy Moore, M.S., who serves as project manager, Kari Mae Hickman, M.S.W., and Julie Cleveland, B.A., who interview subjects, and the volunteer participants and caregivers, who share their insights as they cope with Alzheimer's disease. The quotations in this chapter are from actual transcripts of participant and caregiver statements, which have been edited to protect the identities of participants and for brevity.

REFERENCES

Albert, S., C. Castillo-Castanada, D. M. Jacobs, M. Sano, K. Bell, C. Merchant, S. Small, and Y. Stern. 1999. Proxy-reported quality of life in Alzheimer's patients: Comparison of clinical and population-based samples. *Journal of Mental Health and Aging* 5 (1): 49–58.

Albert, S. M., and R. G. Logsdon, eds. 2000. *Assessing quality of life in dementia.* New York: Springer.

Birren, J. E., and L. Dieckmann. 1991. Concepts and content of quality of life in the later years: An overview. In *The concept and measurement of quality of life in the frail elderly,* ed. J. E. Birren, J. E. Lubben, J. C. Rowe, and D. E. Deutchman, 344–60. New York: Academic.

Brod, M., A. Stewart, L. Sands, and P. Walton. 1999. Conceptualization and measurement of quality of life in dementia: The dementia quality of life instrument (DQoL). *Gerontologist* 39:25–35.

Cella, D. 1992. Quality of life: The concept. *Journal of Palliative Care* 8 (3): 8–13.

Drinka, J. K., J. C. Smith, and P. J. Drinka. 1987. Correlates of depression and burden for informal caregivers of patients in a geriatrics referral clinic. *Journal of the American Geriatrics Society* 35:522–25.

Folstein, M. F., S. E. Folstein, and P. R. McHugh. 1975. Mini-mental state: A practical method for grading the cognitive state of patients for the clinician. *Journal of Psychiatric Research* 12:189–98.

Institute of Medicine. 1986. *Improving the quality of care in nursing homes*. Washington, D.C.: National Academy Press.

Lawton, M. P. 1991. A multidimensional view of quality of life in frail elders. In *The concept and measurement of quality of life in the frail elderly*, ed. J. E. Birren, J. E. Lubben, J. C. Rowe, and D. E. Deutchman, 4–27. New York: Academic.

———. 1994. Quality of life in Alzheimer disease. *Alzheimer Disease and Associated Disorders* 8:138–50.

Lawton, M. P., and E. M. Brody. 1969. Assessment of older people: Self-maintaining and instrumental activities of daily living. *Gerontologist* 9:179–86.

Lawton, M. P., K. Van Haitsma, M. Perkinson, and K. Ruckdeschel. 1999. Observed affect and quality of life in dementia: Further affirmations and problems. *Journal of Mental Health and Aging* 5 (1): 69–82.

Logsdon, R. G., L. E. Gibbons, S. M. McCurry, and L. Teri. In press. Assessing quality of life in older adults with cognitive impairment. *Psychosomatic Medicine*.

Logsdon, R. G., and S. M. Albert. 1999. Assessing quality of life in Alzheimer's disease: Conceptual and methodological issues. *Journal of Mental Health and Aging* 5 (1): 3–6.

Logsdon, R. G., L. E. Gibbons, S. M. McCurry, and L. Teri. 1999. Quality of life in Alzheimer's disease: Patient and caregiver reports. *Journal of Mental Health and Aging* 5 (1): 21–32.

Logsdon, R. G., and L. Teri. 1997. The pleasant events schedule—AD: Psychometric properties and relationship to depression and cognition in Alzheimer's disease patients. *Gerontologist* 37:40–45.

McSweeney, A. J., and T. L. Creer. 1995. Health related quality of life in medical care. *Disease-a-Month* 41:11–71.

Patrick, D. L., M. Danis, L. I. Southerland, and G. Hong. 1988. Quality of life following intensive care. *Journal of General Internal Medicine* 3:218–23.

Pearlman, R. A., and R. F. Uhlmann. 1991. Quality of life in elderly, chronically ill outpatients. *Journal of Gerontology: Medical Sciences* 46:M31–38.

Pearson, J., L. Teri, B. V. Reifler, and M. Raskind. 1989. Functional status and cognitive impairment in Alzheimer's disease patients with and without depression. *Journal of the American Geriatrics Society* 37:1117–21.

Post, S. G., and P. J. Whitehouse. 1995. Fairhill guidelines on ethics of the care of people with Alzheimer's disease: A clinical summary. *Journal of the American Geriatrics Society* 43:1423–29.

Rabins, P., J. D. Kasper, L. Kleinman, B. S. Black, and D. L. Patrick. 1999. Concepts and methods in the development of the ADRQL: An instrument for assessing health-related quality of life in persons with Alzheimer's disease. *Journal of Mental Health and Aging* 5 (1): 33–48.

Reisberg, B., J. Borenstein, S. P. Salob, S. H. Ferris, E. Franssen, and A. Georgotas. 1987. Behavioral symptoms in Alzheimer's disease: Phenomenology and treatment. *Journal of Clinical Psychiatry* 48 (suppl. 5): 9–15.

Roy, D. 1992. Measurement in the service of compassion. *Journal of Palliative Care* 8 (3): 3–4.

Salek, S. S., M. D. Walker, and A. J. Bayer. 1998. A review of quality of life in Alzheimer's disease. Part 2: Issues in assessing drug effects. *Pharmacoeconomics* 14:613–27.

Selai, C., M. R. Trimble, M. N. Rossor, and R. J. Harvey. 2000. The quality of life assessment schedule (QOLAS)—A new method for assessing quality of life in dementia. In *Assessing quality of life in Alzheimer's disease*, ed. S. M. Albert and R. G. Logsdon, 31–50. New York: Springer.

Stewart, A. L., R. Hays, and J. E. Ware Jr. 1988. The MOS short-form general health survey: Reliability and validity in a patient population. *Medical Care* 26: 724–32.

Teri, L., and R. G. Logsdon. 1991. Identifying pleasant activities for Alzheimer's disease patients: The pleasant events schedule—AD. *Gerontologist* 31:124–27.

Teri, L., R. G. Logsdon, A. Wagner, and J. Uomoto. 1994. The caregiver role in behavioral treatment of depression in dementia patients. In *Stress effects on family caregivers of Alzheimer's patients*, ed. B. Light, B. Lebowitz, and G. Niederehe, 185–204. New York: Springer.

Teri, L., P. Truax, R. G. Logsdon, J. Uomoto, S. Zarit, and P. P. Vitaliano. 1992. Assessment of behavioral problems in dementia: The revised memory and behavior problems checklist. *Psychology and Aging* 7:622–31.

Vitaliano, P. P., J. Russo, H. M. Young, J. Becker, and R. D. Maiuro. 1991. The screen for caregiver burden. *Gerontologist* 31:76–83.

Volicer, L., and L. Bloom-Charette, eds. 1999. *Enhancing the quality of life in advanced dementia*. Philadelphia: Taylor & Francis Group.

Volicer, L., A. C. Hurley, and L. Camberg. 1999. A model of psychological well-being in advanced dementia. *Journal of Mental Health and Aging* 5 (1): 83–94.

Walker, M., S. S. Salek, and A. J. Bayer. 1998. A review of quality of life in Alzheimer's disease. Part I: Issues in assessing disease impact. *Pharmacoeconomics* 14:499–530.

Whitehouse, P. J., J. M. Orgogozo, R. E. Becker, S. Gauthier, M. Pontecorvo, H. Erzigkeit, S. Rogers, R. C. Mohs, N. Bodick, G. Bruno, and P. Dal-Bianco. 1997. Quality-of-life assessment in dementia drug development: Position paper from the International Working Group on Harmonization of Dementia Drug Guidelines. *Alzheimer Disease and Associated Disorders* 11 (suppl. 3): 56–60.

Whitehouse, P. J., and P. V. Rabins. 1992. Quality of life and dementia. *Alzheimer Disease and Associated Disorders* 6:135–37.

Wilson, I., and P. D. Cleary. 1995. Linking clinical variables with health-related quality of life: A conceptual model of patient outcomes. *Journal of the American Medical Association* 273:59–65.

Winblad, B., S. Hill, B. Beermann, S. G. Post, and A. Wimo. 1997. Issues in the economic evaluation of treatment for dementia: Position paper from the International Working Group on Harmonization of Dementia Drug Guidelines. *Alzheimer Disease and Associated Disorders* 11 (suppl. 3): 39–45.

Yesavage, J. A., T. L. Brink, T. L. Rose, O. Lum, V. Huang, M. B. Adey, and V. O. Leirer. 1983. Development and validation of a geriatric depression screening scale: A preliminary report. *Journal of Psychiatric Research* 17:37–49.

5

Selfhood and Alzheimer's Disease

STEVEN R. SABAT

*I think the issue is that . . . I am not satisfied with myself because what I want
isn't here. . . . and it makes me angry as well . . . and I guess that
is what is happening now.*
—Dr. M., a 75-year-old former college professor

Alzheimer's disease is most often associated with the dimensions of loss and
dysfunction on neuropathological and behavioral levels. Surely there is
logical reason for such an association. Not only is there evident damage to
brain cells and depletion in a variety of neurotransmitters; it is painfully
clear both to the person with AD and to his or her loved ones that the way
the former copes with the demands of everyday life is deficient in many
ways due to the presence and progress of the illness. It is apparent that the
person with AD experiences losses in a variety of cognitive and behavioral
functions, including the inability to recall relatively recent events, to find
and pronounce desired words while trying to converse, to dress, to read, to
write, to use eating utensils, to drive, and to calculate, among others. Indeed, it has been asserted that the person with AD exhibits paranoia, delusions, hallucinations (Reisberg et al. 1987), diminished ability to think
(American Psychiatric Association 1994), and changes in his or her personality (Hamel et. al. 1990). It is even considered reasonable to assert that

Some extracts in this chapter have been previously published in Sabat 1991, Sabat
1994b, and Sabat 2001. The punctuation and typographical conventions may differ
slightly here.

the person with AD has lost his or her identity, personhood, and self (Cohen and Eisdorfer 1986).

It seems logical to some, as it did to the philosopher John Locke (1956), that one's selfhood, one's identity, is dependent upon one's memory functions, for it is through such functions that the continuous "narrative" of one's life remains intact and available to be recalled. More recently, Oliver Sacks, in just one of his many wonderfully refreshing books, made the connection between selfhood and memory by questioning the existence of the selfhood of two of his patients who suffered from Korsakoff's syndrome (Sacks 1985). Although the symptoms and areas of brain damage associated with Korsakoff's syndrome are quite different for the most part from those associated with AD, a memory dysfunction resulting in problems with recall of relatively recent events is common to both. Nonetheless, Sacks wondered whether his two Korsakoff's patients had experienced a loss of "self."

Although the deficits caused by AD in a variety of functions are patently apparent, it is increasingly clear that the environment in which the person with AD dwells can exert a potent effect upon his or her cognitive and behavioral abilities. Specifically, it has become clear in a number of cases that "excess disability" can occur. Brody (1971), in coining this term, referred to the fact that deficits in a person's behavioral functions can extend beyond those that the extant organic damage would lead one to expect, and Sabat (1994a) related the existence of excess disability in a person with AD to the presence of what Kitwood (1990, 1998) and Kitwood and Bredin (1992) called "malignant social psychology." That is, under conditions in which the person with AD was innocently treated in a way that prevented him or her from maximizing the use of his or her remaining abilities, the person would be characterized as being incapable of demonstrating those abilities. The fact remained, however, that under more optimal social conditions the person with AD who was described by her spouse as being incapable of doing a variety of things at home (helping to set the table or with other household chores, feeding or grooming herself) was able to do those very things at the day care center that she attended two to three days per week (Sabat 1994a).

It is also clear that it is possible for healthy others to facilitate not only routine activities of daily living but also the conversational ability of the person with AD, by (1) giving him or her more time, without interruption, to formulate and express thoughts and (2) using what psycholinguists refer to as "indirect repair" in order to clarify for the listener what the person with AD is trying to say (Sabat 1991a, 1991b, 1999). Indirect repair is the process of checking one's understanding of what another person has said by saying such things as, "Let me see if I understand your point here . . ." and recounting one's understanding. This gives one's conversational partner the opportunity to confirm that understanding by saying "yes" or "no." I call attention to these phenomena to alert the reader not only to the fact of excess disability but also to the notion that its presence or absence may extend well beyond the performance of routine daily activities. In this chapter I attempt to examine various aspects of self and to show how the behavior of healthy others in the diagnosed person's social world can have a profound effect upon aspects of the experience and expression of selfhood in the person who has AD.

In what follows, I attempt to show that (1) there is a self of personal identity, the experience and expression of personal singularity, that remains intact even into the moderate to severe stages of AD as defined by standard tests; (2) there is a self that is made up of mental and physical attributes that, like the self of personal identity, can persist far into the course of the disease; and (3) there are other aspects of the person, the socially presented personae, that can be lost, but such losses are not direct effects of AD but are more directly related to the ways in which the person with AD is treated by healthy others.

Why should selfhood be discussed in relation to persons with AD? Simply stated, in the spirit of what Kitwood outlined in his observations regarding malignant social psychology, along with the observations of Sabat and Harré (1992, 1994), the ways in which persons with AD are viewed and treated by others can profoundly affect their behavior. Thus, if we assume that any deviations from the "norm" in the behavior of the person with AD are due to the effects of the disease alone, we may be making a potentially profound mistake, for we will be ignoring the facts that (1) the social environment can also have a powerful effect upon the behavior of the person with AD and (2) the reactions of the person with AD to the effects of the disease can likewise be a potent factor in his or her behavior. It follows that if we make assumptions about the person with the disease that are based primarily on his or her defects, to the extent that we assume that the person has lost his or her "self," our behavior toward that person will be affected by such interpretations and assumptions and we will treat the person very differently from the ways we would treat them if we assumed the opposite. Thus, derogatory or humiliating comments that might otherwise be made "behind the person's back" are now made in front of the person with AD, based on the assumption that he or she doesn't know, or understand the meaning of, what is being said.

In order to tell this story, I first introduce what has appeared to be an increasingly valuable heuristic device in the attempt to delineate aspects of selfhood, the Social Constructionist approach. It is important to note, however, that I do not propose that such an approach is *the* answer to abiding questions about the nature of selfhood, but rather that this conceptual scheme can help us to understand issues of selfhood for persons with AD as described by them.

The Constructionist Approach: A Framework for Analyzing the Self

The Social Constructionist approach, as seen in the work of Coulter (1981) and Harré (1983, 1991), was partly inspired by the writings of Vygotsky (1965) and Wittgenstein (1953). According to this approach, selfhood is manifested in a variety of ways. In public discourse, for example, it is manifested in recounting autobiographical events, assuming responsibility for one's acts, evincing interest or doubt, objecting to the lack of fairness in situations. To be more specific, there are three aspects of personhood, which I shall refer to as Self 1, Self 2, and Self 3, each of which has unique characteristics.

Self 1, the Self of Personal Identity

The self of personal identity is typically expressed in conversation through the use of first-person pronouns such as *I, me, my, myself,* and *mine* and refers to the continuity of one's singular and unique point of view. Most of us experience ourselves as singular persons. This experience of being one and the same person who has a continuous point of view in the world is one's Self 1. The use of first-person pronouns helps to locate, or index, for others the source of our opinions, beliefs, feelings, and the like. Thus, when a person says, "I am happy," he or she is locating for others the source and

ownership of the feeling of delight. Likewise, the use of first-person pronouns also indexes, or locates, with the speaker what we may call the moral
force of a statement. For example, saying "I'll help you" commits the
speaker to what has been promised.

One's continuous experience as a singular person in the world—one's
personal identity, or Self 1—is not dependent upon one's personal history
or one's ability to recount that history for others. In other words, in principle, a person who had suffered an amnesia such that he or she could not
recall his or her name, age, place of birth, present location, and the like,
could still have an intact Self 1. This is the case because the moment the
person employs first-person pronouns or even uses gestures to indicate "I,"
"me," "my," and the like, he or she is experiencing and expressing his or
her personal identity and is indexing for everyone else the location of his
or her singular, unique point of view in the world. In other words, if a person says, "I don't like that," he or she is locating the source of his or her experienced feelings and expressing his or her personal identity. What this
means is that if a person with AD employs first-person indexical pronouns
in a coherent manner in conversation, he or she is experiencing and expressing an intact Self 1.

Self 2, the Self of Mental and Physical Attributes

Each of us possesses a set of such attributes that differ, in some ways at least,
from those of any other person. Thus, Self 2, the self of mental and physical attributes, is the totality of attributes that a person possesses. Some attributes, such as having attained a particular level of education, vocational
accomplishments, one's sense of humor, one's height, and other physical
features, may have a long history, while others, such as having been diagnosed with probable AD, may be rather new in comparison. Among one's
mental attributes we might find, for example, a facility with languages or
mathematics or a "good memory." Among one's mental attributes we also
find one's beliefs. Thus, one might have particular religious and political
orientations, particular attitudes toward the importance of family or the
meaning of public service.

Self 2 also includes one's beliefs about one's attributes. For example, one
might take great pride in one's accomplishments in one or another vocational pursuit, one's devotion to family, or a particular social cause, and one

may also be rather displeased about other attributes, such as one's tendency to procrastinate, one's weight, or having been diagnosed with probable AD, the latter often being a source of shame and embarrassment. Consequently, another rather new Self 2 attribute of the person with AD may be sadness, even depression. It will be seen that the extent to which the person with AD can manifest a wide range of positively regarded Self 2 attributes may well be related to the extent to which healthy others in the person's social world focus their attention upon the very attributes that arouse negative reactions in the person with the disease. In other words, as healthy others focus more and more attention on the attributes that arouse shame and embarrassment in the person with AD, there will be less and less opportunity for that person to call attention to attributes in which he or she can take pride.

Self 3, the Socially Presented Selves, or Personae

A person may manifest a variety of social selves, each having its own unique set of behavioral patterns, including, for example, the devoted friend, who interacts with others as equals, the department chairperson who acts from a senior position in relation to junior colleagues, the respectful child who acts from a junior position toward his or her elderly parents, the devoted parent who acts from a senior position while helping his or her child with a difficult homework assignment. In each case, the nature and quality of the persona and the accompanying behavior will vary according to the demands of the social situation. As a result, depending upon the social situations in which we encounter a person, we may see only one particular persona, and we may be "surprised" in other social situations to see that same person behave in ways that seem "uncharacteristic." For example, the junior colleague may be taken aback when he or she first observes the department chairperson acting in a "silly" or "giddy" way while playing with young children, for the junior colleague experiences only one of the chairperson's Self 3 personae in the situations that typically occur in campus life.

A very important difference between Self 3 and Selves 1 and 2 is that in order for us to construct a particular Self 3 persona, we require the cooperation of at least one other person. That is to say, it would be impossible for an individual to manifest the persona of department chairperson and the associated cluster of behavioral patterns in the absence of the recognition and cooperation of colleagues, impossible to manifest the persona of devoted parent without the recognition and cooperation of one's child. Thus, any particular Self 3 is continuously created in the course of social interaction.

The fact that Self 3 personae require the cooperation of others will be seen to contribute to the vulnerability of the person with AD. In other words, in order for him or her to manifest Self 3 personae that are sources of pride and self-worth, others must not view him or her predominantly as "the patient" or "demented," with all the negative connotations entailed in those labels. For if others view the person with AD in such a way as to emphasize his or her defects, it will be difficult, if not impossible, for that person to gain the very cooperation that is required to construct a Self 3 other than that of the "burdensome, dysfunctional patient." In instances in which the person with AD is viewed mainly in terms of his or her defects there may well be a loss of Self 3 personae, but such losses would hardly be attributable to the direct effects of the disease itself. Conversely, in principle, it would be the case that given the cooperation necessary to constructing valued, worthy, personae, the person with AD should be able to manifest such personae despite the effects of the disease.

Case Examples

Let us now explore the conversation of specific persons with AD in light of the tripartite constructionist approach to selfhood. In each case, I present transcribed extracts of conversation between myself and a person with AD, and in each case my relationship with that person lasted a minimum of one and a half years, during which time we met at least once a week for more than an hour at a time. These were not "fleeting" encounters. Rather, they were person-to-person relationships, which had a chance to develop and grow over time, like most human relationships that have any enduring quality. My presence in their lives was principally as one who wished to understand their experience of AD and was attempting to offer some help in coping with problems that arose in their lives. In no case was there a "patient-physician" or "client-psychologist" relationship in the formal sense of those terms. Each relationship was person-to-person in nature. In no case have I altered the transcribed discourse of the person with AD, so that errors in pronunciation and syntax are preserved for the reader's benefit. Although I do not claim to be able to generalize from these individuals to all those who have AD, other instances of the phenomena I report have already been noted (Sabat and Harré 1992). As a result, I would assert that what is true of the people discussed here may be true of many others as well.

The Case of Dr. M.

Dr. M. was 75 years old at the beginning of my two-year association with her. She had been diagnosed with probable AD according to NINCDS-ADRDA (National Institute of Neurological Disorders and Stroke–Alzheimer's Disease and Related Disorders Association) criteria (McKhann et al. 1984) four years earlier but had experienced memory problems five years prior to the diagnosis and was considered to be moderately to severely afflicted. She evidenced severe word-finding problems, could not sign her name, and was unable to perform simple calculations, copy a design, or recall the date, month, or year. She was unable to use eating utensils and had striking difficulties with dressing and grooming. She held two advanced degrees (Ph.D. and M.S.W.) and had spent decades of her vocational life as a professor. One and a half years before our association began, her performance on standard neuropsychological tests was said to indicate decrements in memory, abstraction, concept formation, and word finding that were consistent with dementia.

Throughout my association with Dr. M., she evidenced an intact Self 1 by using first-person pronouns to index her experiences, feelings, and beliefs as her own. In the following extract she not only uses such indexicals but does so with regard to her reactions to Self 2 attributes that have resulted from AD. The issue at hand involved her reactions to her severe word-finding problems. It is important to keep in mind that Dr. M. was a person of extraordinary linguistic ability throughout her life, as evidenced in her writings and teaching at the university level.

INTERVIEWER: You're not just any ordinary person who has some problems finding words. You're a person for whom words, words to you are kind of like a musical instrument.

DR. M: Um-hum, um-hum. That's exactly right.

INTERVIEWER: And so the kind of frustration you feel would be greater than for a person whose focus in life was not so literary. That could give you cause for a lot of grief.

DR. M: I think the issue is, that is, for me maybe especially this day for some reason or other, but for last, maybe four years, that I am not satisfied with myself because what I want isn't here. I've, uh, thinking of it and it makes me angry as well as, that is part of the . . . and I guess that is what is happening now. Don't you think?

In this extract we see that Dr. M. uses first-person indexical pronouns to locate as hers the feeling that she is not satisfied with herself because, as a result of AD, she can no longer do what she wants to be able to do. She also indexes as her own the feeling of being angry with herself as a result of her word-finding problems, because to her, as I put it, "words are kind of like a musical instrument." In addition to revealing an intact Self 1 (the self of personal identity), she also reveals intact Self 2 attributes and beliefs about those attributes, for it makes her "angry as well" as being "not satisfied with myself." She is keenly aware of the difference between her present ability to use language (Self 2) and her lifelong, cherished facility with words (also a Self 2 attribute and belief about that attribute). In fact, her beliefs about her relatively new, dysfunctional attributes, which have come in the wake of AD, are very clear, for example, in her comment about her initial reluctance to tell friends and family about her diagnosis: "Why this reluctance to name my malady? Can it be that the term Alzheimer's has a connotation similar to the 'Scarlet Letter' or the 'Black Plague'? Is it even more embarrassing than a sexual disease?" For Dr. M., whose intellectual abilities and beliefs about those abilities, especially in the realm of linguistics, constituted an important part of her Self 2, the weakening of this particular attribute was especially frustrating and embarrassing. We can understand her embarrassment even more vividly when we examine her reaction to being exposed to standard tests.

Her deeply devoted and loving spouse thought at one point that Dr. M. might benefit from speech therapy, and although she went for days of initial testing, she soon decided against continuing. In discussing her reluctance to pursue further speech therapy, she not only showed evidence of an intact Self 1 through her use of first-person pronouns but also revealed an important issue with regard to Self 2 attributes:

INTERVIEWER: It didn't give you the feeling that going back and doing some kind of speech therapy would be helpful to you?

DR. M.: No . . . it wasn't important and I, you know, at this time too, I found that I really don't like to be, uh, talking about what, what's my trouble. It's gotten, I know what my trouble is. And I think that what I would like it, uh, only if there's something that is, uh, a time, a, uh, a time and with a person who there is a real . . . [gestures back and forth with hands]

INTERVIEWER: Back and forth—a relationship.

DR. M.: Um-hum.

The conversation moved on and then I said, "Let me back up for a second because I think I'm missing your point. You don't want your life to be . . . ," which she completed with "Going always to see people to see what's wrong with me."

Here Dr. M. expresses rather poignantly her reasons for discontinuing speech therapy. As a result of her exposure to the standard testing that is clearly a necessary part of speech therapy, Dr. M. encountered numerous examples of her inability to use words as she always had in the past and as she wished to do in the present. Thus, for her, the entire focus of this experience was on Self 2 attributes that stemmed from the disease, which were anathema to her. She also indexes as her own her desire for a real relationship with another person, a relationship not based on Self 2 attributes about which she felt great dismay, frustration, even anger. In other words, the type of social relationship that she could have with the speech therapist was based primarily upon her deficiencies, and this was the very type of relationship that she wanted to avoid as much as possible. Put another way, she wanted to enjoy social relationships that were based more upon the Self 2 attributes that she valued highly. It may be a quiet irony that Dr. M., who was said to be deficient in concept formation on the basis of standard neuropsychological tests given to her two years before this particular conversation occurred, was clearly still in command of the concepts of self-worth and self-respect, which turns out to be an indicator of what Kitwood and Bredin (1992) call "relative well-being."

Self 2 attributes can include those that the individual enjoyed for extended periods in the past, as well as those that are relatively more recent, along with the related beliefs about those attributes. In the case of the person with AD the two can clash, for the person can be very well aware of the deficiencies that have occurred as a result of the disease. This is quite evident in the following extract, in which Dr. M. discusses the effect of her word-finding problems:

DR. M.: I don't know how you go through the various steps, but I want to have a, a feel that when I talk, that when I can, talk, I, I can talk.
INTERVIEWER: Um-hum.
DR. M.: I can't always do that.
INTERVIEWER: Um-hum, well, you're doing it pretty well right now.
DR. M.: No, but when I haven't, we're just talking, uh . . .
INTERVIEWER: Light.
DR. M.: Light, light stuff, and even light stuff are problems because I miss and word and I can't find it.
INTERVIEWER: Um-hum.
DR. M.: And I'm probably able to do it as other people can, but, uh, not it that good, it's not good enough for me.

In order to say, "it's not good enough for me," Dr. M. had to be able to make a comparison between some criterion, perhaps her past facility with language, and her present ability, recognizing that her present ability does not measure up to her personal standards. As she herself said, "Apparently since I was a child I was a good talker . . . now, it's different." In this statement she provides evidence of the existence of Self 2 attributes both past and present along with her beliefs about them. She also uses first-person pronouns to index as her own her experience of her present abilities as well as her beliefs about them.

In another conversation Dr. M. and I discussed the fact that her speech was far more fluent in one-on-one conversations with me than it was when she attempted to speak at her support group meetings. In the following extract there is further evidence of the effect of Self 2 attributes on the sense of self of the person with AD:

INTERVIEWER: You're much more verbal, much more assertive about what you say; you . . . your humor comes out much more. Over there [in the support group meetings], I think you're much quieter, I think maybe—you can tell me if I'm wrong—maybe there you feel more pressure to speak quickly. I'm not sure.

Dr. M.: You might be right that way too . . . too . . . because I spend time before I tell people because I have so much problem with what I really want to see [say]. And so I take all that time and that's why, in part, I'm asking you now about it because I don't feel myself. You know, all my life it seems to me that I said, I did the things I wanted to say and what it means and all that stuff. Uh, and I don't . . . I don't go think this is the right thing, that's the bad thing, uh, I ought to think about it, I . . . I play . . . I played with it.

Interviewer: Um-hum.

Dr. M.: And I never had it that way and this way.

Again, we see Dr. M. using first-person pronouns to index her feelings and actions as her own, thus revealing an intact self of personal identity (Self 1). But as we move through her comments, we understand that she is feeling as though she has to take much more time to speak her thoughts now than she ever did in the past. As a result, she says, "I don't feel myself." She is using as her standard her Self 2 attributes from the past and comparing them with their weakened, present form. Because of the decline in her verbal ability, she doesn't feel like herself: in place of the Self 2 attribute of verbal facility that she so cherished in the past she now has a weakened form of that attribute and a set of reactions to and beliefs about that weakened attribute. She even went on to say, "You know what? Because I don't speak like I used to be, it seems to me that I don't have any good way of speaking." It would hardly be surprising that, given such beliefs about the attribute of her present way of speaking (Self 2), for Dr. M. to also be experiencing great sadness, frustration, and anger toward herself.

Thus far, it should be quite apparent that even though Dr. M. was in the moderate to severe stages of the progression of AD, she still possessed an intact Self 1 and an intact Self 2. I would assert, however, that when Dr. M. said, "I don't feel myself," she was referring not only to the fact that some of her valued mental attributes from the past were now terribly weakened by AD but also to the third aspect of personhood in the constructionist view, Self 3, the various social personae that are publicly presented. This aspect of her experience was made even more apparent when she commented, "Sure, I uh, I can handle myself when I try not to let myself be presented as an Alcazheimer's. I'm very different."

I must hasten to call the reader's attention to four important points here. First, Dr. M., whose academic training was in the areas of sociology and social work, was very well aware of what it meant to be presented as having been diagnosed with AD: it meant that others would view her and react to her mainly in terms of her diagnosis and her defects, which are themselves a source of great embarrassment and sadness to her. Second, she recognized that she is better able to interact with others when she avoids being presented in such a way. Third, when possible, she refuses to be positioned by others as a person with AD. Fourth, and perhaps most important in our attempt to understand the experience of the person with AD who refuses to be positioned negatively by others, it is the case that many, if not most, people are not able to refuse to be positioned primarily as having AD by healthy others and so must endure the effects of such positioning.

I will try to communicate here that among the effects of being identified primarily on the basis of having AD is the great potential for the loss of valued Self 3 personae. Recall that a person's ability to construct and manifest a variety of Self 3 personae depends upon the cooperation the individual receives from others in the social world. In this respect the person with AD is extremely vulnerable because to the extent that healthy others focus upon the Self 2 attribute of AD and its deleterious effects upon other valued Self 2 attributes, while simultaneously paying less heed to those attributes that the person with AD values, he or she will encounter great difficulty in obtaining the cooperation required to construct Self 3 personae that reflect qualities in which he or she takes pride. Put another way, if we view the person with AD as someone who is defective and incompetent, it will be extremely difficult for that person to construct a Self 3 persona other than that of the "burdensome, dysfunctional patient." Such a situation conduces rather easily to the belief that this is all the person *can be*. What is involved here is a radical misunderstanding of the abilities of the person with AD. The acid test of the belief that the person with AD can be nothing more than a "dysfunctional patient" involves giving that person just the sort of cooperation he or she needs to construct Self 3 personae in which he or she may take pride and then observing the effects.

In the case of Dr. M., it became patently clear that she could be far more than simply an "AD sufferer-patient." When our association began, she was very dissatisfied with the support group that she took part in every two weeks. She expressed one reason for her dissatisfaction in the following extract:

DR. M.: Um-hum. I felt, she [the group leader] . . . she told the people that who, uh, had, uh, ability to, uh, come and talk, uh, and see I had a . . . a very neat thing statement and I had to and I couldn't handle it. Um anyhow, they . . . they were talking about how they could make it organized. I had for about, uh, maybe five days, five days of the time, five times had that not . . . they didn't have that. I couldn't put that in them. I knew exactly what they should do and uh . . . and I . . . I . . . at least I don't mean I was perfect. I mean there's a way of bring-ing in and . . . uh . . . and so I say I watched them and I help, I saw what was going on, and I was not a hero. I couldn't I . . . I said nothing. And at the end, the caretaker said, "You have not said anything. What do you think? We haven't heard from you." Now the fact was that I knew that it was something that had been done and that would have and should have been done and that was good and it was good with a good person. I know what to do with it. I had when there were other people being able to make a st-, st-, a stance of, of uh, what could be done, or something like that. But it wasn't my role . . .

INTERVIEWER: Um-hum.

DR. M.: Uh, unless there was someone else, it . . . it was not appropriate at all to to say this . . . I felt I wasn't myself and I couldn't, in my role, I couldn't do, I couldn't have done the, the good thing . . . and the good caretaker said, "Re-member you said you'd talk." And I don't know quite how to handle that . . . see, we don't know each other's backgrounds at all and there were and our experi-ences are different and I don't know how to . . . nobody says, uh, what that's a problem. What do you do, doctor?

INTERVIEWER: Let me see if I understand here. You, you see an oppor-tunity to give some constructive criticism.

DR. M.: Well, ya. It's peoples are not all there at the same time. It's not well organized.

INTERVIEWER: And you have some thoughts about how to organize it.

DR. M.: Ya, but it's not my role.

Although Dr. M. was trained as a social worker and understood quite well what should have been done to improve the organization of the group, two things stood in the way of her taking action: her word-finding prob-lems, about which she felt great embarrassment, and the fact that she be-lieved that it wasn't her role to do so. As a result, she said that she did not want to continue attending group meetings because "I don't get enough" out of the group.

However, she did encourage me to attend a meeting, which led to my being invited back, and eventually I attended the meetings for many months, eventually becoming a co-leader of the group. On many occasions Dr. M. and I would discuss situations that transpired at the meetings, which enabled her to construct, with my cooperation, a Self 3 of "academic/social worker." In the conversation of which the following extract was a part Dr. M. initiated a discussion of an interaction that had occurred between herself and another support group member. She had addressed him, and he had had difficulty understanding what she had said to him. He had seemed to become sad, as if it had been his fault that he hadn't understood what Dr. M. said. Dr. M. had noticed his reaction and feared that she had said something hurtful to him. I told her what I recalled from that interaction, and we spent the better part of an hour taking turns discussing the situation. We reached some measure of closure when I was able to help her understand that she had not, in fact, said something hurtful to the man.

INTERVIEWER: But at first I think he was feeling very uncomfortable because he didn't understand and maybe he was blaming himself for not understanding.
DR. M.: It seems to me, uh, that that's int- . . . interesting and I just love going through things like that and what it seems like and when and it, uh, it's very . . . I like to do it. And I like to do it with you.
INTERVIEWER: Oh, well thank you! It's mutual.

In her comment here Dr. M. makes quite clear that as she did throughout her vocational life, she still loves to analyze the social interactions among people, and she expresses her feeling that she likes to do so with me (Self 2). Although her use of first-person pronouns indexes her feelings as her own (Self 1), and although she expresses her beliefs about analyzing such interactions, it is also important to the present discussion that in order for Dr. M. to construct the Self 3 of "academic/social worker," she required my cooperation. She could hardly have even begun to have such a conversation without a cooperative partner. Indeed, it was in the context of constructing a valued Self 3 persona that Dr. M. could openly discuss Self 2 attributes that were troublesome and frustrating to her.

In still other conversations we had about events transpiring at her support group meetings Dr. M. was able, with my cooperation, to construct a

Self 3 of "colleague/mentor." After my first meeting with her support group, Dr. M. and I discussed my reactions to being invited to return to speak with the support group. The following extract was part of that conversation and is revealing of the Self 3 that Dr. M. was able to construct in that context:

INTERVIEWER: That's how I felt when the group leader asked me if I would come back. Inside my head I was saying, "Would I? Are you kidding? I would love to!"

DR. M.: I knew that! **I knew that, I knew that it gives you just what you're looking for. So uh, and I think it gives . . . gives the group some.** You repeated . . . I mean I repeated what you had said in a sense.

INTERVIEWER: Yes indeed! I think we learn more about what people *can* do [when we observe them] in very rich social settings.

DR. M.: Um-hum, **and you can have it for the next, uh . . . paper.**

INTERVIEWER: That's right!

In the comments that I have emphasized, Dr. M., with my cooperation, constructed a Self 3 persona of "colleague/mentor" in two ways. First, she reveals in her first comment that she understands that there is an important connection between what transpired in the support group meeting and my own research interests, and second, she states, in a way that would be consistent with the role of a senior colleague or mentor, that what transpired in that meeting constituted material that I could use for my "next . . . paper." Dr. M. was thus behaving in ways that are utterly inconsistent with the Self 3 of "burdensome AD patient," for a person restricted to constructing such a Self 3 would neither have been given the opportunity to comment about such connections nor have been engaged in such a way so as to feel free enough to encourage a younger academic as Dr. M. did.

This phenomenon indicates that even though she was described as being in the moderate to severe stages of AD, Dr. M. was still able to construct valued and worthy Self 3 personae. Therefore, *it is important to understand that the cognitive and behavioral abilities that are sampled by the methods of assessment used to define her stage of AD are different from those that could be brought to bear to construct a Self 3 that was a source of great satisfaction to her.* In other words, the Self 2 attributes that provide the data employed to define her stage in the progress of the disease are quite different from the Self 2 attributes that must exist in order for her to construct the worthy and valued Self 3 personae of "colleague/mentor" and "academic/social worker." That our conversations were, in fact, a source of great satisfaction to her can be inferred from what she said to me when her medical appointments precluded one or another of our meetings: "I missed you."

Using the Social Constructionist approach to analyzing selfhood, then, we can readily see in the case of Dr. M. that she had (1) an intact Self 1, or self of personal identity, as she employed first-person pronouns to index her experiences as being her own; (2) a Self 2, or self of mental and physical attributes, which included longstanding attributes and beliefs about her attributes, as well as attributes that derived from the disease itself along with beliefs about those attributes; and (3) the ability to construct, with my cooperation, Self 3 personae that were consistent with valued abilities she had enjoyed throughout decades of her vocational life. These Self 3 personae of "academic/social worker" and "colleague/mentor" were well within her ability to construct, but in order to do so she had to have the cooperation of another person in order to be able to use the abilities she retained.

These observations indicate that despite the plethora of deficiencies that she experienced as a result of AD, Dr. M. was hardly experiencing a loss of self. Additionally, if Dr. M. were to experience a loss of self, that loss would be confined primarily to (1) the Self 3 social personae, which would be derivative of the confines of her social world rather than due to the direct effects of the disease, and (2) the lack of attention given by healthy others to the worthy and valued Self 2 attributes that must be available for her use in order for her to be able to construct such a valued Self 3. Of course, I recognize that some of her losses in the domain of Self 2 attributes (e.g., her word-finding problems) are in fact derived from AD and that she did not "feel like herself" in part as a result of those losses. Still, (1) and (2) above constitute areas in which assaults on aspects of her personhood are determined less by the disease itself and more by the social situations in which she finds herself, for despite her AD-related losses, she was still able to construct Self 3 personae that she valued and in which she found great satisfaction even with a diagnosis of probable AD in the moderate to severe stage.

A Critical Question: Is Dr. M. "Typical"?

It might be tempting to wonder if, given her high level of education and her academic career, Dr. M.'s ability to construct worthy Self 3 personae is "atypical" of persons with AD in the moderate to severe stages of the disease. Surely, having earned advanced degrees made Dr. M. "atypical" of people in general. I would like to propose three responses to such a reasonable question: *First*, there is no "typical" person with AD, just as there is no "average person" or "typical person." There are statistical averages, as well as average test scores for a group of people with AD and for groups of normal control subjects, but there is no average person and no average person with AD. Even when such average scores are used, there is always some degree of associated variance, and even if such variance is not "significant" in the statistical sense, it can be quite significant when we attempt to understand individual people.

Indeed, the stereotype that is based upon even the tacit belief that an average or typical person with AD exists contributes to the tendency to view the person with AD principally in terms of his or her defects because, *second*, the commonalities that may be shown by those who are diagnosed with probable AD are usually their symptoms, their deficits, which is quite in line with a strictly medical approach to understanding the effects of a disease. Most studies in the extant literature are not of the detailed case study variety, in which the symptoms of the disease are examined within the larger context of the life of the person with AD, and it is in that larger context that we invariably find the subtle differences that spell individuality and, hence, variability. Thus, in order to know what is and what is not typical with regard to selfhood among those with AD, we must examine large numbers of individuals in great detail and avoid obscuring their individuality through the use of statistical treatments.

Third, we can examine the conversation, the discourse, of a person with AD whose educational background and vocation are significantly different from those of Dr. M.

The Case of Mrs. D.

Mrs. D. was 70 years old at the beginning of our association and had been diagnosed with probable AD five years prior to that. According to standard tests, she was moderately to severely afflicted (stage 4 on the Global Deterioration Scale [Reisberg, Ferris, and Crook 1984], score of 7 on the Mini-Mental State Test [Folstein, Folstein, and McHugh 1975]), and she satisfied the NINCDS-ADRDA criteria for probable AD (McKhann et al.

1984). When tested, she could not name (via recall) the day of the week, the month, the season, the year, the city and county she was in, or the date. She had a number of sensory-motor problems, such as difficulties in picking up eating utensils when sitting at the lunch table, getting food to her mouth, imitating the movements of the instructor during exercises. She underestimated her age, saying that she was "sixty, sixty-something," when she was actually seventy, and she had difficulties in distinguishing right from left. Her ability to use spoken language was not as compromised as were her recall and her sensory-motor skills, although she did experience frequent word-finding problems and paraphasias. She had been raised in a show-business family and loved to sing and tell jokes. At the time of our association she was living at home with her husband and attended a day care center. I met with her two to three hours per week at her home and at the day care center for approximately one and a half years.

From a Social Constructionist point of view, Mrs. D.'s Self 2 was replete with attributes and beliefs about her attributes from her healthy days through the time of our association. It was in the social situation of the day care center that Mrs. D. was able to construct a Self 3 that was far different from that of "AD sufferer-burden," which she was limited to constructing at home. Her husband, though he loved her deeply, had developed story lines, or narratives, that painted her as delusional and confused. One of her "delusions" that Mr. D. reported stemmed from the fact that often, before he took her to the day care center in the morning, she would ask him to hurry so that she "wouldn't be late for work." Since Mr. D. was unaware that his wife had a job, and given her diagnosis of AD, he believed that her comment signaled a delusion.

As reported previously (Sabat 1994b), I asked Mrs. D. about this situation and her response turned out to be extremely informative on a number of different levels. She explained that because many of the participants at the day care center were sad, she would cheer them up by singing songs and telling jokes. Given her family background, Mrs. D. was a fountain of knowledge of old songs that were familiar to most of the participants, and she would often lead the group in spontaneous sing-a-longs and tell jokes that would provoke hearty laughter. The day care staff members recognized her ability to bring good cheer to others and engaged Mrs. D.'s help in a number of areas, including integrating new participants into the group, providing sympathy and understanding to those who were experiencing particular difficulties, and engaging participants in conversation. Mrs. D. explained: "Some of them are in bad shape, you know, that they couldn't remember a thing. I would try to help them. That's what you have to do almost, if you want to get along . . . I think it's a nice thing to do. Instead of me sitting down with the little I have gone, a little bit, a little higher, and not trying my fellow person . . . as things went by, I would work, you know, with somebody just to keep them happy."

From her behavior and her comments we learn that (1) she used first-person pronouns to index her feelings, beliefs, and experiences as her own, thereby indicating an intact Self 1, the self of personal identity; (2) she revealed intact Self 2 attributes, such as extroversion, a warm personality, a wonderful sense of humor, sympathy for the plight of others, a fine singing voice, as well as beliefs about what she did ("I think it's a nice thing to do"); (3) she was able, with the cooperation of staff members and participants, to construct a Self 3 of what might be called "the life of the party," by which the other participants knew her, and also a Self 3 of "liaison between staff and participants"; (4) "work," as she called it, was to help other participants and the staff in sundry ways, and although she was not a salaried employee, she did have a well-defined set of responsibilities that she carried out with great elan and satisfaction; and (5) contrary to her husband's interpretation, Mrs. D. was not delusional at all, for she did in fact have a job, or role, at the day care center. Of course, if one were to take the word of her spouse as being fact, and not make the effort to examine the social dynamics of her life at the day care center, one would arrive at a very inaccurate picture not only of Mrs. D. but of the effects of AD as well.

One might infer that one of the reasons that Mrs. D. loved going to the day care center, as attested to by her husband, was that in that setting she was able to find the necessary cooperation with which to construct Self 3 personae in which she could take pride, finding a measure of self-worth and satisfaction in being able to help others. Her situation at home was markedly different, for Mr. D. positioned and interacted with Mrs. D. principally on the basis of her being afflicted with AD. As a result, at home she had no "work" to do other than trying to comply with her husband's infrequent requests, and her mood was sullen and withdrawn. Her husband reported, "Mrs. D. used to do everything around the house. Now she doesn't do anything. I have to do everything." Indeed, Mr. D. even did most of her talking for her, and he treated her subjective reports about feeling cold in the house during the winter as being inaccurate and symptomatic of AD since he did not feel chilly in the house. Although he indicated that his wife "loved coming to the day care center," he seemed to be unaware of her reasons for feeling that way. He reported that he did not speak with her about his problems and feelings because "she wouldn't understand." As a result, Mrs. D. could not construct a Self 3 other than that of "burdensome AD patient" at home because her husband focused his attention primarily on Mrs. D.'s Self 2 attributes that were due to the disease and therefore did not provide the cooperation she required to construct a valued and valuable Self 3, which, however, she was able to do at the day care center, where staff members paid a great deal of attention to Mrs. D.'s intact, healthy Self 2 attributes.

Interestingly, her spouse's defining her primarily on the basis of her Self 2 attribute of having AD contributed to his cooperating with her in constructing yet another Self 3 in which she could take pride, the Self 3 of "research volunteer." Mrs. D. spent a great deal of her time volunteering as a subject in research studies at the National Institutes of Health. When she was asked why she did this, she responded, "That was the nicety of it, cause I could have said, 'no' but believe me, if I can help me and my fe [fellow] man, I would do it." Here again, as with the construction of all Self 3 personae, she required the cooperation of others, in this case her husband, for it was he who had to transport her to and from the National Institutes of Health.

Whereas Dr. M. eschewed formal testing situations because such interactions highlighted the decline of her own cherished abilities, Mrs. D. did not place nearly as much weight on her previous intellectual prowess and could, as a result, view such situations as nonthreatening and therefore welcome opportunities to be of help in the search for a better understanding of the disease. In the process, Mrs. D. was able to find yet another way to do something of value for others and thereby add to her own sense of self-worth (see, e.g., Sabat et al. 1999). Reflecting on the stories of these two women, we find that although both might be characterized as being in the moderate to severe stages of AD, and although both demonstrated intact Self 1, Self 2, and Self 3 aspects of personhood, their ways of reacting to particular social situations (e.g., formal testing and group meetings) were quite different. Such a difference in reactions to similar situations casts further doubt upon the validity of stereotyping those with AD as being some sort of homogeneous group that can be defined solely or even primarily on the basis of the diagnosis and related deficits. It is important to remember that those who have AD are persons first, so it is hardly surprising that two persons who have different Self 2 attributes and beliefs about those attributes would have different proclivities and reactions to the situations they confront.

Lessons Learned

Using the Social Constructionist tripartite approach to personhood as a heuristic device, we can see that despite the deficits in cognitive and behavioral function that are used to define persons with AD as being moderately to severely afflicted, the following are true:

1. It is possible to observe the existence of intact Self 1 (self of personal identity), Self 2 (self of mental and physical attributes), and Self 3 (self of social personae) aspects of personhood.

2. The ability of persons with AD to manifest social personae in which they take pride and gain a measure of satisfaction is directly related to the extent to which healthy others give them the cooperation they need in order to do so. Losses in Self 3 in these cases are related, then, not directly to the disease but to the social situations in which persons with AD find themselves.

3. In order to provide the cooperation required for the construction of valued Self 3 personae, caregivers must avoid viewing the person diagnosed with AD principally in terms of the diagnosis and related deficits, thereby restricting him or her to the construction of a Self 3 of "burdensome, dysfunctional patient."

4. Honoring the Self 2 attributes that are valued by persons with AD and helping them to construct valued Self 3 personae can result in the reduction of excess disability—disability that is due not to brain injury but to dysfunctional social interactions—thereby aiding caregivers and those with AD alike in their attempts to cope with the effects of the disease. Reducing excess disability enables the person with AD to use his or her remaining abilities to their fullest extent, thus enhancing interpersonal relationships and communication.

Conclusion

The foregoing seems to indicate that an explanation of the effects of AD cannot be based simply on biomedical and neuropathological factors but must include careful attention to, and understanding of, the social dynamics that exist between caregivers and the persons with AD. Perhaps it is not beyond the pale to suggest that there is a moral issue involved here: do unto others as you would have them do unto you. Those among us who have been diagnosed with AD are persons—they are not "patients" except in relation to their physicians and the special social dynamics involved in such relationships. And so their evident personhood and ability to experience and express different aspects of selfhood must be respected and supported to the fullest extent. To do otherwise would be simply to rub salt into an open wound.

REFERENCES

American Psychiatric Association. 1994. *Diagnostic and statistical manual of mental disorders*. Washington, D.C.

Brody, E. 1971. Excess disabilities of mentally impaired aged: Impact of individualized treatment. *Gerontologist* 25:124–33.

Cohen, D., and C. Eisdorfer. 1986. *The loss of self*. New York: Norton.

Coulter, J. 1981. *The social construction of mind*. London: Macmillan.

Folstein, M. F., S. E. Folstein, and P. R. McHugh. 1975. Mini-mental state. *Journal of Psychiatric Research* 12:189–98.

Hamel, M., D. Pushkar, D. Andres, M. Reis, D. Dastoor, H. Grauer, and H. Bergman. 1990. Predictors and consequences of aggressive behavior by community-based dementia patients. *Gerontologist* 30:206–11.

Harré, R. 1983. *Personal being*. Oxford: Blackwell.

———. 1991. The discursive production of selves. *Theory and Psychology* 1:51–63.

Kitwood, T. 1990. The dialectics of dementia: With particular reference to Alzheimer's disease. *Ageing and Society* 10:177–96.

———. 1998. Toward a theory of dementia care: Ethics and interaction. *Journal of Clinical Ethics* 9:23–34.

Kitwood, T., and K. Bredin. 1992. Towards a theory of dementia care: Personhood and well-being. *Ageing and Society* 12:269–87.

Locke, J. 1956. *An essay concerning human understanding*. 1841. Reprint. Chicago: Regnery.

McKhann, G., D. Drachman, M. Folstein, R. Katzman, D. Price, and E. M. Stadlan.

1984. Clinical diagnosis of Alzheimer's disease: Report of the NINCDS-ADRDA work group under the auspices of the Department of Health and Human Services task force on Alzheimer's disease. *Neurology* 34:939–44.

Reisberg, B., J. Borenstein, S. Salob, and S. Ferris. 1987. Behavioral symptoms in Alzheimer's disease: Phenomenology and treatment. *Journal of Clinical Psychiatry* 48 (suppl.): 9–15.

Reisberg, B., S. H. Ferris, and T. O. Crook. 1984. Signs, symptoms, and course of age-associated cognitive decline. In *Aging*. Vol. 19, *Alzheimer's disease: A report of progress in research*, ed. S. Corkin, K. L. Davis, J. H. Growdon, E. Usdin, and R. J. Wurtman, 177–81. New York: Raven.

Sabat, S. R. 1991a. Facilitating conversation via indirect repair: A case study of Alzheimer's disease. *Georgetown Journal of Languages and Linguistics* 2:284–96.

———. 1991b. Turn-taking, turn-giving, and Alzheimer's disease: A case study of conversation. *Georgetown Journal of Languages and Linguistics* 2:167–81.

———. 1994a. Excess disability and malignant social psychology: A case study of Alzheimer's disease. *Journal of Community and Applied Social Psychology* 4:157–66.

———. 1994b. Recognizing and working with remaining abilities: Toward improving the care of Alzheimer's disease sufferers. *American Journal of Alzheimer's Care and Related Disorders and Research* 9:8–16.

———. 1999. Facilitating conversation with an Alzheimer's disease sufferer through the use of indirect repair. In *Language and communication in old age*, ed. H. Hamilton, 115–31. New York: Garland.

———. 2001. *The experience of Alzheimer's disease: Life through a tangled veil*. Oxford: Blackwell.

Sabat, S. R., H. Fath, F. M. Moghaddam, and R. Harré. 1999. The maintenance of self-esteem: Lessons from the culture of Alzheimer's sufferers. *Culture and Psychology* 5:5–31.

Sabat, S. R., and R. Harré. 1992. The construction and deconstruction of self in Alzheimer's disease. *Ageing and Society* 12:443–61.

———. 1994. The Alzheimer's disease sufferer as a semiotic subject. *Philosophy, Psychiatry, Psychology* 1:145–60.

Sacks, O. 1985. *The man who mistook his wife for a hat*. New York: HarperCollins.

Vygotsky, L. 1965. *Thought and language*. Cambridge: MIT Press.

Wittgenstein, L. 1953. *Philosophical investigations*. Oxford: Blackwell.

6

Social and Family Relationships

Establishing and Maintaining Connections

LISA SNYDER

People in my situation need a lot of companionship and friends.
—Consuelo, age 35, a retired elementary-school teacher

"One of the things about this is, it's in the family and the family has not only me and my wife, but we have our children and the children have their spouses. In other words, this whole thing about Alzheimer's is not just about two people. It's about a whole mess of people. Not only our families, but our extended families and their friends. It gets very involved. But that's the way life is supposed to be" (Henderson 1998, 65).

The speaker is Cary Henderson, a retired history professor diagnosed with Alzheimer's disease. His message acknowledges both the complex impact of AD on family and social relationships and the inherent social nature of human beings. People do not live in isolation, and optimally each individual is engaged in meaningful relationships with others. The fabric of interactions is woven with simple or more elaborate patterns relative to each person's established networks and ability to form new associations over time. For those living with AD, however, the insidious experience of the disease inevitably unravels many of these well-worn and familiar patterns of relationship. It challenges "the way life is supposed to be" with barriers to communication, risks of withdrawal, and threats to the experience of belonging.

Acknowledging the work of Bowlby and, more recently, of Mielsen,

Kitwood (1997) emphasizes the role of familial and social attachments for persons with AD. His pioneering work in person-centered care establishes a dialectical model involving a continuing interplay between both neuropathological and social psychological influences. The progression of AD poses threats to personal identity and environmental familiarity and can result in feelings of anxiety, uncertainty, abandonment, and fear. Modifications in social interactions with those diagnosed can have an impact upon these feelings and affect the condition and quality of their lives. Stable and caring relationships can provide comfort, security, and feelings of inclusion that are threatened by the experience of the disease.

Goldsmith (1996) summarizes the work of European researchers who have investigated client satisfaction with services rendered to them and affirms the theoretical importance of relationship for persons with AD. Findings revealed that clients with Alzheimer's were more concerned about the social aspects of their care than they were about the physical aspects. Recurrent concerns included the desire for companionship, the need to feel valued and to experience a sense of belonging, and the desire to have stimulating activities.

In the United States, Feinberg, Whitlatch, and Tucke (2000) interviewed both caregivers of persons with dementia and care receivers about everyday care preferences and decisions. Their values-and-preferences scale comprised thirty-six items that fell into one of seven subscales. Of the care receivers' six most highly rated values and preferences (rated very important), three—having the primary caregiving family member continue to be the one to assist with current and future care needs; that the caregiver not put his or her life on hold; and that the person with AD avoid being a physical burden to the family—fell into the family/caregiver subscale. A factor analysis of the overall most highly rated values and preferences found that the broader domain of environment/social interactions ranked highest in order of importance, including the preferences of living in one's own home and being with family and friends.

In her exemplary investigation into the effects of AD on marriage, Wright (1993) interviewed thirty couples about the distribution of household tasks and degrees of tension, companionship, affection and sexuality, and commitment in the marital relationship. She concluded that afflicted spouses have a great need for companionship, as well as significant dependency needs; they recognize that their spouse is the most important person in their life. All of the above findings support the primacy of social and family relationships in the priorities of persons with dementia.

Although researchers have acknowledged the significance of social and family relationships in studies of communication patterns, social interactions, and expressions of selfhood in persons with AD (Burgener, Shimer, and Murrell 1993; Hutchinson, Krall, and Wilson 1997; Kelly 1997; Phinney 1998; Sabat and Collins 1999), explorations of the subjective experience of relationships for those with the disease have been lacking. This chapter explores the significance of social and family relationships through the direct written and verbal testimonies of persons with AD and elaborates on the critical themes that surface along the continuum of the disease. Drawing on advice from those diagnosed and my own investigation, I offer recommendations for more effectively evaluating and addressing the relational needs of persons with AD.

Method

I reviewed video footage, manuscripts written by persons with AD, verbatim quotes garnered from the works of other clinicians and documented in written literature, and transcriptions from my own individual and group sessions with diagnosed individuals. Quotations pertaining to social or family relationships were extracted from these references and collected for review. A total of 112 authentic verbalizations from sixty individuals with AD were then divided into meaningful categories or themes. Quotations were collected from twenty-seven men and twenty-six women; the speaker's gender was not provided for seven quotations. Individuals whose age was specified ranged from 35 to 82 years old. There were 3 African Americans, 1 Hispanic, 41 Caucasians, and 11 of unspecified ethnicity.

The following themes were categorized under family relationships: fear or recognition of becoming a burden, role changes, loss of autonomy, mutual adjustments, and family as survival. Themes categorized under social relationships included ambivalence about disclosing the diagnosis, responses from others, isolation and withdrawal, and establishing new supports. Two themes—barriers to communication, and devaluation—applied to either category and described experiences applicable to relationships in general.

Themes

Barriers to Communication

Verbal communication is a fundamental component of interpersonal relationships. For the person with AD, the ability to express and understand language is profoundly affected over the course of the disease and challenges communication. In a qualitative study of five interviewed individuals with AD, Phinney (1998) identified experiences of conversation breakdown as a common theme. People expressed increased discomfort with speaking because of difficulty tracking discussions and finding words. One woman spoke of "things coming out the wrong way" (11). These concerns were reiterated by others with AD. A woman confided to friends in an early-stage AD social club: "I'm aware that I'm losing larger and larger chunks of memory. . . . I lose one word and then I can't come up with the rest of the sentence. I just stop talking and people think something is really wrong with me" (Trabert 1997). A man in his early fifties who was forced to retire from his job as an editor described the irony of his word-finding difficulties to his peers in an AD support group: "For awhile, I'll search for a word and I can see it walking away from me. It gets littler and littler. It always comes back, but at the wrong time. You can't be spontaneous" (Snyder et al. 1995, 694).

Language barriers are exacerbated by real or perceived responses from others. One man experienced significant problems with concentration and aphasia but was able to articulate his distress: "It seems my main trouble is with communication. Sometimes, I'm about to say something that is very important to me and it's nearly impossible to transmit the information because everyone listening has the presumption that what I'm about to say is unscrewed. There's essentially no way for me to convince anybody that although I'm affected by Alzheimer's in many ways, there's still a lot that's up there in my mind that has reason to be communicated!" (Barlow 1997).

Devaluation

These barriers to verbal communication have a significant impact on social and family relationships and affect the self-esteem of persons with AD. In a qualitative analysis of authentic verbalizations from fifteen support group participants, my colleagues and I identified feelings of devaluation in relation to others as a recurrent theme. One woman attested to keeping her feelings private to avoid further threat to her self-esteem: "I know people don't care about me one way or another. You don't want them to know about your problems. It could decrease your sense of value" (Snyder et al. 1995, 694). This experience of devaluation can foster secondary feelings of anger and alienation. A woman interviewed for an illuminating video from the Cleveland Area Alzheimer's Association (1994) stated, "I still would like to be treated like a person, you know, because I'm still a person whether I do it wrong or right . . . I want to feel like I'm somebody, too, worth somebody because a lot of times with this—already with what I have . . . I really don't belong any place."

Henderson (1998) kept a journal of his experiences of AD in which he confesses apologetically to feelings of suspicion and paranoia toward family arising from devaluing experiences: "The feeling of being put on and the feeling nobody loves us, I think those are perfectly normal feelings. . . . I think for a lot of us the feeling of being cheated, or the feeling of being belittled and somehow made jokes of, I think that's one of the worst things about Alzheimer's" (37). Given these barriers to communication and experiences of devaluation, it is not surprising that many individuals value their relationship with a pet. A pet affords an experience of companionship that transcends language barriers. "I sort of think that anybody with Alzheimer's could benefit from a friendly little dog," writes Henderson. "Somebody they can play with and talk to—it's kinda nice to talk to a dog that you know is not going to talk back. And you can't make a mistake that way. She's just a companion who's always there" (13). For others the experience of devaluation is offset by caring for the pet. Interviewed in the Cleveland video, one woman with early-onset AD speaks about her dog: "Muffin doesn't care what kind of a mood I'm in—she doesn't care if I remember her name. All she cares about is being my friend. I needed a little responsibility but not too much because there were so many responsibilities being taken away from me" (Cleveland Area Alzheimer's Association 1994).

Family Relationships

The Fear or Recognition of Being a Burden

While barriers to communication and experiences of devaluation permeate many interactions for persons with AD, others themes are more specific to either family or social relationships. Persons in the early stages of AD often express the fear or recognition of being a burden. There has been a long-standing bias in both the AD literature and support networks that the caregiver suffers more than the patient in this disease. This bias can have repercussions that influence the diagnosed individual's concern about becoming a burden. One articulate woman with early-onset AD writes, "The guilt that is heaped upon the patient is enormous—not intentionally perhaps, but it is there. Through no fault of our own, we have Alzheimer's, which will cause untold misery for our caregivers. More than anything, this picture of misery for your loved ones is hammered into you as you seek advice from health care and legal professionals. . . . There is no question that those days will come when my family will need the support, but I am not incompetent just because a diagnosis was made" (Phillips 2000). In his letter to the public after he was diagnosed with AD former President Ronald Reagan expressed grief over the inevitable impact the disease would have on his loved ones: "At the moment, I feel just fine. . . . Unfortunately as Alzheimer's disease progresses, the family often bears a heavy burden. I only wish there was some way I could spare Nancy from this painful experience" (Reagan 1994).

Whether because of a prevailing bias or because they are acutely aware of the impact of the disease on loved ones, some individuals with AD make reference to their spouse's need for respite. A man in his early sixties stated: "It's tougher for a wife with our disease because we sometimes repeat things. We get angry at ourselves and this carries through to them. . . . So my wife has all of my aggravations and all of her aggravations. . . . She has her own business. Her work is her therapy to get my problems out of her mind" (Bachrach 1997, 1). A 75-year-old woman noted her growing dependency and discussed the impact of this on her husband: "It seems like Joe's having to do too much, but I can't do anything about it. I try to get him to go down in the afternoon and play pool and get away for a few hours because otherwise he's with me constantly. . . . I depend on Joe for everything. I'm isolating him as well as myself and I'm not being fair to him" (Snyder 1999, 24). And in his journal Henderson writes: "The caregivers are doing their darndest—they want to be like any other people, and they deserve their moments and their times—their times away from us, because it can be very tedious. We can be very tedious. I can be very tedious, and I'm aware of that" (Henderson 1998, 82).

Some individuals with AD express little concern over being a burden and derive feelings of comfort and security from receiving care. A 56-year-old man stated, "In my life I've done a lot of letting people take care of me, so

I'm managing fine. . . . I was always the kind of kid who liked getting his hair cut or going to the dentist. I'm a little strange, but it's helping me now with Alzheimer's. I don't feel like I am a burden" (Harris and Sterin 1999, 251). Others are so impressed with their spouses' capable coping and exemplary organizational abilities that they see little outward evidence of their stress. As a result, they do not understand the extent of the added burdens in their caregivers' lives.

Concern about being a burden can also be tempered by a degree of insight. Although many persons with AD express some awareness of memory and functional impairment, the extent of their insight is highly variable and can diminish as the disease progresses (Mangone et al. 1991; McDaniel et al. 1995). Research suggests that impaired awareness of memory deficits may influence the degree of caregiver burden (Seltzer et al. 1997), and it is not uncommon for those diagnosed to express limited or fluctuating understanding of a spouse's increased responsibilities. For example, one man with moderate impairment became indignant when his wife referred to herself as a "caregiver" and insisted that he needed no care whatsoever. As his wife gently gave examples of the numerous tasks she had assumed since his disability, as well as his need for assistance with personal care, he begrudgingly acknowledged her new responsibilities. Clinicians have noted, however, that some individuals in more advanced stages of AD do remain aware of the impact of their disease (Goldsmith 1996; Kitwood 1997; Snyder 1999). A man in his mid-seventies who has significant functional and cognitive impairment feels remorse over his wife's increased responsibilities: "[She] has to do all of the driving, thinking, and putting things together. Instead of my doing things for her, now she's the one who jumps in and gets things done. I wish that I could do more so that the burden wouldn't be on her shoulders. . . . Since Alzheimer's, there are so many things that I can't do" (Snyder 1999, 85).

In their suggestions to family members participants of the Eastern Massachusetts Alzheimer's Association Support Group acknowledge the variability of their own insight and provide an important summation: "Try to understand that there are some days when I think there is nothing wrong with me. There are other days that nothing works right" (Silverio and Koenig-Coste 1997).

Role Changes

As care responsibilities increase, there are subsequent role changes for both the person with AD and his or her significant other. One Italian American man feels the change in his marital relationship acutely: "There are times when I have a difficult time doing things, and I ask for her help. I guess that's different from what it used to be. Years ago, I was the macho man. I was the guy who did everything. Now, she does most things and that I don't like. But it's something that has to be done" (Tilleli 1996, 2). Harris and Sterin interviewed a 70-year-old woman who articulated the delicate balance in these changing roles: "We used to be on equal footing with each other, a marriage of two accomplished people. Now he is 'caregiver' and I am a 'caregiven.' There must be a fine line between sensible adjustment to an essential level of dependence on others and on their memories as compared to a total surrender of all independent thought and action" (Harris and Sterin 1999, 246).

While some role changes result from shifts in ability and decision-making authority, three men interviewed by me (Snyder 1999) described a more generalized regression into a parent-child relationship. This role change evoked feelings ranging from demoralization and ambivalence to comforting surrender. Accustomed to being a competent provider in his marital relationship, one of the men sometimes rebels against the shift: "Sometimes I give [my wife] a hard time just to be nasty. I guess it's because I'd like to be doing things myself instead of having someone telling me to do this or do that. I'm a little boy now. I have a mommy to take care of me. It's not a very good feeling. I'd much rather be out there doing something else" (85). Another man, with early-onset dementia, found the shifts destabilizing but also recognized a certain grace in the process. Discussing his relationship with his sons, he stated, "They used to learn from me and now I have to learn from them. I don't really like it. I feel like it's topsy-turvy but that's the way it has to be. . . . I feel so stupid when I have to ask for help" (43). In a second interview, two and a half years later, he reflected on the greater simplicity in his life: "I'm becoming more childlike now. I enjoy the things children enjoy. I don't have the same responsibilities. I can do what I want" (51). An African American man accustomed to a matriarchal family structure derives comfort from a degree of surrender, "I'm blessed to have a wonderful daughter. . . . I can be a bit more at ease in my thinking because she takes care of things and she knows how to do it. . . . I depend upon her. . . . I'm in my baby phase now, so to speak. So sometimes I call her 'my mumma'" (103).

Loss of Autonomy

Although persons with AD respond in varying ways to role changes, many speak about threats to their freedom and independence. These shifts are felt most acutely with losses in privileges, responsibilities, or decision-making authority. The complex issue of driving illustrates the pain and enforced surrender that often accompany these losses. One woman stated, "What hurts is people telling you that you can't do something when you know you can. I lost my driver's license . . . I just felt like I might as well give it up. I couldn't handle all these people fighting about me having a license. Maybe I'm wrong to even try to do anything other than have people take care of me. But, somehow that doesn't suit me, and I think that's why I miss driving" (Snyder 1998). Another woman who lives alone found multiple threats to her autonomy once she was diagnosed with AD: "There are a lot of people who help you in the beginning. That's their job. There are people who very early in this process said you must get someone to do your checkbook. I wasn't at that point yet. It was very insulting to me to be told, 'Never mind what you think. This is what I think you should do.' There is a lot of that attitude in these well intentioned people" (Snyder and Yale 1997, 1). A woman interviewed in the Cleveland video (Cleveland Area Alzheimer's Association 1994) uses metaphor to describe threats to her decision-making authority: "I'm not a loaf of bread that you can pick up and put there or pick up and put there. We will talk about it. I will listen, but you must talk with me about it so that I can make an informed decision— it's my decision."

When persons with AD feel diminished or threatened by a family member's authority, they can become argumentative or defensive. One 73-year-old woman vented her frustration to members of her support group, "My daughter can be overpowering and overprotective. I have to push back sometimes." A woman diagnosed in her fifties writes in her diary, "The worst problem I have is agitation . . . I've also had some unreasonable temper tantrums directed at my poor George. I hate myself for it, but can't stop them and I think I'm acting normal" (Tennis 1992, 10). These struggles, though not limited to the AD experience, are complicated by memory loss and require that both parties adapt to changing dynamics in their relationship.

Mutual Adjustments

Some persons with AD describe examples of mutual adjustment as each party in the relationship learns to cope with the disease. One woman newly diagnosed with AD described a common problem for spouses: "Sometimes when I forget something, Kurt has to get hold of himself and not get all uptight about it. Obviously he's having to learn this over a period of time. It irritates me that he gets ticked off over something that I've forgotten and every once in awhile I blow up. I'm sorry about it, but I just forget things" (Snyder 1999, 117). Two years later both partners had made difficult but positive adjustments: "I'm learning to be dependent on him. He's also more accustomed to the memory problems now. When I forget things, he reminds me and he's not nasty about it" (126). Another woman described a similar adjustment process in her support group meeting: "[My husband] wanted me to shape up. He didn't want to think I had Alzheimer's. He was scared. He has stopped asking me, 'Don't you remember?' and I'm so proud of him." Finally, a male group member summed up the adjustments both he and his wife have made in managing the routines and responsibilities of daily living: "Everything is OK as long as I don't interfere with her schedule."

Although researchers have explored changes in marital intimacy and sexuality (Ballard and Poer 1993; Kuhn 1994; Vanden Bosch 1995; Wright 1993), there has been little investigation into the experience of those with the disease. One 68-year-old woman diagnosed with AD interviewed by Feinberg, Whitlatch, and Tucke (2000) stated, "You haven't asked me anything about sex . . . sex isn't like it was early in our marriage. There's nothing written in any of the Alzheimer's literature about sex—I guess they think it doesn't happen" (87). Wright reported that when she interviewed couples about affection and sexuality within the marital relationship, some spouses with AD overreported the frequency of sexual contacts or claimed to be sexually active when they were not. Some attributed declining or absent sexual relations to aging. Others were acutely aware that their spouse no longer wanted sexual relations and expressed feelings of rejection or anger. "It's this condition," said one man. "Oh yes, I'm still interested. . . . But . . . [hostility in his voice] she don't want these hands on her" (81). These complex, personal issues can create feelings of tension and loss for both partners in the relationship.

Prosopagnosia, the loss of recognition of familiar faces, is thought to be a symptom of late-stage AD. However, this symptom is also reported by persons with moderate impairment and can be very troubling when experienced in deeply familiar family relationships. One man recalls about riding in the car with his son, "I really wasn't sure who this guy was who was driving me. We had been talking, but it wasn't making much sense to me. . . . But as I turned to look at him, I suddenly realized by the profile that it was Tom. . . . It was such a shock to me because for awhile, I didn't even know who he was" (Snyder 1999, 94). A woman in the Cleveland video who occasionally is unable to recognize her husband says, "I know that I love him and he loves me—I have this thought 'I love this person, but I don't know who in the heck you are'" (Cleveland Area Alzheimer's Association 1994).

It is not uncommon for persons with AD or family members to fear that the inability to recognize familiar faces will be a sign of real devastation and severance from core relationships. Although such incidents can be very disturbing for all involved, they can be transient and may happen more often and earlier in the course of the disease than caregivers realize.

Family as Survival

Persons with AD often express a reliance on family for basic survival and well-being. In a support group session a husband acknowledged his wife's significance by stating, "It would be a disaster if something happened to Joyce. I'd just get along." Others rely on a family member's deep and longstanding relationship to patch and mend their increasingly fragmented identities. Henderson (1998) writes about his wife: "I'm afraid of losing contact. She's the only one who really understands me and I'm hard to understand" (28). Referring to his profound aphasia, another man noted, "Mostly I try to joke about it, or if there is a family member near by, I hope that they can interpret. I rely so much on Kathleen and the boys to decode what I want to say" (Snyder 1999, 44).

Perhaps the threat to survival is felt most acutely upon the death of a primary caregiver. One widow reflected, "My husband's death a year and a half ago was a big kick in my memory. When Harry was here, half of the time when I was having problems, he could help me through and get me back on track. . . . I have had to get used to the loss of somebody who understands me" (Snyder 1999, 66). A recently widowed man noted that his peer support group was now central to his life: "It's encouragement for me. My wife died and I went real low, but I had the group. . . . She did everything for me so that was a big blow" (Young 2000).

THESE GENERAL THEMES concerning family relationships do not encompass every dimension of the AD experience. They do provide a framework, however, for exploring commonly expressed concerns and experiences of those with the disease and can help to normalize these issues for persons with AD and their families.

Social Relationships

The progressive symptoms of AD will undoubtedly affect the diagnosed person's social interactions and relationships. For those who have led more private or reclusive lives, an increased dependency on others or a care-giver's need for respite will likely thrust them into new social interactions. Other persons with the disease have extensive and valued preexisting social relationships that undergo significant adjustment or deterioration over the course of the disease. The following themes reflect issues commonly faced by individuals in reconciling their relationships with friends and society.

Ambivalence about Disclosing the Diagnosis

Persons with AD may deliberate about disclosing their diagnosis. Some individuals (and family members) doubt or deny the diagnosis, which contributes to ambivalence. Others are selective in their disclosure or may conceal the news in order to maintain their own self-concept. In their examination of the subjective experience of AD, Cotrell and Shultz (1993) distinguish between felt and enacted stigma. Felt stigma derives from the person's own embarrassment or shame over his or her illness. This stigma is illustrated in the comment of a 62-year-old man interviewed by me in 1993: "I don't care who knows or doesn't know. I don't try to hide it. Well, yes I do. I do try to hide it. You make a mistake or something and you try to hide it. I think it's natural. You don't want to appear to be less than you want to be. You want to appear as strong as you could be." A man featured in the Cleveland video reiterates this caution: "You ask whether I tell business people? Well I do a lot of . . . not research . . . but advisory things—how to do this in business and how not to and so forth. And no, I don't tell them. They would have no faith at all, would they?" (Cleveland Area Alzheimer's Association 1994).

There is often a discrepancy between what the person with AD thinks others know about his or her condition and what others have actually noticed. Some think they can hide their symptoms or are unaware that others already are alert to their memory problem. One woman acknowledged her diagnosis in our Alzheimer's support group but saw no need to tell her bridge group: "I'm not aware that they're aware of anything different." Some persons disclose the diagnosis when their symptoms become too difficult to disguise. As one man stated, "Why shouldn't I tell people about Alzheimer's? Why hide it? Otherwise they'll think, 'What is he doing?' I didn't tell people in the beginning. It wasn't until the Alzheimer's became more prevalent—when I couldn't do things that I had done previously" (Snyder 1999, 87).

Some individuals do not experience the concept of felt stigma and readily disclose their diagnosis to heighten public awareness. A small but growing number of persons with mild impairment are participating on panels at AD conferences or fundraisers. Others use day-to-day opportunities to increase public sensitivity. One young-looking woman diagnosed in her early fifties is a powerful example: "I tell everybody! It's nothing to be ashamed of. People need to know that we're just like them. The other day, I was in Nordstrom's and I was in line to buy my dress. The cashier was making mistakes and joking, 'Oh no, I must have Alzheimer's!' When I got up to the register, I looked at her and I said, 'I do have Alzheimer's.' I think she was pretty embarrassed that she had joked about it" (Snyder and Yale 1997, 2).

Responses from Others

Cotrell and Shultz (1993) suggest that in contrast to the subjectivity of felt stigma, *enacted* stigma results from the responses of others, who may devalue or retreat from the person with AD based on their own fears or feelings of discomfort. These responses can have a direct impact on a decision to disclose the diagnosis. One man writes that although his family and "true friends" responded with sincere understanding and caring, those relationships existing more on the periphery of his life underwent dramatic changes. "Their perceptions of me ranged from my being intellectually suspect and unreliable to my being physically lame. Others simply tiptoed out of our lives. I felt totally depleted, powerless, and enraged!" (Dubiner 2000, 10). Davis

(1989) notes a similar response when he declared his need to retire from the ministry: "As soon as my diagnosis was announced, some people became very uncomfortable around me. I realize that the shock and pain are difficult to deal with at first. It was strange that in most cases I had to make the effort to seek out people who were avoiding me and look them in the eye and say, 'I don't bite. I am still the same person, but I just can't do my work anymore'" (100). Another woman is sympathetic to her friend's silence: "I've told them about Alzheimer's disease. They are very quiet. They don't know what to say. I don't know what to say. . . . But they are saddened and moved and you just have to swallow it. . . . I don't expect them to respond any more than I could have responded two years ago" (Snyder 1999, 67).

Some individuals describe the demeaning experience of being ignored. Conversation in the doctor's office or in a social setting is deferred to the caregiver. A woman in the Cleveland video states: "Some people when my husband and I are together, they refer to me as her, not us or them or you two. It's like I'm there but they can't see me. . . . And it's so aggravating—I want to stick my tongue out and say, 'I have Alzheimer's but I can still comprehend and speak for myself most of the time'" (Cleveland Area Alzheimer's Association 1994).

Withdrawal and Isolation

Negative responses from others can lead to withdrawal and isolation. In her study examining the subjective experience of forgetfulness among elders Cromwell (1994) noted that when some individuals can no longer cover up or compensate for their memory failures, they withdraw from social situations. One research participant stated: "I lose track, yes, so I quit the game. . . . I had to give up a lot of jobs . . . because I can't handle it. . . . I gave up all those things because I felt I don't qualify and I don't want to expose myself" (456). In correspondence submitted to me for the newsletter *Perspectives* Raymer (2000) shared a similar sentiment: "When I am alone it is easier. I can do what I want at my own pace . . . around other people I feel that I pretend."

Persons with AD may also withdraw from relationships because of overstimulation experienced in social settings. Davis (1989) writes that "in larger groups I go into such overload that I have to withdraw and leave the group early. I still need social contact, but it must be limited to just a few people at a time and with little stimulation" (104). Others withdraw because they fear the unpredictability or judgment of others. For example, Rose (1996) writes, "I am becoming more and more withdrawn. It is much easier to stay in the safety of my home where Stella treats me with love and respect, than to expose myself to people who don't understand, people who raise their eyebrows when I have trouble making the right change at the cash register, or when I am unable to think of the right words when asked a question" (32).

Although individuals are at risk for physical withdrawal from society, some also describe an internal feeling of isolation. Henderson (1998) writes, "I think one of the worst things about Alzheimer's is you're so alone with it. Nobody around you really knows what's going on. And half the time, most of the time, we don't know what's going on ourselves" (55). A man interviewed by me supports Henderson's experience and remarks: "A lot of people have no idea what this disease is all about—no idea what we go through and the things that we feel we're losing" (Snyder 1999, 93). These feelings of isolation can be accompanied by an increased suspiciousness of others that leave the person with AD at even greater risk of withdrawal. Killick (1999) spoke with a man who described this painful dilemma: "It's very lonely, I'm telling you. . . . Although you're here, you can't get into company. You get this thing in your head and it switches off, and you're left nowhere. It's just like switching the light out, and it's terrible. . . . I was the most happy-go-lucky fellow. I used to go down to the club and the pub and drink whisky. Now I **don't** want to go out. And I don't want anyone coming in here. I weigh people up. I'm watching them. In my position, the way that I feel, I don't have trust. And I never was like that" (160).

These experiences of alienation can be particularly acute for those with AD who live alone or have working caregivers. Limited means of transportation and a shrinking social network leave these individuals at even greater risk for isolation and withdrawal.

Establishing Connections

Although many persons with AD report adequate activity and social interaction—often in sharp contrast to caregivers' report that they do very little and rely heavily on the caregiver for companionship—others report the value of specialized social programs. Essential support services for caregivers are well developed in many communities, but programs devoted to the direct needs of persons with AD, while increasing in number, are still sparse. Some persons with AD are acutely aware of this discrepancy. Noting the array of support services being directed to her husband, one newly diagnosed woman told her counselor, "I feel like my leg has been amputated and my husband is being fitted for the prosthesis." An energetic man diagnosed in his mid-fifties noted that persons with AD risk isolation because there are limited activities to choose from: "The worse thing in Alzheimer's is that people don't get out. And there has to be better things to get them out. I don't want to vegetate" (Snyder 1999, 50).

Creative community programming can help to reduce the risk of withdrawal and isolation. One newly diagnosed woman who wanted to join a support group said, "People may deny that they have Alzheimer's disease because they don't have the opportunity to talk with other people who are sympathetic and understanding, and who will help them along in the whole process. That's a sad state of affairs. Anyone who has this diagnosis needs to have others with whom to talk" (Snyder 1999, 120). The need for peer support and for a remedy for feelings of isolation was reiterated by a participant in a group for younger persons with AD in Grampion, in northeastern Scotland: "Having this illness is a lonely experience, even when you have a close family who gives you a lot of love. There is a part of me that they can't reach or understand, but when I'm with my buddies I don't have that lonely feeling because they can understand me" (Duff 1998, 5). Another man also noted the distinction between his family and his peers: "A group like this is easier than talking with family. You don't have all of the interruptions—can't get into discussion as in-depth with family because they are all so busy" (Snyder et al. 1995, 694). Others value co-participation in couples programs. A participant in the Forget Me Not Club, a social support group for couples in Nova Scotia, explained: "There is such a wonderful warmth, closeness, and feeling of not being 'different' from other couples" (Grant 1999, 5).

Community programs for persons with AD can also offset feelings of devaluation. Henderson (1998) laments, "Sometimes we miss being important—miss being needed" (74). The Alzheimer's Family Care Center, in Chicago, Illinois, combines supervised volunteer work at local community agencies with support and recreational activities to create a meaningful sense of purpose for those involved (see chapter 11 in this volume, by Jane

Stansell). One participant stated that "the greatest feeling that I feel is that I know what my problem is, but I'm able to help somebody who needs help" (Swanson, Levi, and Matano 1999).

Lessons Learned

Although the quotations in this chapter illustrate a wide range of responses to aspects of social and family relationships, they are presented as illustrations of general themes and cannot encompass the unique experiences of every person with AD. However, the process of conducting interviews and opening avenues for dialogue can teach us valuable lessons as we help individuals and families reconcile relationship issues.

When working with persons with AD it is helpful to inquire about past patterns of interaction in both family and social relationships. Although the progression of the disease often alters well-established personality traits and interpersonal behaviors, some core qualities may remain unchanged. When possible, it is helpful to obtain separate histories from the person with AD and the caregiver and to inquire about existing family and social networks, current experiences with these relationships, and the impact of AD on interactions with others. Some persons with the disease will be forthright in their comments and grateful for an opportunity to discuss these issues. Others will have limited response due to protection of personal privacy, inhibited awareness of their condition, or the need to defend themselves against potentially painful topics. Separate interviews afford the opportunity to compare different persons' impressions and to determine potential barriers and bridges to communication between the person with AD and the caregiver.

Conjoint interviews are equally valuable as they afford the opportunity to observe patterns of interaction and to open up dialogue between the parties. It is important to note whether the caregiver assumes a dominant role in the discussion or answers for the person with AD even though the latter is capable of responding. Note the parties' level of patience, frustration, or denial as they interact with each other and discuss various dimensions of the disease. Tread lightly and respectfully and avoid confrontation. The primary goal of an interview is to experience the world from each person's vantage point regardless of the degree of clarity or distortion and to test the possibilities for or obstacles to more open discussion of AD. In the words of a retired social worker with AD, "The main issue is to help people to be open about Alzheimer's—not to privatize it, especially within the family. . . . [Too many health care professionals] don't really accept the significance of illness for people. They know the diagnosis, but they don't take the time to find out what it truly means for that person. . . . It's important to be both sympathetic and curious and to have a real interest in discovery about who the person is. You have to really be willing to be present with the person with Alzheimer's" (Snyder 1999, 123–24).

Although the clinician must assess each person's family and social-relationship history, there is often a paucity of community services available to address each individual's unique circumstances and needs. We need an array of innovative program options for mildly affected persons so that a foundation of new relationships and experiences can be established and built upon throughout the continuum of the disease. This affords persons with AD an experience of belonging in their communities and compels others to include those with disabilities into the complex fabric of society. One man with AD reminds us of a fundamental principle: "As Alzheimer's patients, we need to be strong and not be pushed out of people's minds. We are real, and smart, and can be a part of the world we live in" (Liebow 2000).

Although individuals in the earlier stages of AD are often able to verbally articulate their reflections and feelings, as the disease advances communication in relationships becomes far more challenging. Expressions may become more symbolic or may shift from verbal to more behavioral or gestures. People may continue to experience similar feelings but express them differently as their confusion increases and their capacity to articulate decreases. The person with more moderate to severe AD may communicate through delusions, confabulation, or elaborate storytelling, all of which can convey important themes to the attentive listener (Crisp 1995). We must begin to listen early on in the course of AD for themes in communication in the hope that this will enhance our understanding and facilitate a continued relationship as the disease progresses.

The environment's significance in fostering or inhibiting relational interactions must not be underestimated. McAllister and Silverman (1999) looked at the process of community formation and the maintenance of community roles among residents with dementia in both a residential AD facility and a traditional nursing home. They determined that dementia alone was not a barrier to the development of community and relationships. Environmental and programmatic conditions were most significant in promoting or undermining the potential for community formation for residents. In her exceptionally well written chronicle of her mother's last years in a special home for residents with AD, Joyce Dyer (1996) observes in great detail the elaborate gestures, interactions, and sometimes unspoken indicators of varied relationships among the residents. She describes the last day of her mother's life, marked by frequent visits from residents who came to pay their last respects: "All afternoon Alzheimer's residents stopped to pay tribute, and say goodbye. They sensed something was wrong. They were walking. Annabelle was not. They were making loud sounds and screams. Annabelle was silent. So one by one, they called" (134). Although all the residents were severely affected by AD, their gestures, comments, and offerings all indicated an awareness of and sensitivity to one of the most profound transitions in a relationship.

Conclusion

In Kitwood's extensive investigation of the experience of dementia and the effects of the social environment on well-being he asks the fundamental question, "What do people with dementia need?" His response is five essential components to personal and social relationship: comfort, attachment, inclusion, occupation, and identity (Kitwood 1997, 80). The quotations in this chapter all speak to these themes and provide insights into the concerns and experiences that arise in each of these domains. Kitwood risks oversimplification in stating that these five categories all stem from a primary, all-encompassing need—the need for love. The invaluable, multifaceted experience of love cannot always transcend the day-to-day challenges and traumas of AD. Yet, when challenging periods dissipate into the satisfying moments that can be encountered throughout the disease, love can prove to be the sustaining thread that weaves one moment into the next and maintains the fabric of relationship. Tim Brennan (1999), a gifted writer living with AD, closes this chapter with a lesson he asks that we learn: "Someday those who care for a person with Alzheimer's may be faced with what appears to be an unsolvable problem. Caregivers may try everything they have been taught but nothing works. So, they touch the arm of the person with Alzheimer's and speak softly and gently. Because of the patient's apparent distress, the caregiver may hug the person with Alzheimer's or give a kiss and tell the person that he or she is loved. One day, if the caregiver is lucky, a revelation occurs. That person learns that the last thing we ever lose is love. Our memories may be gone. Intellect and logic may have diminished. We may have forgotten your name and where we are, or what we are doing. But we remember love."

REFERENCES

Bachrach, R. 1997. Doing my best. In *Perspectives: A Newsletter for Individuals with Alzheimer's*, ed. L. Snyder, 3 (1): 1–2.

Bahro, M., E. Silber, and T. Sunderland. 1995. How do patients with Alzheimer's disease cope with their illness? A clinical experience report. *Journal of the American Geriatrics Society* 43:41–46.

Ballard, E. L., and C. M. Poer. 1993. *Sexuality and the Alzheimer's patient*. Durham, N.C.: Duke University Medical School, Joseph and Kathleen Bryan Alzheimer's Disease Research Center.

Barlow, D. 1997. A communication barrier. In *Perspectives: A Newsletter for Individuals with Alzheimer's*, ed. L. Snyder, 3 (2): 6.

Brennan, T. 1999. A message of love. In *Perspectives: A Newsletter for Individuals with Alzheimer's*, ed. L. Snyder, 4 (2): 7.

Burgener, S., R. Shimer, and L. Murrell. 1993. Expressions of individuality in cognitively impaired elders: Need for individual assessment and care. *Journal of Gerontological Nursing* 19 (4): 13–22.

Cleveland Area Alzheimer's Association. 1994. *Alzheimer's disease: Inside looking out*. Terra Nova Films, Chicago.

Cotrell, V., and R. Shultz. 1993. The perspective of the patient with Alzheimer's disease: A neglected dimension of dementia research. *Gerontologist* 33 (2): 205–11.

Crisp, J. 1995. Making sense of the stories that people with Alzheimer's tell: A journey with my mother. *Nursing Inquiry* 2:133–40.

Cromwell, S. L. 1994. The subjective experience of forgetfulness among elders. *Qualitative Health Research* 4 (4): 444–62.

Davis, R. 1989. *My journey into Alzheimer's disease*. Wheaton, Ill.: Tyndale House.

Dilworth-Anderson, P., and B. E. Gibson. 1999. Ethnic minority perspectives on dementia, family caregiving, and interventions. *Generations* 23 (3): 40–45.

Dubiner, M. 2000. Thoughts and comments. In *Contexts: A Forum for Medical Humanities*, ed. J. B. Walsh, 8 (3): 9–10.

Duff, S. 1998. Alzheimer Scotland—action on dementia: Younger person's group in Grampian, northeast Scotland. In *Early Alzheimer's: An International Newsletter on Dementia*, ed. I. Gatz, 1 (2): 4–5.

Dyer, J. 1996. *In a tangled wood: An Alzheimer's journey*. Dallas: Southern Methodist Univ. Press.

Feinberg, L. F., C. J. Whitlatch, and S. Tucke. 2000. *Making hard choices: Respecting both voices*. San Francisco: Family Caregiver Alliance.

Goldsmith, M. 1996. *Hearing the voice of people with dementia: Opportunities and obstacles*. London: Jessica Kingsley.

Grant, M. 1999. Alzheimer forget-me-not club. In *Early Alzheimer's: An International Newsletter on Dementia*, ed. I. Gatz, 1 (4): 4–5.

Harris, P. B., and G. J. Sterin. 1999. Insider's perspective: Defining and preserving the self of dementia. *Journal of Mental Health and Aging* 5 (3): 241–56.

Henderson, C. 1998. *Partial view: An Alzheimer's journal*. Dallas: Southern Methodist Univ. Press.

Hutchinson, S., S. Krall, and H. Wilson. 1997. Early probable Alzheimer's disease and awareness context theory. *Social Science and Medicine* 45 (9): 1399–1409.

Kelly, M. F. 1997. Social interaction among people with dementia. *Journal of Gerontological Nursing* 23 (4): 16–20.

Killick, J. 1999. Dark head amongst the grey: Experiencing the worlds of younger persons with dementia. In *Younger people with dementia: Planning, practice, and development*, ed. S. Cox and J. Keady, 160. London: Jessica Kingsley.

Kitwood, T. 1997. *Dementia reconsidered: The person comes first*. Philadelphia: Open Univ. Press.

Kuhn, D. R. 1994. The changing face of sexual intimacy in Alzheimer's disease. *American Journal of Alzheimer's Care and Research* 9 (5): 7–14.

Liebow, P. 2000. The support group. In *Contexts: A Forum for Medical Humanities*, ed. J. B. Walsh, 8 (3): 13–14.

Mangone, C. A, D. B. Hier, P. B. Gorelick, R. J. Ganellen, P. Langenberg, R. Boarman, and W. Dollear. 1991. Impaired insight in Alzheimer's disease. *Journal of Geriatric Psychiatry and Neurology* 4:189–93.

McAllister, C. L., and M. A. Silverman. 1999. Community formation and community roles among persons with Alzheimer's disease: A comparative study of experiences in a residential Alzheimer's facility and a traditional nursing home. *Qualitative Health Research* 9 (1): 65–85.

McDaniel, K. D., S. D. Edland, A. Heyman, and CERAD Clinical Investigators. 1995. Relationship between level of insight and severity of dementia in Alzheimer's disease. *Alzheimer's Disease and Associated Disorders* 9 (2): 101–4.

Phillips, J. 2000. *A personal view of living with early-onset Alzheimer's disease: Opening a door to understanding*. Toronto: Sunnybrook and Women's College Health Sciences Centre.

Phinney, A. 1998. Living with dementia from the patient's perspective. *Journal of Gerontological Nursing* 24 (6): 8–15.

Raymer, L. 2000. Reflections and observations of living with early-onset Alzheimer's. Unpublished.

Reagan, R. 1994. Letter to my fellow Americans. *San Diego Union Tribune*, Sunday, 13 November.

Rose, L. 1996. *Show me the way to go home*. Forest Knolls, Calif.: Elder Books.

Sabat, S., and M. Collins. 1999. Intact social, cognitive ability and selfhood: A case study of Alzheimer's disease. *American Journal of Alzheimer's Disease* 14 (1): 11–19.

Seltzer, B., J. J. Vasterling, J. Yoder, and K. A. Thompson. 1997. Awareness of deficit in Alzheimer's disease: Relation to caregiver burden. *Gerontologist* 37 (1): 20–24.

Silverio, E., and J. Koenig-Coste. 1997. *Suggestions from people with Alzheimer's disease for the family.* Cambridge: Alzheimer's Association, Massachusetts Chapter.

Snyder, L. 1998. A conversation with Bobby. In *Perspectives: A Newsletter for Individuals with Alzheimer's,* ed. L. Snyder, 3 (3): 7.

———. 1999. *Speaking our minds: Personal reflections from individuals with Alzheimer's.* New York: W. H. Freeman.

Snyder, L., M. P. Quayhagen, S. Shepherd, and D. Bower. 1995. Supportive seminar groups: An intervention for early stage dementia patients. *Gerontologist* 35 (5): 691–95.

Snyder, L., and R. Yale. 1997. Disclosing the diagnosis: Who and when to tell. In *Perspectives: A Newsletter for Individuals with Alzheimer's,* ed. L. Snyder, 2 (4): 1–3.

Swanson, N., G. Levi, and T. Matano. 1999. A volunteer program for persons with early-stage dementia. *Early Alzheimer's: An International Newsletter on Dementia,* ed. I. Gatz, 1 (3): 10.

Tennis, L. 1992. The diary of Letty Tennis. In *The Caregiver,* ed. L. Gwyther, 12 (3): 10. Durham, N.C.: Duke University Medical School, Joseph and Kathleen Bryan Alzheimer's Disease Research Center.

Tilleli, D. 1996. Reflections. In *Perspectives: A Newsletter for Individuals with Alzheimer's,* ed. L. Snyder, 2 (2): 1–3.

Trabert, M. 1997. The DRC club. In *Perspectives: A Newsletter for Individuals with Alzheimer's,* ed. L. Snyder, 2 (3): 7.

Vanden Bosch, J. 1995. *A thousand tomorrows: Sexuality, intimacy, and Alzheimer's disease.* Terra Nova Films, Chicago.

Woods, B. 1999. The person in dementia care. *Generations* 23 (3): 35–39.

Wright, L. 1993. *Alzheimer's disease and marriage.* Newbury Park, Calif.: Sage.

Yeo, G., and D. Gallagher-Thompson, eds. 1996. *Ethnicity and the dementias.* Washington, D.C.: Taylor & Francis.

Young, T. 2000. *Alzheimer's disease: Voices from the journey.* Mayo Alzheimer's Disease Research Center, Rochester, Minn. Film.

7

Meaningful Communication
throughout the Journey
Clinical Observations

DOROTHY SEMAN

Listen with the ears of your heart.
—Sue Sweeney, 76 years old

This chapter addresses the issue of meaningful communication with people with dementia. *Meaningful communication* is defined here as engagement on deeper levels involving feelings and meanings and grappling with issues related to self-esteem, one's relationship with others, and one's place in the world. Thus, the focus here is on a holistic and global approach to communication, trying to capture those nuggets that seem to contain a depth of meaning and allow the humanity of the person with dementia to shine through.

The data consist of quotations from men and women who have been diagnosed with dementia observed from my perspective as a reflective practitioner. This orientation has emerged from daily clinical practice—from three decades as a nurse clinician, including thirteen years caring for persons diagnosed with AD and related dementias. It is based on the premise that all behavior has meaning and that one has to look below the surface to fully understand it.

Some quotations are lighthearted and convey the spontaneous humor of the moment. Others reveal a struggle to come to terms with the impact that dementia and the people in their lives have on those living with the disease. Some of the material recognizes distress and the enduring capacity of persons with AD to provide comfort and support to others in need. In order to understand the needs and feelings of persons with AD, it is necessary to pay attention to the nuances and subtlety of their communications and to looking at the complex relationships they have with their environment.

Background

There are four basic sources of information about communication involving persons with AD: psychometric testing, the caregiving literature, the lay press, and the communication of individuals diagnosed with AD. The first type consists of data reported from formal psychometric testing, which make up part of the initial diagnostic evaluation; the items that generated the data are then repeated on follow-up mental status testing as a way of evaluating the progression of the disease. The initial diagnostic evaluation and subsequent follow-up testing measures the common neurolinguistic changes flowing from the complex range of neuropathologies that develop in many persons with AD over time. These symptoms include a wide range of impairments in the structure and content of language, resulting in problems in expression and comprehension. This area of inquiry has been widely noted by neuropsychologists, speech and audiology specialists, and neurologists (see Lubinski 1991).

This assessment is typically done in accordance with protocols that use standardized formal testing procedures. It may be conducted in a clinic or in a nursing home or hospital setting. If it is conducted in a public place, such as a bustling hallway in a hospital or a high-traffic corridor or activity room in a residential care setting, with the attendant distractions, the person being tested may not be able to perform at his or her highest level of capability because of anxiety or sensory overload. A premium is placed on the objective measurement of performance in several areas of functioning, done in the artificial universe, away from the person's familiar environment. The assessment protocol is typically administered by a polite but unfamiliar and dispassionate technician or professional. The manner of testing is usually carefully proscribed and may not have obvious relevance to the person being tested. The procedure is based on the Western medical model, focusing on potential problem areas and "scoring" the number of correct answers against the total number of benchmarked correct answers in writing, manipulating geometric images, short- and long-term recall, attention span, and so on. These data provide an objective baseline description of cognitive functioning in a number of critical domains when there are no environmental or interpersonal cues or supports available to enhance functional performance. In combination with other diagnostic tests, formal psychometric testing assists the practitioner in making a differential diagnosis. This initial comprehensive assessment serves as a reference point against which the direction and degree of change in future performance can be measured periodically. Despite limitations, it may be useful in determining eligibility for research protocols, as well as the potential impact of pharmacological and nonpharmacological treatments.

A second major area in which communication is discussed is caregiver-focused, more practical and clinically useful literature. This body of practical information evolved from the trial-and-error efforts of clinicians who learned to work effectively with persons with dementia. The material provides guidelines, principles, tips, and techniques that may help caregivers with the routine activities of personal care and activities that can provide structure to the day (Rau 1993). A number of publications suggest ways to communicate about specific activities that lead to "task completion": bathing, dressing, eating, and assistance in the bathroom (see, for example, Robinson, Spencer, and White 1989; and Rader 1995). These books, pamphlets, and videos on communication and dementia provide a foundation for good basic daily care. In the past several years there has even been a shift to a more person-focused and relationship-focused approach to caring for persons with dementia, always placing the person first (Bell and Troxel 1997; Kitwood 1997; Zgola 1999).

A third area in which communication involving persons with dementia is approached is metacommunication. The metacommunication is conveyed, intentionally or not, in all forms of media, particularly television and newspapers. Persons with dementia are typically portrayed and described as hapless and helpless victims. The lay press commonly uses terms like *living death* and *unending funeral* to describe persons with AD. This theme of illness and abject dependency is often perpetuated by pictures on brochures, photographs and language used in the solicitations of Alzheimer's associations, and marketing materials of pharmaceutical companies and other purveyors of health care products and services.

The fourth approach, the paradigm this chapter advocates, is largely un-addressed in the literature on communication. This approach focuses on the words spoken or written by people with dementia as a way of discover-ing and describing who they are as individuals. Several books have begun to address this gap, including Kuhn (1999) and Snyder (1999).

This approach requires one to "be with" a person with dementia, to give them our undivided attention and emotional presence. Such availability for meaningful communication requires dedicating all of our senses to the person or the group—listening, actually hearing, observing, and demon-strating our connection to the individual or group. It involves the ability to share silence and to "hold" the dialogue gently, absorbing it, supporting it, responding to it, connecting others in turn at the level at which they can and want to relate. It involves the capacity to do the parallel, related work of supporting the individual and the group in a way that facilitates their communication without exerting too much control over them. It in-volves letting them know that they have been heard and trying to elicit what, if anything, is required of us—supplying a missing word, a hug, an empathic response, information, a word of encouragement or hope, an hon-est answer, a laugh, a segue into another, less stressful activity.

This chapter is not intended to provide an exhaustive catalogue of themes, nor does it attempt to analyze or theorize. The intent is rather to offer a more balanced and comprehensive way of thinking about commu-nication with persons who have dementia. My hope is that it will expand the present biomedical paradigm to make it more inclusive and encom-passing, that it will challenge clinicians and researchers to rethink their currently narrow expectations of people with AD and their relationship with them. This perspective is absent from most of the literature. If our communication with persons with AD is limited, our understanding of them and of the experience of AD will necessarily be diminished.

About the Data

The voices presented here have been garnered from daily interactions with diagnosed men and women attending an adult day program designed for persons in all phases of dementia. The individuals have progressive and ir-reversible dementias, primarily AD, and some have dementia resulting from vascular causes, Parkinson's disease, or a dementia of mixed etiologies.

The communication upon which this chapter is based—the seeing, the hearing, and the understanding—comes out of the day-to-day interactions, in groups or one-on-one, both in the day care setting and during home visits prior to admission to the adult day program. Both the comments and the manner in which they are presented exemplify what cultural anthropologists call a "participant-observer approach." I see these data as representing a form of experiential learning, information discerned in a context and reflecting the subtlety and texture of that context. The comments are woven into the fabric of daily life, the rich and varied strands that create a living tapestry. That tapestry is the richer because persons with dementia are interconnected with others in varying circumstances and virtually always in public spaces.

It is my hope that the reader will be challenged to consider possible correlations between the content of the comments, the feeling tone that they simultaneously convey and evoke, and the living environment in which these comments occurred. In a sense, if we are to have meaningful communication, we must look at the individual, the dyadic relationships, and the community environment in which these comments were made. Communication is best understood as a complex set of interactions, not isolated or bracketed transactions occurring in a vacuum. The sense of place is a vital part of the message. Our understanding of the subtlety of communication is only just beginning to be understood.

For the most part, the words of these men and women were captured in the immediacy of the moment, pen and paper always at hand to accurately record the eloquent communication, often characterized by surprising clarity and meaning. Some smaller bits of the material were transcribed from tape recordings made in meetings of support groups, held weekly over a number of years in the same adult day program. Some of the words were written in a common staff book gently titled "The wit and wisdom of persons with dementia." It is common for staff in health care settings to keep an incident report log or notes of events occurring during their shift, which typically reflect negative behaviors or events. Staff felt that noting the "aha" events would enable staff to think about and foster the kind of climate that generated these rich and expressive interchanges.

The materials and formulations that emerged were not intended as formal research. The intent was to help me and other day care staff to increase our sensitivity and skill by listening more carefully and more fully and then using that information to enhance our interactions. Efforts were made to record and share with other staff comments that took us by surprise, touched us, or taught us, comments that provided us with important insights.

This communication informed our understanding of those individuals and continues to guide the way care is provided. Notably, people are divided into discrete clinical groups tailored to their abilities and losses. The communication was sometimes verbal, occasionally symbolic. Sometimes the comments were made directly, and sometimes they were overheard, at times spoken aloud to no one in particular. Sue, a very wise woman with dementia, suggested that staff "listen with the ears of your heart" if they really wanted to understand what people need. Sue Sweeney, a 76-year-old woman in the middle stage of Alzheimer's disease, said in response to my asking whether I could quote her, "Yes, and tell them my full name. I want them to know that a real person is saying these things and feeling these things."

Methodological Concerns

There are limitations to this methodology. Practicing professionals are socialized early in their undergraduate work to look askance at anecdotal reports, and rightly so: there are too many variables, known and unknown, that affect the integrity of those "nonscientific" reports. One cannot generalize meaning without further inquiry. On the other hand, professionals must find a way to incorporate the many useful contributions from those who see, hear, or otherwise have a deeply intimate knowledge about persons with AD based on encounters in daily care. This intimate knowledge has largely remained outside the scope of most researchers. So though these clinical observations were not designed as a qualitative study that scientifically and systematically collects in-depth data on people's lives in their social context, they capture an essential part of the AD experience that is often missed.

Examples of Meaningful Communication

The materials presented here were among hundreds of comments I heard that make one question the prevailing view that a person with AD loses the capacity for conceptual thinking and appropriate affective responses, becomes fully self-absorbed, and so on. This characterization seems to fall upon the individual as a mantle at the time of diagnosis. The comments presented below reveal an enormous range and depth of inner life and the capacity to relate deeply to one another.

On Spirituality, Religion, and Man's Humanity to Man

In a routine exercise group right before lunch near the Jewish holiday of Roshashana there was some discussion about the upcoming religious observance. Anne, a quiet, elderly Lutheran woman, 93 years old, in the middle stage of AD, suddenly spoke in a language that sounded like Hebrew: "Baruch ata Adonai eloheinu melech ha-olam asher kideshanu be mitzvo-tav vetsivanu al ahilat matzoh." The staff member was speechless, and Ruth, a 90-year-old Jewish woman in an advanced stage of AD who was usually silent, sat up and took notice, following the conversation closely. The staff member expressed her surprise and asked Anne what she had just said. Anne spoke of learning this Hebrew prayer in Europe before the war. She then spoke in words that sounded almost like a Shakespearean soliloquy:

> My grandfather told us since we were living across the street from a synagogue, we should come to know and understand our neighbors. He insisted that we understand and respect those of a different faith and belief than ours. "The Jews," he said, "are no better than you. And you—none of us is better than the Jews. Bad things are happening all around us. The Jews are being taken away, and they don't ever come back. Today when I go to town, I'm going to bring an old blanket to cover Mr. Abrams and bring him back with me. He is old and alone. And he cannot run away from them. They will catch him and kill him for sure if they find him. I'm going to lay him in our barn between the two cows. I want you to bring him food, when you go out to feed the cows. You must never tell anyone about this . . . no one! If word gets out, they will kill him and all of us along with him." So that's why I remember this prayer. I don't exactly know what it means, but it is a special prayer for the Jewish people, and so I keep it in my mind, because this is what my grandfather told us, and taught us to do.

The entire group was suddenly intently focused on Anne as she told this moving story about the prayer that issued forth from her. Ruth went over to Anne with tears in her eyes. She kissed Anne, told her that she was so lucky to have such a brave, courageous, wonderful grandfather, and thanked her for telling that story to everyone.

A few weeks later, an Orthodox Jewish man named Arthur joined the adult day center. When I asked Anne to say the prayer for Art and tell him about it, she did so exactly as before. Art was stunned by her saying the prayer in Hebrew. He translated the Hebrew prayer into English: "Praised be Thou, our Lord, our God, King of the universe, Who bringest forth sustenance from the earth."

For the next several weeks our prayer before lunch was said in Hebrew by Anne, a Lutheran. With great pride and pleasure, Art said the prayer in English so that we could all understand it. It was very moving on each occasion. Within a few weeks, Art's wife moved him to a nursing home because his dementia, as well as his metastatic bladder cancer, had progressed.

Ed was a quiet, gentle man with a warm smile who attended the day program five days a week for nearly three years. On a daily basis his wife was able to see the warm bond he shared with the other participants in the programs. When he died quickly after a sudden cardiac problem, his wife invited the persons from his group to join the family at the church service the morning of his funeral. A few of his friends from the group, accompanied by several members of the staff, said a few of the formal prayers that were part of the religious service. They sat in a front pew and filed past his casket along with the other mourners. A few touched his hand as they passed; others bowed their heads in prayer. They said goodbye as friends do, indistinguishable from the other mourners in their shared sorrow. We talked about Ed back at the day program over lunch, remembering things about him that had touched us.

On Compassion and Empathy

In an exercise group, there was often some friendly conversation among the members. Unexpectedly, Blanche, a participant with advanced dementia who was normally friendly and cheerful but had been unable to speak coherently for several years, began to speak in earnest, but with profound dysarthria. She seemed to have something she wanted to say, but only word fragments came out. A fiercely proud and independent woman, she was persistent in her repeated efforts, but she knew her speech was not coming out clearly. Her face flushed, she clenched her fist in determination and frustration. The man and woman on either side of her offered warm and supportive expressions of encouragement, and the staff attempted to assist Blanche, but to no avail. Blanche's face flushed red again in embarrassed frustration. Charlotte, who also has advanced dementia and is virtually deaf, was seated across the room. Charlotte's family described her as paranoid and uncooperative but compassionate. Although she could probably hear nothing of Blanche's language, she seemed well aware of Blanche's distress. Charlotte's mounting empathic concern was evident. She rummaged carefully through her own purse—through rubber-banded napkins, straws, and other collectibles—and finally, after much focused, persistent effort, located a rumpled tissue. She walked over to Blanche, gently brushed her tear-streaked cheeks, and knelt to cradle her head and comfort her. This simple act of kindness soothed Blanche. The gentleman who sat next to Blanche offered his seat to Charlotte so she could sit next to Blanche and then quietly moved to the seat Charlotte had vacated. After a few moments Blanche pulled herself together, nodded her thanks to the woman who had assisted her, and managed to extend the best hug she could, given her severe apraxia. There was unambiguous communication between these two women with advanced dementia and those of us who had witnessed this most profound human exchange. The two women held hands briefly, and then the group resumed its activity.

Eugene had seen staff frequently redirect another gentleman, Ray, who tended to have profound apraxia and visuo-spatial perception problems. Ray had a lot of motor restlessness and was constantly on the go. He would often slowly walk into the wall and be unable to "turn himself out of that situation." Once this happened when the staff member was busy caring for someone else. Eugene, who was incontinent and had little coherent speech but a cheerful demeanor and a good heart, looked at the staff member as if to say, "I know what to do." The staff member simply smiled and nodded back at Eugene. Eugene then put his arm around Ray and gently guided him back into the room where he could walk about freely, patting him on the back as they reentered the open space of the room. Eugene then turned and smiled broadly at the staff member. His accomplishment was evident, and he almost beamed when the staff member expressed thanks and appreciation for his help.

On Insights about Living with AD

One day Marion was walking about the unit with a staff member and a visitor. She always had held high-profile jobs and had given tours to important people herself—many years ago. She offered spontaneously to the staff member and visitor: "I don't know why people say that I'm living with Alzheimer's disease. Alzheimer's is living with me!"

Morris, who had moderate vascular dementia, appeared far more impaired than he actually was. His physical condition added to the first impression of very profound impairment. He had suffered several strokes. He drooled almost continuously, stuttered when he began to speak, was fully incontinent, and walked with a very ataxic gait because several of his toes had been amputated after he suffered from diabetic gangrene. When a staff person asked group members what the hardest part of having dementia was for them, he was thoughtful for about five minutes, listening and thinking. He then said in slow and halting speech: "The hardest part for me is not being able to remember poetry. I have always loved poetry. My favorite poem is 'Thanatopsis.'" When a staff member inquired further about the poem, Morris said, "It's a poem about death, but it makes me think about life." When the staff member inquired who the poet was, Morris thought a while and then replied with some certainty that it was William Cullen Bryant. The staff member checked this and discovered that Morris was right. The staff member was able to locate the poem and copied the poem for him later that week. Morris recited it to the group, haltingly but proudly, through his tears. "This makes me feel so good . . . to say these words . . . to know I can still have them when I forget them." Morris kept the copy of the poem, which became increasingly dog-eared from many readings. A book of poetry was located for him to peruse at his leisure, which he did. When he read poetry, he said, "I fly like a butterfly, but I don't sting like a bee," a reference to the famous African American boxer Cassius Clay, perhaps better known as Muhammad Ali.

One morning Sue said, "A lot of people, hearing they've got Alzheimer's say, 'Why me?' Well, I say, why not me? I've had a good life. . . . No regrets. . . . We've all got to have something, so why not just take what you've got and be grateful for you had so good for so long. . . . There's no pain with this. A lot of people truly suffer, like with cancer. So what if I forget? Hell, I can just ask some-

one to help me and they will. They have and they will. It's all about helping yourself and each other."

Betty walked into a staff member's office one day and said:

Can I talk to you now, before I forget? This is very important. It comes to me now
very clearly, just what I want to tell you about . . . to let you know how I feel . . .
because sometimes you'll ask . . . and I think you really mean it . . . you'll ask,
"Betty, how are you feeling?" So here it is: A few days ago I was at the stove cooking chili. My daughter—I have two, you know—she was saw me cooking. Well,
she came by and she reached in front of me while I'm at the stove. Let me show
you how it happened, and let me ask you if I was wrong to feel the way I do.
[Betty gets up and demonstrates to the staff member] She reaches right across
my belly and turns off the stove, as if I wasn't there . . . as if I was stupid . . . as
if I didn't matter. . . . It really hurt my feelings badly. She could have just said,
"Mom, that chili smells just great and I'm starving." Or she could have said,
"Mom, you're the one who taught us how to make that delicious chili, let's have
some." So that's what I'm wanting to get at. . . . At this age, you hate to be ignored or chastised without words. . . . You hate to be made to look like a fool,
even if you are one sometimes. . . . We don't forget intentionally, you know. . . .
It just happens to us. It could happen to you some day, but I hope not. . . . So it's
these little things that grind you down to practically nothing. . . . It's not so much
the forgetting that wears you down, but how others treat you.

Once, after spilling a few things in quick succession, an older woman
was overheard singing softly to herself, somehow creating and having some
small comfort in the company of a kindred spirit, "The old gray mare, she
ain't what she used to be . . ."

Zelda, incontinent, withdrawn, speaking in sentence fragments if at all,
had a limited attention span. She generally walked about hurriedly with no
particular destination in mind. She could not tolerate touch, which made
caring for her very challenging. She could not sit to eat, and she ate very
little of the finger foods that she could eat as she walked about. When the
day program received a donation of stuffed animals, Zelda eagerly looked
through the assortment in a random, frenzied fashion and located a brown
bear with one missing eye. Within a few days Zelda seemed to have befriended this well-worn, soft brown bear. She would sit and rock the bear
as if it were a child. She was tender, cooing and cuddling, and her "baby

talk" was quite coherent. She began to "feed" the bear, coaxing him along at mealtime saying, "You'll have to eat so you'll be nice and strong," and then demonstrating to the bear how to eat. In this way Zelda's appetite and food intake gradually increased. Her whole demeanor softened, and she gradually became much more approachable. One of the staff overheard her saying to the bear in one of her cuddles: "I love you, you know, because you're broken just like me."

On the Journey of Aging

During a visit to the home of Marion, a potential client, a staff member admired a painting there. The painting, which had been done by Marion's mother-in-law, was of a vase of lilacs sitting on a windowsill, overlooking the backyard. Most of the blooms were fresh and healthy, but one was drooping slightly and becoming brown around the edges. Marion noted the lingering look of the staff member. "Yes, I like that painting too. . . . It reminds me of myself. . . . I recognize I'm fading. There's nothing much to do but accept that it's your time. It comes to us all, though you hate for it to be so, just the same."

After the sudden death of Princess Diana, of the United Kingdom, and Mother Theresa, the day program staff led the group in a thoughtful discussion on grief and sadness and loss. During the group activity that followed, Millie, a strong and spirited woman, suddenly began to sob heavily. At length she spoke of how old and ugly she had felt since breaking her hip about a year earlier:

I used to be the fastest waitress in the place. Just about everyone who came in said they wanted to wait for one of my tables to come open. . . . I tried to be cheerful. . . . You try to let your problems go for a while to put your customers' needs first. . . . Now I walk so bad and look like such a fool . . . I can feel my granddaughter's eyes just piercing my back when it's time to go in the morning. I go as fast as I can go, but it's never good enough. I can tell by her eyes that she would like me to just move quicker. . . . No one wishes that more than me. If I push myself harder, I worry that I'll fall again and that just frightens me to death. . . . [sobbing] If I go away again [to the hospital], I'm sure they'll forget me. . . . [sobbing more loudly] There's not much left of me as it is now . . . and now I'm acting like a bigger baby.

Others in the group offered words of consolation and support. Then Impy spoke very forcefully: "I don't remember your name, but I've always liked you, as a dear friend. I thought I should mention that when I first started to get old, I hurt my foot really bad and it held me down for a long time. It changed me a lot. . . . I think that these kinds of things that happen. . . . Well, I don't exactly know why, but I think it's God's way of teaching us how to live a new kind of life. We can do it, honey. We just have to be strong, and not give up, and the most important part, is to help each other."

On Humor

Ben had always exhibited a wonderful sardonic wit when he came to the day program. A practicing attorney for years, he was famous for his dry wit. Now he often spoke in meandering sentences, with elegant style and syntax but many jumbled and misplaced words. One of the group activities he participated in was not going particularly well. There was a fair amount of restlessness, not much cohesiveness. The staff's skill was not up to the challenge of several new group members, along with some distracting jackhammering going on just outside the group room. After a time, Ben said in a stage whisper, "Tempus figit." The staff, familiar with the Latin phrase but not sure what Ben was saying, asked Ben what that meant. He replied: "You notice I didn't say 'Tempus fugit,' time flies; I said 'Tempus figit,' time is I not flying . . . everyone is fidgeting."

Wally was part of a lively discussion about first cars. Not known for bragging, he waxed eloquent about how he was the envy of his neighborhood. He said he was the first guy on his block to have a car. He smiled as he recalled warmly, "Yeah, back then, for a while, I was a real big shot." Another man in the group said to Wally, "Well, you may have been a big shot then, but you're half shot now." Everyone had a hearty laugh, Wally most of all.

On another occasion, two women, both named Sue, were joining the group, adding to the several other Sues already in the group. After a few minutes a gentleman suggested, "Why don't we just rename the place Sioux City so it will be easy for us all to remember?"

On Building a Sense of Community and Belonging

Participants at the center welcome new participants with a variety of spontaneous greetings, such as "Welcome to the bracelet club"; "You may be new
here, but you're no stranger to us"; "This is a friendship club more than anything.
You can do what you want, and people can help you do it. You can get help if
you need it and give help if you've got it to give"; "We learned to laugh at ourselves and sometimes cry with each other"; and "It so easy to 'be' here. There's
no way to say how good it feels when you know you are wanted and needed. It's
a home for all times, good and bad. You feel like you belong, and you don't have
to be perfect because none of us really are that perfect anyway."

Lessons Learned

Many of the most extraordinary and insightful comments are made under
the most ordinary circumstances. The sacred and the mundane seem to be
woven together inextricably. Thus, we cannot simply go through our daily
work "on autopilot." We must maintain a level of openness, attentiveness,
and mindfulness that enables us to help the person with dementia communicate what they wish to communicate.

There are a number of clinical and communication skills that staff or
family members may use to encourage and support this kind of communication. One of these is the ability to listen attentively, expressed in the jar-
gon of mental health as "listening with the third ear." This skill has everything to do with seeking out the emotional message or need, which may or
may not be conveyed in words. The emotional availability of the caregiver
must be conveyed in ways that the individual with dementia can understand. One's demeanor must clearly express empathy and concern for the
well-being of the person. In essence, one must demonstrate a willingness
to be, in the words of the Alzheimer's Association, "someone to stand by
you," that is, someone who will not abandon the person with AD but will
assist, value and appreciate, and seek to understand him or her, , someone
who will relate to the person as a multidimensional individual who is not
defined by his or her diagnosis; someone who will share in the ups and
downs of the person's current life experiences, conveying a sense of equality and presenting himself or herself as a familiar and enduring presence.

Sometimes the clinical work involves giving cues, facilitating a process or activity, responding to the individual's need or wishes in the here and now. At other times it may require that the family or staff learn how to interpret the person's behavior and respond to his or her needs. Very often this involves the ability to understand an individual's unique behavior in a given situation since the individual may not be able to verbalize his or her needs. A caregiver may sometimes be able to facilitate this communication through his or her actions; at other times what is called for is knowing enough to stand aside and allow these magical moments to unfold.

To summarize, then:

- If we look at people with AD as multifaceted human beings, their diagnosis will not define the scope or terms of the relationships.
- People with AD have a capacity to communicate with their peers and staff on many different levels. Staff members have an obligation to facilitate that process.
- The medical model is not broad enough to provide therapeutic care for persons with AD. It is preferable to use a more holistic or humanistic model, one that frames care in terms of the person with AD rather than in terms of the disease, a bio-psycho-social-spiritual approach that treats what is alive and essential as well as what is frail and halting.
- We must look at relationships as the primary vehicle of care for persons with AD; these relationships are, by definition, reciprocal in many ways.
- Because of some limitations imposed by the disease, staff members must assume the mantle of gentle stewardship on behalf of the persons entrusted to their care.
- We must read widely in the arts, ethics, and spirituality, as well as the literature of related health and social sciences. In addition to a philosophy of care, a philosophy of life is essential because AD challenges us to consider what it means to be truly human and what we owe our fellow human beings.

Conclusion

This chapter does not present any elegant clinical concepts. However, perhaps the voices presented here, along with the voices presented in other chapters, will allow us to broaden our expectations about the potential for enhanced communication with persons with AD. As a first step, the reader is challenged to look at the data and consider their potential implications for all practice settings. Second, the reader is encouraged to look within himself or herself to discover his or her own level of comfort and commitment to engage more fully with the essential human who has AD. The prevailing medical model guides our communication to focus on what has been lost rather than on what remains. A more humanistic, person-centered paradigm will remind us that caring for persons with AD is an art as well as science and that the two perspectives enrich each other. We must work toward developing the clinical models of communication and the practical clinical skills needed to facilitate the kind of communication that will keeps persons with dementia connected to themselves, to one another, and to the communities to which they belong. By doing so, we can help them maintain their full humanity and foster our own in the process.

REFERENCES

Bell, V., and D. Troxel. 1997. *The best friends approach to Alzheimer's care*. Baltimore: Health Professions Press.

Kitwood, T. 1997. *Dementia reconsidered: The person comes first*. Philadelphia: Open Univ. Press.

Kuhn, D. 1999. *Alzheimer's early stages: First steps in caring and treatment*. Alameda, Calif.: Hunter House.

Lubinski, R., ed. 1991. *Dementia and communication*. Philadelphia: B. C. Decker.

Rader, J. 1995. *Individualized dementia care: Creative compassionate approaches*. New York: Springer.

Rau, M. T. 1993. *Coping with communication challenges in Alzheimer's disease*. San Diego: Singular Publishing.

Robinson, A., B. Spencer, and L. White. 1989. *Understanding difficult behaviors*. Ypsilanti: Eastern Michigan Univ. Press.

Snyder, L. 1999. *Speaking our minds: Personal reflections from individuals with Alzheimer's*. New York: W. H. Freeman.

Zgola, J. 1999. *Care that works: A relationship approach to persons with dementia*. Baltimore: Johns Hopkins Univ. Press.

Connecting to the Spirit

JON C. STUCKEY

*It's never going to be written in a prayer book, but my prayer is,
"God, you gave this to me, help me deal with it."*
—Cynthia, a 57-year-old retired schoolteacher

Evidence of the resiliency of the human spirit is embodied in the journey of Alzheimer's disease. From a clinical standpoint there is nothing positive about AD. The disease takes away memories, personalities, and the ability to communicate with one's social world. It may bring on financial hardship and difficult legal issues that only exacerbate an already stressful situation. And yet, even amidst this devastation the hope that emerges among those who have been diagnosed bears testament to the capacity of the human spirit to rise above the ravages of the disease.

AD can be so devastating to persons suffering from their disease as well as their families that it completely undermines spiritual well-being. It leads to such questions as, "Where is my mother now that we can no longer communicate?" "Is she trapped in the quagmire of her memory loss or is she at peace?" "Why is this happening?" "What purpose is there in having Alzheimer's disease?" As in other times of uncertainty, the human tendency is to look to a divine or spiritual realm for answers. The added layer of complexity in the experience of AD is that at some point the person with the disease can no longer effectively communicate his or her feelings. Consequently, it becomes very difficult to find a reliable window through which to view the subjective experience of AD.

That is not to say that connections cannot still be maintained to the spirit. In the first section of the chapter I explore the theology of AD. Many have written about the apparent discrepancy between a benevolent Supreme Being and something as devastating as AD. Next, I discuss the spiritual care of persons with AD, reviewing evidence that persons remain "spiritual" beings long after they have ceased to be "cognitive" beings. The thoughts and feelings on religion and spirituality presented here are those of people with dementia themselves, drawn from the work of others and from informant data from a community dialog series held in Cleveland, Ohio. I conclude the chapter with a review of the clinical and practical lessons learned from the study in Cleveland, as well as a discussion of the underlying hope and meaning evidenced by making connections to the spirit amidst dementia.

The following working definitions of *religion* and *spirituality* are offered to help draw distinctions between the two constructs. *Religion* is a particular doctrinal framework that guides sacred beliefs and practices in ways that are sanctioned by a broader faith community or organization. It is a system of beliefs and practices that helps structure how people worship. *Spirituality* refers to experiences that connect persons with sacred and meaningful entities and emotions. These experiences create and sustain a personal relationship with a higher source of power, defined according to that person's own beliefs. These definitions are consistent with prevailing work in the field (e.g., Ellor and Bracki 1995; Koenig 1995). This chapter focuses mostly on spirituality rather than on religion per se. However, at times religion and spirituality are closely linked.

The Theology of Alzheimer's Disease

At the very heart of spiritual care for persons with AD is the need for the individual to reconcile his or her religious beliefs with the diagnosis. In the book *When bad things happen to good people*, Rabbi Kushner (1981) notes that when people are confronted with tragedy or extreme stress, they tend to turn against God or against their religious beliefs. Although this is certainly not true in every case, people often report feeling abandoned by God. This chapter focuses mainly on the positive aspects of religion and spirituality as they relate to AD. But that is not to say that there is not a negative side.

Persons with AD, like persons with any disease, may feel resentment about having the disease. "Am I being punished?" they might ask. Keck (1996) notes that AD is a "theological disease" because it strikes at the very core of who we are. The loss of our memories leaves us paralyzed, trying to figure out how we connect to those around us and to the divine. Dyer (1996) writes poignantly about her mother, who was in the throes of Alzheimer's disease. Someone in the nursing home in which Dyer's mother resided was trying to comfort her mother by reading from the Psalms. Dyer writes: "The psalmist cannot, dare not, advise her any longer with words. He cannot touch her. He, too, even he, would fall silent in her presence. She would heal him of his arrogance. Still him forever. Heal him and still him forever and forever" (15). The ethos that rises from Dyer's words cuts to the very core of this disease. Religious platitudes may only serve to worsen how we feel, not make the situation better.

Indeed, as noted by Hopkins (1997), religion can be a barrier to finding peace in stressful life events, particularly if family or friends imply that one's sufferings are either a test or a punishment from God. Taken to extremes, this view may lead people to believe that the condition of AD could have been reversed if only they had prayed hard enough or lived a "better" life, which in turn may lead to guilt, anger, or alienation.

Sapp (1997) makes an interesting point when he writes that all humans have "spiritual Alzheimer's disease." That is, we are constantly forgetting evidence of God's grace in our lives and rarely acknowledge any role of the divine in our own accomplishments. In this respect all humans are connected along a continuum of dementia that begins with everyone having spiritual dementia and ends with those who have both spiritual dementia and cognitive dementia.

What, then, can be done to bridge the gap between religion and theology, on the one side, and those affected by AD, on the other? The theological debates surrounding illness and disease are ongoing. We have no ready explanations for the theological rationale for AD. However, persons with AD who have been given spiritual care, that is, care that focused on connecting them to sacred and meaningful entities and emotions, have been shown to respond in significant and positive ways. Consequently, it is vital that we preserve connections to spiritual well-being by fostering and nurturing the spiritual care of those with AD and related dementias.

Spiritual Care

In this new era of "rethinking Alzheimer's care," Fazio, Seman, and Stansell (1999), along with others (Bell and Troxel 1999; Castleman, Gallagher-Thompson, and Naythons 2000; Kuhn 1999), have led a shift away from a defeatist approach to AD to one that celebrates to the greatest extent possible the personhood of those with dementia. Kitwood (1997) writes that validating personhood emphasizes dignity and individuality. Implied in many of these models of care are the value of the human spirit and the need to address issues of religion and spirituality as they relate to dementia. In other words, by focusing solely on the physical aspects, for example, symptom management, we neglect other areas that also require care in the dementia experience, namely, spiritual well-being.

Several books and journal articles focus on how to engage persons with AD in worship or how to minister to them. Clayton (1991) argues for a "right-brain" approach to worship, that is, one that focuses less on intellectual skills and more on music, aroma, and touch. Richards (1990) emphasizes that early memories are often preserved in persons with AD and can be triggered using religious symbols that may have had important meaning in past years.

In her book *Forget Me Not: The Spiritual Care of Alzheimer's Disease*, Everett (1996) notes that traditional religious services employ an abundance of cognitive-based expressions of faith (e.g., reciting scripture, listening to homilies or sermons, responsive reading). She suggests that worship can and should be a multisensory experience, using touch, music, and even nature as pathways of connection to someone with AD.

Indeed, the senses are an important tool in worship. Anecdotal and, to a limited extent, empirical data bolster the connections among the senses, memory, and spirituality. Many families and nursing home staff members have recounted to me instances of persons with AD who had not spoken for years spontaneously singing the words to a religious hymn or participating in a sacred ritual. Research in music therapy has underscored the value of using music in the care of persons with AD (Clair 1996; Groene et al. 1998).

Empirical data also have suggested a link between memory and the sense of smell. Research consistently demonstrates that persons with AD have a reduced capacity to detect odors (Moore, Paulsen, and Murphy 1999; Nordin, Monsch, and Murphy 1995). However, the use of aromatherapy among persons with dementia suggests that odors can trigger a calming ef-fect (Brooker et al. 1997). Drawing on the sense of smell to evoke emo-tional and spiritual responses can be a powerful way to maintain connec-tions to the spirit even in advanced stages of AD.

Spiritual care and support of persons with AD are as important as phys-ical or emotional care and support. It should not be assumed that a loss of cognitive capacity will necessarily be accompanied by a loss of spiritual ca-pacity or need. Clinicians and families should be encouraged to use what-ever means possible (e.g., senses, reading, or music) to maintain a connec-tion to the spirit of persons with AD regardless of the stage of the disease.

The Subjective Voice

Nowhere is the power of the human spirit more poignantly and profoundly expressed than in the words of persons with AD. With the growing inter-est in and recognition of AD as a major public-health issue, the voice of the diagnosed has emerged. One of the earliest contributions to the area of spirituality and AD was written by Reverend Robert Davis (1989). Even though much of the book was written with the assistance of his wife, it is often cited as the first book in which a person with AD expressed his or her feelings about the disease and its impact on his or her spiritual well-being. Davis writes: "I know that the Lord is with me. That knowledge has always given me inner peace. He has always had a purpose for me. I trust that this [AD] is a part of that purpose" (13).

Throughout his account Davis speaks about how his faith sustained him even when the disease began to affect his capacity to reason. The issue here is not that religion or spirituality takes away the pain and trauma associ-ated with a diagnosis of dementia but that participating in religious or spir-itual practices and rituals can help sustain both the person with AD and his or her caregivers in the face of cognitive decline.

In her moving account of persons living with AD, Snyder (1999) touches on several aspects of spirituality. The pervasiveness of hope in her book gives light to a common thread in many stories of AD, namely, per-sons asking, "How can I make the best of this?" There is Bill, who "was edit-ing the verbose narrative of his life into haiku-poems whose paucity of words revealed not so much a poverty of language as the richness of each given word" (52). Or Betty, who identified "pragmatism" as her religion and who was adamant that AD did not wholly define her. And there is Consuelo, who notes, "As anyone would, I've wondered, 'Why me? I'm a good person, so why is this happening to me?' But only God knows. I'm not angry, but I feel helpless because God can't answer my questions with a human voice. But I realize he knows what he's doing and he'll take care of me" (146).

Snyder's book was not written as a book on religion and spirituality, yet the theme of spirituality is woven throughout the book. It speaks to how people try to make sense out of AD. It speaks about hope, which appears to be the greatest contribution of supporting the religious and or spiritual well-being of those with AD and related dementias. That is, religion and spirituality offer hope and help people cope. The work of Pargament and his colleagues (Pargament 1998; Pargament et al. 1990) has focused extensively on religion and coping. Pargament has called for an incorporation of the religious dimension into research on coping because of the consistency with which he has found persons to rely on their religious practices during times of crises, such as following a diagnosis of AD.

The Cleveland Community Dialogue

In the fall of 1998 the University Alzheimer Center, affiliated with the University Hospitals of Cleveland and Case Western Reserve University (CWRU), led a community dialogue series on religion, spirituality, and AD. The dialog was held in partnership with the Cleveland Area Chapter of the Alzheimer's Association, the Fairhill Center for Aging, and the Center for Biomedical Ethics at CWRU. The purpose of the dialogue was to focus attention on religion and spirituality in dementia care and to respond to and acknowledge the emerging interest in spiritual well-being for the cognitively impaired.

We invited more than fifty clinicians, researchers, ethicists, clergy leaders, and family members to participate in the conversations; thirty-nine accepted. The professionals included physicians, nurses, social workers, sociologists, psychologists, ministers, and rabbis. Religions represented included Protestant, Catholic, Jewish, and Unitarian, among others. Eighteen percent of the participants were nonwhite.

The first session of the dialogue series focused on the subjective experience of AD. Four persons who had been diagnosed with AD spoke about how they had incorporated their religious and spiritual views into their experience with AD. The Cleveland Area Chapter of the Alzheimer's Association arranged for the four speakers. These individuals were not chosen because they shared any major demographic characteristics. Two were men, and two were women; two were Catholic, and two were Protestant; three were white, and one was black. Rather, in the course of discussing their disease at a meeting of a support group for the newly diagnosed each had mentioned how he or she had incorporated various religious and spiritual views into the AD experience.

Beatrice

When Beatrice spoke at the community dialogue, she emphasized the importance of integrating persons with AD into the congregation. Beatrice, who was in her late sixties, had been diagnosed at 65. She lived with her husband, and had two grown children who lived outside of the area. Beatrice had left her own church because she did not feel welcome there after her symptoms became noticeable. However, even at her new church she remained isolated. She had chosen not to share her diagnosis with either the minister or other members of the congregation. "I go to church by myself, and I feel a little awkward because for years my husband went with me. He doesn't anymore, and then it's a little awkward. I mean, I just go to church and go home."

Beatrice's situation highlights what Rabbi Richard Address calls the "caring congregation" (1991). "Establishing a Caring Community or congregation begins and ends with deeds . . . deeds of loving-kindness motivated by a fundamental understanding that as human beings, created in a divine image, we share each and every one of us, in the process of creation. By reaching out to and being involved with others, we meet and confront the very presence of the divine" (196).

Persons with AD, people like Beatrice, would benefit greatly from a "caring congregation." Rather than simply designating a time for coming together to worship, churches should encourage congregants to look out for persons who come to services alone and leave alone. The very essence of humanity that draws people to religion and spirituality is somehow intertwined with a desire to help others in need of support. Places of worship are ideal settings for not only worship but also reaching out to others.

In addition, Beatrice spoke about the worship service itself. Others have written about worship services designed for persons with dementia (e.g., Richards 1990). Beatrice noted that she preferred the older hymns in Christian worship. "Well, I think they do a good job there with the old songs— those that you have known when you were a child. Some of the new ones I sometimes don't care for because they're not as pretty as the older ones. I like the old ones because it makes me very frustrated when they bring a song in that I've never heard. I realize they can't play the same songs all the time, but I like the old songs."

Beatrice also shared how she felt about prayer. Many of the participants spoke about prayer and the role that it played in their expressions of spirituality. Through prayer Beatrice was able to express feelings that she was not able to share even with her family. In this way she gained a level of peace and strength that otherwise might have been unattainable.

> I never [pray] out loud, but I do it in the car when I've been frustrated. I will call for the Lord to help me do what I should do and not be angry. And I think it's hard on the people that I live with to have to put up with me because I can't remember anything. And so, I pray silently to myself . . . I've never thought of [God answering] because I don't expect it. I just think that maybe he can move things that will help me. But I don't really think of him talking to me. I just talk to him to try to get [rid of] the burden I have. I guess if everybody in the world does that, he's pretty busy!

Paul

Paul was 48 when he spoke at the community dialogue session. He had been diagnosed with a rare form of dementia and had been forced into early retirement. His two sons were still in college, and his wife was working full-time. Paul felt lost when he first heard his diagnosis. However, he spoke about an experience that helped him accept his situation.

> When I was working, everything was the job, coming home, having dinner, going to bed, getting up the next morning, going to work. It was like a rat race in a way. But now, you have time to reflect on the values of life. It's a different sense

of being, a sense of self-worth. But I think it's a better feeling. When I was going through this, you almost feel like jumping off a cliff because you've lost the ability to do your job.

But then I had a vision when I was sleeping one time. I saw this bright light to the left of me, and I turned and I looked and I was kind of scared. And then I looked to my right and there was a bright light there. And then I heard this voice say, "Don't worry, everything will be alright. I will take care of you." And from that day on, I woke up and I said, "I'm going to accept this disease." And my wife says, "My goodness, you've changed." I said, "I'm going to accept it and live with it and go on from here and enjoy life." Some people might say it was just a vision or a dream or something. But it put everything in perspective for me. From that point on, I have been more calm, more caring, and everything has just seemed to fall in place.

Paul's experience of a "vision" could be interpreted as a hallucination, a symptom not uncommon in dementia. Nevertheless, what is most compelling about the vision is not whether it actually occurred but that it led to Paul's acceptance of the disease in a way that probably would not have been possible without the vision. Not a particularly religious or spiritual man before his diagnosis, Paul became both deeply spiritual and connected to a higher purpose for his life.

We as human beings do not know what's in the cards for us. There's only one person [that does], and that's God. And everything happens for a reason, and he knows best what's going to happen in our life, and you have to have your faith in him. I think that for people that do not have that, it's really a sadness. Faith really is the all-healing factor when you look at it. God comes to play in everybody's life. Like I said, before I had this happen I was just a workaholic. And now this made me realize that we have to take each day as it comes and deal with it and God knows what's best.

Cynthia

Cynthia had been a member of a convent but had left the order after thirteen years. Her diagnosis with AD led her to retire from teaching at age 57. She spoke about how her religious beliefs helped her cope with her situation.

My first reaction was denial: This isn't going to happen to me. I taught school. I taught children how to think. I have given them ways to remember and so that's not going to happen to me. So I just refused to accept this. And I cried about it when I couldn't remember things. I became angry; I was angry at God. This is not the way it's supposed to be. But then all of a sudden I just began to realize this is the way it is. There's nothing I can do about it. I can't change myself. I can't do those memory techniques, all of those things that I was going to do to get myself back. And once I came to that realization that this is it, kid, deal with it—I did. I cry a lot. I still do, as you can see. But, it's a way of dealing, too. [Now] I don't get angry. I cry. I don't throw things around. I just sit and sulk a little bit and then I feel better.

Cynthia is supported and cared for by her friend Selma. The two women were in the convent together years ago and have remained friends. For Selma, Cynthia's illness has become part of her own faith journey. She believes that it is her calling in life to care for Cynthia, and she bases this belief on a story from the Bible: "I feel in Cynthia's life I'm a Simon of Syrene [the man who carried Christ's cross on the way to the crucifixion]. I stand back. What Cynthia needs help with today, she may not need help with tomorrow. So my role changes every day, depending on her good days and bad days. I kind of stand back. And if I see she has trouble and she's getting frustrated, then I step in just like Simon did. When Christ fell, Simon stepped in. The hardest part for me is to be sure I don't step in too soon because I don't want to take away whatever independence Cynthia can maintain."

The friendship of the two women demonstrates another kind of spirituality, the spirituality that comes from being connected to another person. Cynthia has a very positive outlook on her disease, but she has been buttressed by Selma's support. "It's never going to be written in a prayer book, but my prayer is, 'God you gave this to me, help me deal with it.' And that's how I cope with it. I can't change it. I will accept it and I will make the best of what I can do."

Gregory

Gregory had been a minister at a local African American church for the past forty years. At the time of the community dialogue session he was still the minister, but his memory problems prevented him from fully carrying out his responsibilities. Gregory's religious training came through in an almost melodic tone as he expressed his reliance on God. "I was taught at home and in seminary that the Lord has a design and his design includes having what you need. The only obstacle that can keep him from using it is you not asking. For he said, 'Ask and it shall be given, seek and you shall find, knock and the door shall be opened.' And when he says shall, that's what he means. Because when he is determined to do something, there is no power in heaven or on earth that can stop him."

Gregory's religious memory, that is, his memory of passages of scripture and hymns, was like an old friend, one that could be called on for support and strength at any hour of the day or night. On the one hand, it appeared that Gregory had lost the capacity to fully understand what he was saying. On the other hand, there is no way to verify whether he understood or not. Moreover, his demeanor the entire evening expressed a peace that comes from knowing things will be all right. "The Bible says 'Seek ye first the kingdom of heaven and His righteousness and all things shall be added unto you.' And, faith, the Bible says, is the substance of things hoped for and evidence of things not seen. And when you've had some spiritual encounter that exposes you to a need to pray and you have got an answer, your problem has been solved. As an old song used to say, 'You can learn to stretch out on His word,' and that means trust Him for everything that you think you have a need for."

Hope and Meaning

In the end, the discussion of spirituality and AD is a discussion about hope and meaning. Farran, Herth, and Popovich (1995) write about hope as a multidimensional construct that includes spiritual, relational, and even rational elements. The hope addressed here is both spiritual and relational. It is spiritual in that both the diagnosed and caregivers speak about a hope for the future that is often based on an afterlife. They hope for a time of being whole again, and they hope for a time when they will be reunited with friends and family members who have already died. However, there is also a striking relational aspect to hope that characterizes many experiences with AD. A caregiver once explained to me that he was praying every day about his wife. He no longer prayed for her to become well. He has resigned himself to the fact that she would die from AD. He simply prayed that he would outlive her because he wanted to be the one to care for her until she died.

Spirituality and AD also deal with meaning. Caregivers report on the meaning they derive from the experience (Farran et al. 1997). However, there is a deeper meaning: the meaning of what it is to be a person. A colleague of mine shared the story of a woman with advanced dementia in a nursing home. If cognitive capacity were the defining criterion of personhood, then this profoundly demented woman would scarcely qualify. The residents were grouped together in a circle, and my friend, who was the nursing home chaplain, suggested that they imagine what it would be like if Jesus were in the room. "Wouldn't it be great if we could all go over to him and give Jesus a hug?" my friend asked. The woman with advanced dementia, who had spoken little if anything of coherence for several months, said, "No. If Jesus were here, he would come over to me and give *me* a hug." Her spontaneous insight into the grace of Christ was profound and dispelled any challenge to her personhood.

There have been some disturbing unintended consequences of portraying AD as the "disease of the century." The intended consequences are, of course, to increase the level of awareness of AD and to increase the amounts of money available for research. Characterizing AD as "losing a million minds" has created an important and necessary sense of urgency: unless we eradicate this dreaded disease, we will be consumed by it from a public health standpoint.

However, the unintended consequences of such approaches on behalf of persons with dementia are to negate positive aspects, outlooks, and definitions of AD that resist using such terms as *terror, tragedy,* and *victims* to refer to the disease or those diagnosed with it. This is not to say that AD does not devastate the diagnosed and their families. However, even within the AD experience persons can flourish. They can participate in relationships. They can offer and receive gifts and blessings. They can teach and inspire. They can worship. They can love and be loved.

It is almost as if AD becomes a gateway to spiritual well-being and not a barrier. Davis (1989) writes that "perhaps the journey that takes me away from reality into the blackness of that place of the blank, emotionless, unmoving Alzheimer's state is in reality a journey into the richest depths of God's love that few have experienced on earth" (120).

Lessons Learned

When individuals receive a diagnosis of AD, they do not automatically lose their capacity for participating in worship and maintaining meaningful connections to their social and sacred worlds. It is incumbent on those of us in caregiving or supportive roles to provide as many opportunities as possible for religious and spiritual expression. The Cleveland community dialogue elicited several guidelines to keep in mind when offering spiritual support to persons with AD.

GUIDELINES FOR MAINTAINING CONNECTIONS TO THE SPIRIT AMIDST ALZHEIMER'S DISEASE
- Include traditional hymns and sacred readings in the worship experience; avoid long homilies or sermons and unfamiliar songs or lyrics.
- Include touch in the worship experience or as part of communication.
- Integrate those with AD into the worship experience to the greatest extent possible; do not isolate them in the back of the place of worship or make them feel unwelcome because of their behavior.
- If you are a minister, rabbi, or other clergy person, dress in a way that is expected of clergy from the particular religious background of those with whom you are interacting.
- Include nature as a worship experience; for example, take walks or listen to the sounds of the outdoors.
- Teach clergy and laity how best to interact with persons with AD.
- Engage persons with AD in conversation even if they cannot visibly reciprocate.
- Learn about and be sensitive to the specific religious tradition of those with AD with whom you are interacting.
- Maintain regular contact through frequent follow-up visits, particularly if the individual has limited opportunities for interaction with others.

Much more remains to be learned about the connections among religion, spirituality, and AD. For the small gains in insight and understanding regarding Judeo-Christian traditions that have been realized, even less is known about Eastern, Muslim, and other non-Western faith traditions.

It is clear, however, that religion and spirituality are important capacities that must remain available to persons with AD, even until the end of life. They can help to bring meaning to an otherwise meaningless situation. They offer pathways to powerful positive aspects of this disease. They can help bring comfort to both the diagnosed and their families. And they can help sustain persons with AD as they journey down the unknown path of separating from one's mind and memory.

Religion and spirituality are not universal tools and cannot be called on in the same way that medications or other therapies can be called on to help persons manage and cope with disease, but they do have significant power, albeit ephemeral. Whenever possible and appropriate, persons with AD should be given opportunities for worship throughout the dementia experience. Indeed, it is perhaps in the experience of dementia that we gain a purer understanding of the capacity of both humanity and the divine.

REFERENCES

Address, R. 1991. The caring congregation. *Journal of Psychology and Judaism* 15:195–200.

Bell, V., and D. Troxel. 1999. The other face of Alzheimer's disease. *American Journal of Alzheimer's Disease* 14:60–64.

Brooker, D. J., M. Snape, E. Johnson, D. Ward, and M. Payne. 1997. Single case evaluation of the effects of aromatherapy and massage on disturbed behaviour in severe dementia. *British Journal of Clinical Psychology* 36:287–96.

Castleman, M., D. Gallagher-Thompson, and M. Naythons. 2000. *There's still a person in there: The complete guide to treating and coping with Alzheimer's*. New York: Putnam.

Clair, A. A. 1996. The effect of singing on alert responses in persons with late stage dementia. *Journal of Music Therapy* 33:234–47.

Clayton, J. 1991. Let there be life: An approach to worship with Alzheimer's patients and their families. *Journal of Pastoral Care* 45:177–79.

Davis, R. 1989. *My journey into Alzheimer's disease*. Wheaton, Ill.: Tyndale House.

Dyer, J. 1996. *In a tangled wood*. Dallas: Southern Methodist Univ. Press.

Ellor, J. W., and M. A. Bracki. 1995. Assessment, referral, and networking. In *Aging, spirituality, and religion*, ed. M. A. Kimble, S. H. McFadden, J. W. Ellor, and J. J. Seeber, 148–60. Minneapolis: Fortress.

Everett, D. 1996. *Forget me not: The spiritual care of persons with Alzheimer's*. Edmonton, Alberta: Inkwell.

Farran, C. J., K. A. Herth, and J. M. Popovich. 1995. *Hope and hopelessness: Critical clinical constructs*. Thousand Oaks, Calif.: Sage.

Farran, C. J., B. H. Miller, J. E. Kaufman, and L. Davis. 1997. Race, finding meaning, and caregiver distress. *Journal of Aging and Health* 9:316–33.

Fazio, S., D. Seman, and J. Stansell. 1999. *Rethinking Alzheimer's care*. Baltimore: Health Professions Press.

Groene, R., S. Zapchenk, G. Marble, and S. Kantar. 1998. The effect of therapist and activity characteristics on the purposeful responses of probable Alzheimer's disease participants. *Journal of Music Therapy* 35:119–36.

Hopkins, D. D. 1997. Failing brain, faithful God. In *God never forgets: Faith, hope, and Alzheimer's disease*, ed. D. K. McKim, 21–37. Louisville: Westminster John Knox.

Keck, D. 1996. *Forgetting whose we are: Alzheimer's disease and the love of God*. Nashville: Abingdon.

Kitwood, T. 1997. *Dementia reconsidered: The person comes first*. Buckingham: Open Univ. Press.

Koenig, H. G. 1995. Religion and health in later life. In *Aging, spirituality, and religion*, ed. M. A. Kimble, S. H. McFadden, J. W. Ellor, and J. J. Seeber, 9–29. Minneapolis: Fortress.

Kuhn, D. 1999. *Alzheimer's early stages: First steps in caring and treatment*. Alameda, Calif.: Hunter House.

Kushner, H. S. 1981. *When bad things happen to good people*. New York: Schocken.

Moore, A. S., J. S. Paulsen, and C. Murphy. 1999. A test of odor fluency in patients with Alzheimer's and Huntington's disease. *Journal of Clinical and Experimental Neuropsychology* 21:341–51.

Nordin, S., A. U. Monsch, and C. Murphy. 1995. Unawareness of smell loss in normal aging and Alzheimer's disease: Discrepancy between self-reported and diagnosed smell sensitivity. *Journals of Gerontology: Psychological Sciences* 50:P187–92.

Pargament, K. L. 1998. *The psychology of religion and coping: Theory, research, practice*. New York: Guilford.

Pargament, K. L., D. S. Ensing, K. Falgout, H. Olsen, B. Reilly, K. Van Haitsma, and R. Warren. 1990. God help me (I): Religious coping efforts as predictors of the outcomes to significant negative life events. *American Journal of Community Psychology* 18:793–824.

Richards, M. 1990. Meeting the spiritual needs of the cognitively impaired. *Generations* 14:63–64.

Sapp, S. 1997. Hope: The community looks forward. In *God never forgets: Faith, hope, and Alzheimer's disease*, ed. D. K. McKim, 88–103. Louisville: Westminster John Knox.

Snyder, L. 1999. *Speaking our minds: Personal reflections from individuals with Alzheimer's*. New York: W. H. Freeman.

Building Resilience through Coping and Adapting

PHYLLIS BRAUDY HARRIS AND CASEY DURKIN

*I came to that realization. I don't even know at what point I finally said to myself,
this is the way it is, deal with it. I still have my creativity.
Memory ain't so good but* [my] *creativity is there.*
—Ms. Pope, a 61-year-old retired schoolteacher

The word *Alzheimer's* has become synonymous with loss. Many chapters in
this book document the multiple losses that individuals diagnosed with this
type of dementia undergo (see in this volume the chapters by Killick, Phinney, Sabat, and Snyder). Losses in autonomy, self-esteem, and respect and
changes in social roles and family relationships are just a few of the losses
individuals with AD experience. Yet, some people are able to face and meet
the awesome challenge of living with AD, discovering and developing ways
of coping and adapting to the multitude of changes it brings to their lives.
This chapter through qualitative research introduces the reader to people
who are *living*, not dying, with Alzheimer's disease. You will hear their
words and learn about their accomplishments and struggles. Specifically,
this chapter focuses on these people's strengths. It examines the coping
strategies they have developed that have allowed them to live meaningful
lives.

In the research on AD a major theoretical framework for understanding
the caregiving experience has been the stress and coping model (Aneshensel et al. 1995). This theoretical model, extending the transactional cog-

nitive model of stress described by Lazarus (1966) and Lazarus and Folkman (1984), was first proposed by Pearlin et al. (1981) and was further developed in Pearlin 1989 and in Pearlin et al. 1990. The theory is organized
around three domains: the stressors, the difficult problems caregivers deal
with in caring for their family member with AD; the outcomes, the mental and physical health care problems the stressors cause for the caregivers;
and the stress mediators, factors such as personal, social, and financial resources that can act as buffers and lessen the magnitude of the stress on
the caregivers. Coping is one of the key personal mediators in this model.
As defined by Pearlin and Schooler (1978), *coping* is the action that
people take in an attempt to lessen or avoid the impact of life's problems.
In this model, the person with AD is seen as a stressor, not as a person
with strengths that might be used as a resource to lessen the stress on both
parties.

Research on the subjective experience of persons with AD is an emerging field (Cotrell and Schulz 1993; Downs 1997; Fazio, Seman, and Stansell
1999; Keady and Nolan 1994; Kitwood 1990, 1993a, 1993b, 1997; Kitwood
and Benson 1995; Lyman 1989; Snyder 1999; Woods 2001). Consequently,
there has been limited research on the coping and adapting behaviors of
individuals with AD. Yet, since coping is situation-specific (Pearlin 1989),
it behooves health care professionals interested in providing more person-
centered dementia care to include in studies of stress and coping the coping of people with AD, which has been largely disregarded. In the early
stages of AD many coping skills are still intact and can be mobilized.

Cohen and Eisdorfer (Cohen 1991; Cohen, Kennedy, and Eisdorfer
1985) were the first to suggest that people in the early stages of AD could
learn to cope with the stresses of living with the disease. Bahro, Silber, and
Sunderland (1995) discussed the coping of seven individuals with mild to
moderate probable AD but focused on defense mechanisms, discussing the
negative coping responses, such as denial, minimizing, somatization, dis-
placement, and self-blame. They discussed only one person who was aware
of her diagnosis, both cognitively and emotionally, and coped adequately
(according to their definition) by appropriately exhibiting mourning behaviors. However, persons with AD can maintain insight into their conditions and use positive coping behaviors.

Keady and Nolan (1995a, 1995b) developed the Index for Managing
Memory Loss (IMMEL), which assessed specific positive coping behaviors

used by individuals with AD to live with the disease. They included in their forty-two-item scale such coping behaviors as routines, accepting memory loss and finding ways of overcoming it, writing in a personal diary, using lists and other memory aids, staying in familiar surroundings, humor, information seeking, constant repetition to oneself to help one remember, and practicing relaxation techniques. The data from which this scale was developed were based on qualitative interviews with ten individuals with dementia and their caregivers.

Our study built on the emerging area of research that examines the coping and adapting behaviors of people with early-stage AD, people who in Keady and Nolan's model of the dementia experience would be described as in the maximizing stage of the disease (1995b). People can face adversity, learn coping behaviors, and build resilience even in the early stages of AD (McMillen 1999). In a previous study Harris and Sterin (1999) outlined a typology of five different coping patterns, positive as well as negative, that people with early-stage AD use to live with the disease. In this chapter we focus on the positive coping behaviors (instrumental coping and cognitive restructuring) that these individuals use, examining in more detail their large array of coping strategies, some of which support the previous research of Keady and Nolan but also extend this area of research. The present study sought to answer the following major research questions: (1) What are the positive coping behaviors that people with early-stage AD use? (2) How do these coping behaviors play a role in successful adaptation to living with AD? and (3) What lessons can be learned from their experiences that would be helpful to health care professionals, persons with AD, and family members?

The Study Design

Because this is a new area of inquiry in which there has been limited research, we used a qualitative methodology that resulted in a descriptive study. This methodology provides an in-depth understanding, using the words of persons with AD to explain their experiences of living and coping with the disease. From such grounded data further measurement scales and models of coping can be developed.

This study was based on in-depth personal interviews, participant-observations of early-stage support groups, and participation in two national focus groups on early-stage AD. The majority of the data for this chapter are from the interviews. Through contacts with a local chapter of the Alzheimer's Association, twenty-two people with early-stage AD were interviewed. The researchers did not administer the Mini-Mental State Examination (MMSE) themselves. Diagnosis was made by the geriatric-assessment units of local hospitals, and then persons with AD and their families were referred to the Alzheimer's Association's early-stage programs. The persons with AD had been diagnosed within the four years immediately prior to the study. The caregivers of nineteen of the persons with AD were also interviewed; the remaining three interviewees were living independently, two with no local caregivers. All twenty-two were in the early stages of the disease, but a nonrandom purposive sample ensured inclusion of a fairly wide range in demographic characteristics such as race and ethnicity, gender, marital status, socioeconomic status, educational level, urban/rural locations, and work status.

There are many limitations to a qualitative study. The twenty-two persons with AD in the study certainly were not a representative sample of people in the early stages of AD. We used a cross-sectional system of data collection to examine a dynamic process, the impact of living with a dementing disease. However, qualitative research makes no claim to be representative of the population it is examining. The purpose of this methodology is to present a more in-depth, diverse, and complex picture of a phenomenon that has been previously reported and to identify possible variables that need to be tested and confirmed in larger, representative studies.

The demographic profile of the sample was as follows. Fifteen of the twenty-two people with AD were female, and seven were male; two males and two females were African American, and the rest were Caucasian. The mean age was 71; however, the participants ranged in age from 54 to 84. Their occupations were quite varied, from factory workers and housewives to lawyers and professors. As indicated by the occupations, their educational levels also varied greatly. Two people had only completed the eighth grade, and eight individuals had advanced degrees. Five individuals were living alone, one with a child, one with a longtime friend, and the rest with their spouses. Seven lived in rural areas. All twenty-two had been diagnosed with probable AD two years earlier on the average. Thirteen of the nineteen caregivers were spouses, one was a son, three were daughters, one was a friend, and one was a cousin; in all, there were eleven female and eight male caregivers. The caregivers ranged in age from 38 to 85, the mean age being 66. The spousal caregivers had been married from six to sixty-three years, or thirty-eight years on the average. Two of the caregivers had not finished high school, and of the seventeen who had, eight had finished college. Their occupations ranged from part-time cake decorator or assembly-line worker to physician or owner of a large chemical company; ten caregivers were retired.

Seventeen of the interviews were conducted in the participants' homes by two researchers, one of whom had been recently diagnosed with AD. All the interviewees were made aware of this, and all were eager to discuss their experiences with this researcher. The last five interviews were conducted by a clinician, as the researcher with AD felt she was no longer able to handle the rigor of the interview process. Separate informed-consent forms were designed for the persons with AD and the caregivers. At the beginning of the interviews the consent forms were discussed, the overall purpose of the project explained, and any questions answered. All participants in the study understood the purpose and their roles and were eager to participate. No one refused to sign a consent form.

Each of the interviews took approximately two hours, spread over three sessions. In the first session the two interviewers, the person with AD, and the caregivers (except as noted above) met together for an hour and a half. Then the researcher with AD or the clinician met alone with the person with AD while the other researcher met with the caregivers. Since one of the researchers had been diagnosed with AD, there was a strong possibility of researcher bias in that she might overidentify with the issues being discussed or steer the conversation in a certain direction. She was certainly not an objective interviewer. Nevertheless, since this study examined the subjective experience of living with dementia, her in-depth understanding of this experience and her research background helped to offset the bias. In addition, the other researcher was aware of this possible bias and took charge of the interviews in order to keep them on target if this should happen. This was one of the reasons why all the interviews were taped and transcribed and then compared with the field notes. There were no noticeable differences between the data obtained from the interviews completed by both interviewers and those obtained from the interviews completed by the diagnosed researcher. Follow-up telephone calls were made to persons with AD or family members to resolve any discrepancies in the interview information.

In the first interview a set of predetermined topics, developed from the research questions, were integrated into the interviews, which were conducted as conversations. Thus, the resulting data comprise the individuals' responses to topics, as well as data resulting from issues they chose to discuss during the interviews. Major topics included in the interviews were: (1) the impact of living with progressive memory loss—reactions to the diagnosis, changes in lifestyle, the most difficult aspects, the roles it was important to keep, losses, and reactions of others; (2) one's concept of self—defining events, accomplishments, autonomy, impact of AD, and external factors that had an impact; (3) coping strategies and behaviors— helpful and least helpful strategies, factors that influenced one's willingness to develop strategies, strengths and assets, and empowerment issues; and (4) marital and family relationships—AD's impact on the relationship of the diagnosed person with his or her spouse and/or children, and the meaning of the term *caregiver*. During the individual interviews the caregivers and the persons with AD were given the opportunity to discuss in more detail the topics described above or to address any other issues they thought were relevant. Most often both the caregivers and the persons with AD raised additional issues and concerns. This chapter focuses mainly on the section of the interviews that covered coping strategies and behaviors.

Using the analytical strategy suggested by Glaser and Strauss (1967), we separately read the transcripts to develop substantive codes for each interview. The codes were then grouped into themes that emerged from the narratives and issues identified through the interview guide. There are limitations to this methodology, as noted above. The information is based upon a small, nonrandom cross-sectional sample of people in the early stages of a progressive disease. Their situation can change on a daily basis, so generalizability is very limited. However, from these narratives comes a better understanding of the issues and complexities persons with AD grapple with as they cope with the disease.

Findings

The analytical framework from which these narratives were examined was organized around common themes of successful coping and adaptation to early-stage AD that emerged from the data. This chapter focuses on the innovative coping strategies that have not been emphasized in previous research, strategies that go beyond setting routines, gathering information, making lists as a memory aid, keeping a sense of humor, and a supportive family. It is noteworthy that the people who adapted successfully used multiple coping strategies.

Acceptance and Ownership

Among the people with early-stage AD whom we interviewed, those who were coping positively were able to face the reality of their diagnosis and sought no one to blame for it. As one 84-year-old woman said, "Who can you blame? I do though tell my children [who live out of town], 'Don't be deluded by the fact I can have a normal conversation with you, that's just an illusion.' It doesn't give them a hint of what is really wrong." A 61-year-old woman stated, "I came to that realization. I don't even know at what point I finally said to myself, this is the way it is—deal with it. I still have my creativity. Memory ain't so good but [my] creativity is there." And a 71-year-old man explained, "Always deal with the reality of what is, not what could have been, or should have been, but what it is. I mean I've got this problem, it ain't going away. I don't agonize over it. I gotta fault. I recognize that and I cope with it. The thing to do is learn how to cope the best. Deal with it."

Disclosure

Telling friends, family members, neighbors, and acquaintances that they had been diagnosed with probable AD was a powerful release and coping strategy for many of the people interviewed. One 54-year-old woman with early-onset AD explained, "I tell everybody, you have no choice on this. You were dealt all of this. You deal with it or you would be dead. You are in control of something [telling people], even if it is only that. What someone with this diagnosis can do is let people know, 'I have Alzheimer's disease, and I need help in this area of my life, but leave me alone in **this** area.' I told everyone. It's helpful to understand what is going on. Then they don't look funny at you and say, 'Oh, poor thing.' You avoid all that stuff that people are afraid to ask. Don't really embrace it, but don't be afraid of it, and talk about it." And another woman,

74 years old, stated, "Everybody knows, everybody knows it, I think that helps. I think they thought I must be contagious at first, but it didn't last long."

Positive Attitude and Self-Acceptance

Individuals who were coping successfully were able to face AD with a positive attitude and to accept themselves. A 67-year-old woman stated, "I don't feel ashamed I have memory loss. I don't feel that way. I've got it! I'm going to work with it." One 61-year-old woman explained, "I'm not going to give up. I'm going to live until I die. Until my time is up, I'm going top my cup. That's me. I'm going to live my life as long as God gives it to me, or as long as he let's me know I'm living it. I've told my children that you don't need to feel sorry for me. I am who I want to be. What a shame it would be to live the rest of your life in regret." Another woman, also 61, when asked how she felt about herself, replied, "Yes, I very much so [feel OK about myself]. You know, I'm not threatened by anything. . . . I'll take challenge, but nothing that threatens. And that's been working."

Role Relinquishment and Replacement

Persons with AD who had to relinquish social roles because of dementia but replaced them with new roles or adapted previous roles faired the best. A 56-year-old businessman forced to retire because of AD explained, "I never really had a successful career, and now it's like I have a full-time job again— to be a good patient."

A 73-year-old woman discussed giving up her role as a reading teacher and as the one who held her family together. She described this as a relief and said that now she was enjoying life more. "I was in total control, in the classroom, and with raising my family and supervising my husband. I just sort of gave it up. I'm not sure that I did it intentionally, it just sort of happened. I don't even worry about that. So those dolls in those chairs are getting dirty, so let them get dusty, one of these days I'll get to them." Her son interjected, "Mom was always a source of strength for me and she has a great attitude." His mother continued: "I work in my garden. Get me out of the house and get me a garden. I put the vegetables over here by the driveway and that's my big love, it really is. My problems don't interfere with that. I don't want to live down because of this [the diagnosis]. I can either make it or break it. I don't have the mentality to be down."

Innovative Techniques and the Use of Technology

The individuals whom we interviewed were very creative in finding techniques for dealing with their dementia. One man used traveler's checks instead of regular checks because he could no longer write checks. With traveler's checks, he just had to sign his name, and if he lost them, they were replaced. The same individual carried a key chain that had a small digital recorder attached to it, which allowed him to tape what he needed to remember and carry it with him. Another man and his wife used Caller ID to track all the telephone calls to their home. Thus, if he forgot any phone messages left while his wife was at work, there was a backup in place, which eliminated much stress and frustration for both of them.

Other innovative techniques related to daily living and maintaining independence are an information center and a guide for meal planning or cooking. One person's doctor suggested that she and her caregiver maintain a central source of information, a specific *location* where the person could locate things she might need. After starting with a chair that soon overflowed, they purchased a stereo cabinet with glass doors. The woman keeps all her important papers there, along with her volunteer work. She no longer has to look in various rooms but has trained herself to always go to her information center. "We went through the routine of spending three hours a day trying to find a piece of paper, and that doesn't happen anymore." This same woman and her caregiver designed a guide for meal planning and cooking. They broke down all the steps for putting together their favorite meals and wrote them on pages that they laminated and placed in a binder. If a recipe gets dirty in the process of cooking, they can just wipe it clean. The woman with AD now finds it easier to prepare daily dinners following these step-by-step, reusable instructions.

Perhaps the most creative use of technology was a 61-year-old woman's use of a palm-size computer to keep her on schedule and organize her day. "I have a real problem remembering appointments. So I have a computer, which reminds me that I have an appointment [it buzzes]. I can download from a regular computer, and I can take this with me. If I have something I need to do, I've got to put it in there so I can work around it. When it buzzes, I open it up and check it. It also has a calculator and a word processor. I can write notes to myself [and not have notes all over the house]. I couldn't learn it immediately. I keep working at it. Basically, I did what I could figure out, but then went into depth a little more each day."

Fluidity

Being able to go with the flow of the disease also allowed the individuals to manage the daily stresses of dementia. They all talked about their good days and their bad days, which they accepted and worked with. One 84-year-old woman said, "I'm easygoing. I don't let it bother me." Another woman stated, "One day I am articulate and the next day I can't quite grasp what I want to say. I'm on a roll right now. I'm on a high. I'm very productive at this moment, so I am going with it. There are days I can't do anything at all."

Connection with Past Activities

Finding meaningful uses for skills the persons with AD had developed before their diagnosis was a common theme in a number of the narratives. A 74-year-old former professor said that though her memory problems prevented her from continuing to work, she was able to use her research skills to help design a study that examined the changing concept of self in early-stage dementia. "I could never have imagined that my last project would be the study of my own disease. I was making scrambled eggs out of broken ones. However, as an old saying goes, 'If it works, don't knock it!' I am now on both sides of the fence at once; studying the disease I live with daily."

A 71-year-old retired real-estate agent discussed his volunteer work, an extension of the work in community organizing that had been a central part of his life. He is a spokesman now for the local chapter of the Alzheimer's Association and recently received citywide recognition when he was awarded one of the city's Most Valuable Volunteer Awards.

As I look back on my life, I've been involved in a lot of organizations, and for the most part I've been having a very active part in the organization and often in a leadership role. I was student body president in junior high school, and also in senior high school; I was president of my college fraternity. I was director of Operation Equality, dealing with segregation and discrimination in housing. Okay, I wish it were not the case that I have Alzheimer's, but I accept the fact. Saying "poor me" is not going to make it better. I have transferred my desire to participate into doing things with the Alzheimer's Association. I've become a spokesperson for them. I enjoy that. I can give them insights. I enjoy this teaching because it gives me a sense of making a contribution.

Altruism

As the words of the retired real-estate agent just mentioned illustrate, the ability to still be productive members of society and give back to their communities was a very meaningful coping behavior for people interviewed. A 73-year-old woman echoed his thoughts when she explained about helping others through her support group and through the clothing drive at her church, "If somebody recognizes that maybe you could help somebody out and it's sort of uplifting. It makes you feel like you're something more than nothing." The doctor of another woman suggested tutoring or volunteering when she gave up teaching grade school following her diagnosis. "I'm still a teacher and that's great. Because I can do it I have great satisfaction, and the people are glad when I come. . . . It just makes me feel good to know that I can do things and people are responding to me. They aren't just doing it because they are being kind to me."

Taking a Proactive Stance

Taking a proactive stance occurred in a number of different ways. Some people with dementia use "energy efficiency" in managing their lives. One man explained: "Now, I can do one of two things. I can admit the fact that I've got a problem, moan about it, and groan about it, but it's not gonna make it any better. Therefore, I always consider myself as proactive. I say, how do you minimize it? So, I lay out the strategies and do the things that make me as efficient as I can be under the circumstances."

A 56-year-old man explained that since he has more energy in the morning, he does chores and activities requiring the most energy in the morning rather than in the afternoon, when he feels fatigued. For example, he found that when he attempted to accomplish more complicated tasks (be they cognitively complex or physically straining tasks, such as mowing the lawn) in the afternoon, he was far more vulnerable to disorganization and other symptoms of AD. This proactive stance allowed many of the people we interviewed to maintain control over parts of their lives. As one 67-year-old woman stated, "There are little tricks you learn. Once you get used to the idea that you're not a free agent anymore, there's lots of things you can work out to make life manageable and keep some independence."

Anticipatory Adaptation

Anticipating future needs allows persons with AD not only to become familiar with the next challenge but to begin to integrate new behavior. This anticipation helps the person adopt a realistic view of the disease, giving him or her a chance to plan and thus to exercise and maintain control. For example, one 61-year-old woman with early-onset AD stated: "It probably won't be much longer that I won't be able to drive. I'm very productive at the moment. . . . I'm doing what I can do because the day will come when I can't do anything." An 84-year-old woman shared, "I suspect that my ailment is going to get worse, and when it does, I'll have to live differently." She and her children are discussing plans for her to move closer to them and live in an assisted living facility.

Holistic Practices

Some people with AD reported enjoying learning new relaxation techniques, such as reiki, t'ai chi, meditation, yoga, and guided imagery. One 85-year-old woman attended a t'ai chi class at a local senior center twice a week. One man who practiced t'ai chi found that it had a profound calming effect on him, so much so that the teacher taped a video of the t'ai chi exercises so that he could use it on days when he was feeling very agitated.

Spirituality

For a number of the individuals we interviewed, their spiritual beliefs were a source of comfort and support, especially on their bad days. As one 73-year-old woman put it, "I can only go so far. This is all I can do, and I put it in someone's hands. It works for me. Believe in yourself and the doctors and a God and let go of your fears."

A woman with early-onset AD expressed those same thoughts when she explained, "I can't do anything on my own. God is always with me. I deal with what I can deal with and when I can't I say, 'Okay, here it is. You are going to be up all night anyway, go ahead and work it out.' My mom used to have a prayer. She really had a hard life raising all us 13 children. She use to say, 'Lord, I ask not for lighter burdens, just broader shoulders with which to bear.'"

Another woman shared, "You've got to believe that there's someone there to help you. . . . from the beginning I said, 'OK God, you gave me this, you've got to help me deal with it' and he said, 'OK, I'll help you out,' and he's been doing it, you know."

THUS, THE RANGE of positive coping behaviors employed by persons with early-stage AD, from acceptance and disclosure to taking a positive stance and spirituality, help these individuals to meet the challenges of living with dementia by increasing their resilience in the face of the external and internal stresses of AD. They provided them with a sense of control over a devastating illness, hope, and the will to continue the struggle of living.

Lessons Learned

Tables 9.1 and 9.2 show practice implications based on the positive coping strategies identified in the study. Table 9.1 recommends action steps that family members can take, and Table 9.2, action steps that health care professionals can take, to assist persons with AD in coping with the impact of the disease on their everyday lives. Both family members and health care professionals play an important role in encouraging and supporting people with early-stage AD in this process, which will help them adapt as successfully as possible to their disease, therefore promoting resilience.

Conclusion

This chapter advocates instilling a person-centered perspective into the stress and coping paradigm. Such a change enables persons with AD to be seen by others not as stressors or care receivers but as people with strengths and positive coping strategies that can be mobilized to give them the resilience they need to deal with the disease. The three research questions

Table 9.1. Ways for Family Members to Help Persons with AD Develop Positive Coping Strategies

Coping Strategy	Action Steps
Acceptance or ownership	• Secure accurate information on etiology of AD • Discuss these facts with the person with AD • Offer opportunities for counseling and support groups • Accept and own the fact that *your* family member has AD • Acknowledge that the person with AD can be a partner in making decisions
Disclosure: telling significant people	• Talk with the person with AD about sharing the diagnosis with family and friends • Anticipate out loud what any potential reactions may be and how to respond
Innovative techniques and use of technology	• Support the use by the person with AD of all tools and support systems, including beeping key chains, pocket digital tape recorders, electronic organizers, Internet support networks, etc. • Use e-mail to keep all family members apprised of the current situation. If a long-distance family member, use e-mail to stay in regular contact with the person with AD and/or a paid helper. • Use the Internet for family support networks and up-to-date information
Positive attitude or sense of self	• Focus on and reinforce the strengths of the person with AD • Work with the person with AD to compose a list of accomplishments in his or her life and then read it regularly • Accept that memory loss is a part of the *family's* life as well
Role relinquishment and replacement	• Don't take away roles/tasks the person with AD is still capable of performing • Assist in creating alternative and meaningful roles • Support the success of these roles • Be understanding of failures
Connection with past activities	• Assist in creating and exploring opportunities for using the lifelong skills or passions of the person with AD

Table 9.1. (*continued*)

Coping Strategy	Action Steps
Altruism	• Support the person with AD in volunteer activities in which that person feels that he or she is contributing and being appreciated • Address ways in which all family members can ensure success (e.g., transportation, joining in the activity if necessary)
Spirituality	• Try not to introduce the person with AD to "new" religious services that may have a contemporary approach (*comfort is derived from past practices*) • Provide support (e.g., transportation)
Using proactive skills	• Allow the person with AD to be involved in all levels of planning his or her future • Discuss the desires of the person with AD and arrange for a living will and a durable power of attorney for health care • *Use the competency of the person with AD*
Fluidity	• Understand and be aware that disorganized periods may occur in the midst of a good day • Be able to adapt to the needs of the person with AD as the disease changes
Anticipatory adaptation	• Encourage the person with AD to think ahead about inevitable lifestyle changes and how he or she can be in control of these changes, such as driving, living arrangements, etc. • Anticipate and negotiate situations when family members will need to intervene
Holistic practices	• Explore classes at local community centers and senior centers for both the person with AD and the family member

that guided this study are grounded in this perspective: What are the positive coping behaviors that people with early-stage AD use? How do these coping behaviors play a role in successful adaptation to living with AD? And what lessons can be learned from their experiences that would be helpful to persons with AD, family members, and health care professionals?

Table 9.2. Ways for Health Care Professionals to Help Persons with AD Develop Positive
Coping Strategies

Coping Strategy	Action Steps
Acceptance or ownership	• Assure the person with AD that he or she is not to blame for the disease • Assist in obtaining accurate information with hope • Allow time for questions and discussion of physician's recommendations • Provide opportunities and a safe environment for expression of feelings, including anger, guilt, blame, hopelessness, and humiliation • Make referrals to local chapter of the Alzheimer's Association for education and early-stage support groups
Disclosure: telling significant people	• Help the person with AD and his or her family to move toward acknowledgment of the disease • Follow *Fairhill Guidelines on Ethics of the Care of People with AD* (Post and Whitehouse 1995) • Suggest keeping a journal • Develop opportunities during appointments to practice new skills for talking about the disease
Innovative techniques and use of technology	• Supply information on Internet support networks and medical sites (i.e., ADEAR, National Alzheimer's Association) • Offer educational meetings and handouts on how to use these "tools" • Encourage use of tape recorder to record meetings with health care providers (where appropriate) so the person with AD can re-listen to information • Use conference calls with long-distance family members during meetings
Positive attitude or sense of self	• Assess and assist in identifying the strengths of the person with AD • Provide educational programs on discussion and development of positive coping strategies • Evaluate and treat for depression and/or anxiety
Role relinquishment and replacement	• Address feelings related to loss of career and/or social roles • Reframe loss as a relief and an opportunity, not a failure • Refer for possible inclusion in clinical drug trials

Table 9.2. (*continued*)

Coping Strategy	Action Steps
	• Provide opportunities for the person with AD to do meaningful volunteer work or join early-stage adult day care or clubs
Connection with past activities	• Discuss and design possible meaningful activities related to past that uses skills still present • Follow up on previous referral to Alzheimer's Association
Altruism	• Use the person with AD in educational programs as a panelist or speaker • Provide opportunities for the person with early-stage AD to mentor those newly diagnosed • Use persons with early-stage AD as volunteers at all levels of social-service programs—to help with mailings or general office work, or to act as hosts at educational programs • Help the person with AD identify and integrate new feelings of self-worth

Spirituality	• Understand that the person with AD may develop a greater connection with his or her spiritual roots and support this
	• Provide training for clergy of all denominations on topics such as:
	  –memory loss;
	  –what to expect; and
	  –how to provide comfort and support to the person with AD and the family throughout the course of the disease

Using proactive skills	• Treat the person with AD as a capable person and partner in the treatment planning process • Recommend the Alzheimer's Association Safe Return Program as a way to maintain and protect one's independence • Encourage the person with AD to take a proactive stance
Fluidity	• Caution the person with AD and family members that confused and/or disorganized moments or periods are possible on the "best of days" • Discuss ways of managing and regaining control after experiencing a stressful situation

(*Continued*)

Table 9.2. (*continued*)

Coping Strategy	Action Steps
Anticipatory adaptation	• Initiate discussions with the person with AD and the family on difficult topics to encourage proactive planning • Encourage the person with AD to think ahead about inevitable lifestyle changes and how he or she can be in control of these changes
Holistic practices	• Suggest alternative practices as complementary to medical treatment, including relaxation, t'ai chi, yoga, reiki, guided imagery, etc.

This chapter moves us closer to answering these questions. Listening to people with early-stage AD discuss their experiences in coping and adapting to the disease enabled us to identify twelve unique coping strategies that extend the knowledge in this area, strategies such as acceptance or ownership, disclosure, use of technology, positive attitude, role replacement and relinquishment, connection with past activities, altruism, spirituality, proactive skills, fluidity, anticipatory adaptation, and holistic practices. Using these coping behaviors gave people with AD some resilience to meet the challenges of living with this devastating disease. It provided them with some tools to gain a small measure of control over an ever-changing experience, which resulted in periods of hope, productivity, a sense of self-worth, and the ability to still be a contributing citizen. It allowed them to maintain meaningful lives. Based on the positive coping strategies, we were able to identify action steps that health care professionals and family members can follow to help people with AD live with this disease. But this chapter is above all a testimony to the strength, resilience, and courage of persons with AD who actively face this challenge and from whom we have much to learn about living.

ACKNOWLEDGMENTS

The research on which this chapter is based was supported in part by grants from the Cleveland Foundation and John Carroll University. The authors gratefully acknowledge the support and assistance of the Cleveland Area Alzheimer's Association.

REFERENCES

Aneshensel, C. S., J. T. Mullan, L. I. Pearlin, C. J. Whitlatch, and S. H. Zarit. 1995. *Profiles in caregiving: The unexpected career.* San Diego: Academic.

Bahro, M., P. Box, E. Silber, and T. Sunderland. 1995. Giving up driving in Alzheimer's disease: An integrative therapeutic approach. *International Journal of Geriatric Psychiatry* 10:871–74.

Bahro, M., E. Silber, and T. Sunderland. 1995. How do patients with Alzheimer's disease cope with their illness?: A clinical experience report. *Journal of the American Geriatrics Society* 43:41–46.

Cohen, D. 1991. The subjective experience of Alzheimer's disease: The anatomy of an illness as perceived by patients and families. *American Journal of Alzheimer's Care and Related Disease and Research*, May/June, 6–11.

Cohen, D., G. Kennedy, and C. Eisdorfer. 1985. Phases of change in the person with Alzheimer's Disease. *Journal of the American Geriatric Society* 32:11–15.

Cotrell, V., and R. Schulz. 1993. The perspective of the patient with Alzheimer's disease: A neglected dimension of dementia research. *Gerontologist* 33:205–11.

Downs, M. 1997. The emergence of the person in dementia research. *Aging and Society* 17:597–607.

Fazio, S., D. Seman, and J. Stansell. 1999. *Rethinking Alzheimer's care.* Baltimore: Health Professions Press.

Glaser, B., and A. Strauss. 1967. *The discovery of grounded theory.* Chicago: Aldine.

Harris, P. B., and G. J. Sterin. 1999. Insider's perspective: Defining and preserving the self of dementia. *Journal of Mental Health and Aging* 5:241–56.

Keady, J., and M. Nolan. 1994. Younger onset dementia: Developing a longitudinal model as the basis for a research agenda and as a guide to interventions with sufferers and carers. *Journal of Advanced Nursing* 19:659–69.

———. 1995a. IMMEL: Assessing coping responses in the early stages of dementia. *British Journal of Nursing* 4:309–14.

———. 1995b. IMMEL 2: Working to augment coping responses in early dementia. *British Journal of Nursing* 4:377–80.

Kitwood, T. 1990. The dialectics of dementia: With particular reference to Alzheimer's disease. *Aging and Society* 10:177–96.

———. 1993a. Person and process in dementia. *International Journal of Geriatric Psychiatry* 8:541–45.

———. 1993b. Towards a theory of dementia care: The interpersonal process. *Aging and Society* 13:51–67.

———. 1997. The experience of dementia. *Aging and Mental Health* 1:13–22.

Kitwood, T., and S. Benson. 1995. *The new culture of dementia care*. London: Hawker Publications.

Lazarus, R. S. 1966. *Psychological stress and the coping process*. New York: McGraw-Hill.

Lazarus, R. S., and S. Folkman. 1984. *Stress, appraisal, and coping*. New York: Springer.

Lyman, K. 1989. Bringing the social back in: A critique of the biomedicalization of dementia. *Gerontologist* 29:597–605.

McMillen, J. C. 1999. Better for it: How people benefit from adversity. *Social Work* 44:455–68.

Pearlin, L. I. 1989. The sociological study of stress. *Journal of Health and Social Behavior* 30:241–56.

Pearlin, L. I., M. A. Lieberman, E. G. Menaghan, and J. T. Mullan. 1981. The stress process. *Journal of Health and Social Behavior* 22:337–56.

Pearlin, L. I., J. T. Mullan, S. J. Semple, and M. M. Skaff. 1990. Caregiving and the stress process: An overview of concepts and their measures. *Gerontologist* 30:583–94.

Pearlin, L. I., and C. Schooler. 1978. The structure of coping. *Journal of Health and Social Behavior* 19:2–21.

Post, S. G., and P. J. Whitehouse. 1995. Fairhill guidelines on the ethics of the care of people with Alzheimer's disease: A clinical summary. *Journal of the American Geriatrics Society* 43:1423–29.

Snyder, L. 1999. *Speaking our minds: Personal reflections from individuals with Alzheimer's*. New York: Free Press.

Woods, R. T. 2001. Discovering the person with Alzheimer's disease: Cognitive, emotional, and behavioral aspects. *Aging and Mental Health* 5 (supplemental): S7–S16.

Part 3

Experiences with Formal Services

The Experience of People with
Dementia in Community Services

CHARLIE MURPHY

It gets you out of your home—to leave your four walls behind.
—Woman attending a day care center

Traditionally, community services for people with dementia have been seen as primarily offering respite to the family caregiver. Such services were a form of caretaking. The thinking was that since nothing could be done to alleviate the medical aspect of the dementia, nothing could be done at all. Consequently, the family caregivers and not the individual with dementia were seen as the main users of such services. Only the former's viewpoint was sought when such services were being evaluated. This picture has now changed dramatically. Services are acknowledging that the individual with dementia is the main recipient or user. Allied to this development is the recognition that people with dementia are well placed to comment on the services they receive.

This chapter looks at the experience of individuals with dementia in two service settings: a day care project and a befriending (friendly visiting) program. Both of these services operate in the central region of Scotland. As part of an overall evaluation of these two services, fifteen people with dementia were interviewed about the service they received. Among the issues examined in the day care study were why people attended; what they thought of specific activities offered at the center; and the benefits, if any, of attendance. In the study of the befriending service we examined the individual's understanding of the befriending relationship and the benefits, if any, of having a befriender. In both studies the responses of the individuals with dementia were compared with the responses of family caregivers, where relevant.

The chapter also includes discussion of some of the lessons learned in relation to the ethical and practical research issues involved in collecting the views of people with dementia about the services that they receive, as well as how such views might have an impact on service improvement. The implications of the findings for service delivery are also commented upon.

Background on the Two Service Evaluations

The day care project has been running since 1992. The idea for the service developed from a group of family caregivers and former caregivers in the Stirling area of Scotland. This predominantly rural area, popular with tourists, is approximately forty miles northwest of the capital, Edinburgh. A subsequent partnership between the local branch of Alzheimer Scotland Action on Dementia, the local Baptist church, and the social work department led to the establishment of the service as a resource for both family caregivers and people with dementia. The project was overseen by a management committee. That committee commissioned me to carry out the evaluation. The committee members remained directly involved in the design of the evaluation, deciding what they wanted to examine and measure.

It was decided that the evaluation would investigate the success of the project from the perspectives of the person with dementia (the individual member), the family caregiver, and outside agencies (i.e., professionals who had made referrals to the project). The perspective of the person with dementia, which is the main focus of this chapter, was gathered via two separate methods. First, the members were questioned directly in face-to-face interviews; nine members were interviewed for this evaluation. Second, an observational method called Dementia Care Mapping (DCM) (Kitwood and Bredin 1992), was used to see how members fared at the project.

The service started off as a drop-in location in the center of town for people with dementia and their family caregivers. In a café-like environment it offered access to advice and information, peer support for family caregivers, informal activities for the person with dementia (and the caregiver), and a respite opportunity for the caregiver if the person he or she cared for chose to remain at the center without the caregiver. In short, the center was designed to introduce people with dementia and family caregivers to the idea of formal support services in a nonthreatening manner. Over time the center has evolved into something more akin to a day center, although it has maintained much of the flexibility of the drop-in center. Members are not "expected" each week; family caregivers can still spend time at the center (and consequently feel more involved with, and included by, this service than with others that their relative receives); and a high ratio of workers to members has been maintained (roughly one to one).

The second evaluation study looked at a befriending (friendly visiting) service for individuals with dementia. Increasingly, services for people with dementia need to be more responsive to specific needs and tailored to the requirements of individuals. Service providers have to explore the use of more original models of service delivery. This program was an example of such an innovative, flexible response. The program covered a large, predominantly rural area and specifically targeted individuals with dementia. In this it was very unusual among befriending schemes—the only one of its kind in Scotland at the time. It had a part-time paid coordinator and twenty to thirty volunteers at any one time.

The demand for an evaluative study was sparked by the impending arrival of the hundredth referral to the program. Similar to the first study, this evaluation sought the views of service recipients, family caregivers, and professionals who had referred individuals to the service. A total of six service users were interviewed. As with the previous study, there was an observational aspect, although this was much smaller in scale and could not be as formalized as the DCM approach. Also, it was constrained by the one-to-one nature of the relationship. The main difference between the two methods was that volunteers (i.e., befrienders) were also interviewed for the befriending evaluation since it was felt that their role was central to the successful running of the program.

Although the two evaluation studies described above provided the core material for this chapter, three additional sources are referred to. The first is a small-scale survey of users of a day center in the Leith area of Edinburgh, Scotland, for which I acted as an adviser, referred to here as the Leith study. In this survey a community-education student placed at the Development Project, which managed the day center, interviewed eight users of the day center. The second source is a programmatic evaluation conducted by me. This evaluation examined a series of short-term reminiscence projects delivered in various settings across Scotland, three of which involved people with dementia. Seven people with dementia were interviewed at two day centers that hosted a reminiscence project, one in Glasgow and one in the south of Edinburgh. Finally, in October 1998 a major conference was held in Edinburgh for staff and volunteers at the area's twenty-plus dementia day centers in the voluntary sector. Two service users from a day center in North Edinburgh were interviewed at the conference about their experiences of services. Reference is made to some of their comments.

The Day Center

The first challenge in trying to interview the people with dementia who attended the center was to find someone to carry out the interviews who was both independent of the center and yet somehow familiar to the members. It was felt that familiarity would help the individuals with dementia to feel relaxed in what could have been a potentially threatening situation. Fortunately, a freelance arts worker who had previously done some freelance work at the center was available. She was very experienced in interviewing people with dementia for reminiscence work. It was decided to carry out the interviews at the center itself. Not only would this offer an immediate orientation cue to the interviewee but it would be less disruptive than scheduling interviews at members' homes. The interviews took place in a quiet room at the center on successive Thursdays over a three-week period. This arrangement allowed members a clear option to refuse—they could simply remain in the main day care area. At the same time, it gave the interviewer the option to try again in case the member had simply been too tired on the first occasion. On average, the interviews lasted forty-five minutes. All were tape-recorded, permission having been obtained from the individual in advance.

The interviews with members of the day center were carried out using a semistructured format with a small number of open-ended questions to initiate discussion. Nine members agreed to take part in the interviews, and three refused. The interviews attempted to address:

- why members attended the center;
- what they thought of the different activities that went on during their time at the center;
- whether members felt that attending the center was of any benefit to them; and
- how members would change the center.

The average age of those interviewed was 79.5 years, with the youngest aged 58 and the oldest, 91. All but one of the interviewees were female. The group included a florist, a nurse, a cashier, three factory workers, and three housewives. All those interviewed were in the early to middle stages of dementia; no specific diagnosis had been obtained. Seven interviewees had been attending the program on a weekly basis for over a year, while one male and one female attender had joined in the previous three months.

Members' Reasons for Attending

When asked why they attended the center, members gave a range of reasons. The most common response related to the stimulation offered, including some references to specific activities. More than half of those interviewed spoke about their need for stimulation: "Because it takes me away from the ordinary routine. I like doing different things."

The companionship of others and their enjoyment of being at the center also featured prominently, with nearly half of interviewees mentioning each of these reasons: "I enjoy meeting folk and listening to their conversation and sort of mixing it along with your own." One can only speculate on whom the speaker was alluding to when she said "with your own." Did she mean people of the same generation, people from the same social background, or was she acknowledging her own special needs resulting from her dementia?

Another member spoke more directly about such needs when he was asked why he attended. His words reveal a clarity of insight into his illness and the possible role that day care services can play for him: "Well, I started off, I didn't know what it was about or anything, and now I'm beginning to see what it is. The folk concerned, they know there's no betterness and they're making the best out of it, make it as good as you can, take things as they come. . . . The wife says the same thing, you want the company and folk in the same boat as you, sort of style."

Table 10.1. Members' Reasons for Attending
the Day Center ($N = 9$)

Reason for Coming	Number of Members
Company	4
Enjoyment	4
Stimulation	3
Activities	3
Getting out	2
Support	1

This member describes his initial confusion about coming to such a place, which must be common to many introduced to the concept of formal day care. He goes on to recognize the need for those working in such situations to maintain members' existing skills and to understand and accept the nature of the disability. He also appears to echo the comments of the previous interviewee about being "among your own" with his reference to "the same boat." This theme of service users' insight also arose at the Edinburgh conference referred to earlier. The male user who spoke about the day care he attended said, "It gives me what I want. . . . You meet people like myself. . . . It suits my temperament."

Table 10.1 summarizes the reasons the nine interviewees gave for attending the day center. The emphasis on companionship was reinforced by the results from the Leith study, where more than half of the respondents also spoke of the need for companionship. At the Edinburgh conference the female user who spoke described this graphically, "It gets you out of your home, to leave your four walls behind." Social isolation is not associated simply with advancing years. It can often be the result of the difficulties that friends and extended family have in coming to terms with a person's dementia. The consequence is a reduced social network.

The Family's Response

The question why members attend the center was also raised with family caregivers when they were interviewed for the evaluation. Their responses can be summarized as: activities/stimulation (5 caregivers), company (4), an outing (2), lunch (1), and security (1).

We can see that the family caregivers shared their relatives' grasp of their need for company and for stimulation. Interestingly, many family caregivers talked about "activities," yet this word was not used by most members. At the same time, family caregivers did not mention the "enjoyment" referred to by nearly half of the members. Could this disparity be because the members could not recall much detail about their time at the center? In some day care situations members complete daily diaries to take home, which then help family caregivers to understand the experience their relatives have had at the center that day. However, it is more likely that the lack of correspondence is related to caregivers' anxieties and feelings of guilt about relinquishing care. Such feelings might make it difficult to believe that their relatives actually enjoy being at the center.

Notice also that two caregivers focused on caretaking aspects of the day care—providing lunch and providing security. The center's "caretaking" function was acknowledged by only one member. And his lucid comments above—"make it as good as you can"—emphasized the facilitatory nature of the caretaking role: care workers (volunteers) were *enabling* him to do the best that he could, not doing "for" him.

Members' Verdicts on the Activities Program

In talking about the activities program the interviewer used a checklist of activities to prompt the members' opinions about the program. This list included items that some might not regard as formal activities, such as lunch, afternoon tea, and "just chatting," since the principle of seeing everything as an activity was being emphasized (Archibald and Murphy 1995).

The responses to the interviewer's mention of specific activities were categorized as positive, neutral, or negative based on whether the respondent spoke positively about the activity, simply acknowledged that it took place, or made a negative comment about it. Also, there were some non-responses—no discernible reaction to the mention of an activity.

Generally speaking, the informal activities generated the most positive reactions. These included things such as lunch, singing, reminiscing, just chatting, and afternoon tea—activities a person might be expected to take part in in his or her own home. More structured activities, such as dominoes, quizzes, craft activities, and drawing and painting, fared less well. The one exception to this was exercising to music, which was the second most popular activity overall.

The individual comments on specific activities are most illuminating. The informal activities are considered first. About lunch and afternoon tea there were no negative responses at all. Among the positive comments was the following reflection on the day center's providing lunch. "That [lunch] gets people together, and the food is pretty good, and I've never heard any complaints about it." The day at the center starts with lunch, hence the comment about "getting people together" seems particularly relevant. Also, this sentiment can be related back to the earlier references to "company" among the major reasons people attended the center.

Two separate comments on "just chatting" reveal the power behind a central aspect of day care that could too easily be taken for granted: "I think talking to somebody else is a great thing" and "It's nice to have a chat with somebody for a wee while. When you live [by] yourself, you are glad to talk to anybody." That approximately half of individuals with dementia in the United Kingdom who live in the community are living alone provides an important context for these remarks.

Of all the activities listed, singing was rated the most popular, while reminiscing was the only informal activity to have a negative comment made about it. One female member stated, "I don't bother about that now." Perhaps this was a defensive statement, made because she had difficulty recalling even longer-term memories, or it may be an acknowledgment of her failing mental abilities.

Most of the formal activities received at least one negative comment. Craft activities were the least welcomed by the people surveyed. "It was quite interesting, but you needed somebody to guide you" and "I tried that . . . but I was never very good at it, no[t] really" were two of the comments. One senses that these two individuals were being confronted with tasks they are no longer able to perform and that they did not want to highlight their dependence on other people. A comment on old-time dancing was more direct: "No, I'm not too great at the old-time dancing. I haven't the puff."

Pressure to perform when doing activities such as the above seemed to make some people uncomfortable. As one respondent put it, "I must have my mind clear to do the thing right. I don't like pretending to do it, I like to do it right."

At the same time, members can gain a real sense of achievement from doing an activity with an end product: "I really do love baking" and "I love painting. These are things that I'm really interested in, painting." The conclusion one is drawn to is the need for activities programs to be determined by the needs of individuals, not by those of the group. It can be too easy to impose a group "ethos" on the activities program and not notice, or not care, that certain individuals are not gaining from the experiences. The above quotations should caution practitioners against such a uniform approach.

The most popular formal activity was exercising to music. One member remarked humorously, "I think it does me good sometimes because it takes the wrinkles out of my bones." Another showed insight into the skills of the volunteers and careworkers during this activity: "They're making it so everybody can do it." Thus, recognition is given to the range of abilities of those attending the center.

Taking part in quizzes and playing dominoes are two very common activities in dementia day care centers. This survey elicited some polarized responses to these activities, particularly with respect to quizzes, for example, "I think they are quite good for you because they keep your mind up enough to want to think about them. I think that's good for you" and "Well, you don't get everybody with those things in their head."

One fascinating reflection on the activities program came from a woman who talked about taking part in the activities to please the workers: "I would do anything like that if they wanted me to do it. . . . They're doing things to help you, so why not us try to help them?" Thus the notion of the caregiver and the cared for at day care gets very nicely turned on its head. How many careworkers would entertain the idea that members are helping them?

In summary, the most popular activities were singing, exercises, reminiscing, and just chatting. Here popular activities are defined as those to which more than half of the respondents responded favorably.

Did Members Feel That Attending the Center Was of Any Benefit to Them?

Whether members felt that attending the center benefited them was a more overarching question than how members felt about individual activities. Eight out of the nine members interviewed said that attending the center benefited them. One woman responded positively: "Oh yes, definitely. I have had depression . . . and I feel that it's taking me out and you sort of haven't time to think, you're getting away from being miserable. It's good, it bucks you up a bit."

The man who previously gave "making the best out of it" as the reason he attended the center summarized the benefits thus: "I feel that it is doing something different because it's other people and they don't take it the same way as your own family takes it." He appears to be referring to the fresh approach that volunteers and careworkers can adopt since they do not deal with the illness twenty-four hours a day. Again there is the insight into the individual's need for help and family members' need for a break. This insight emerged in the Leith study, in which one man commented that he enjoyed attending "because sometimes it is a break for my wife."

Overall, the members described the benefits as follows: raising self-esteem; having something to look forward to or prepare for in the weekly routine; feeling good inside; feeling comfortable; overcoming depression; combating loneliness; and being free to be oneself without the expectations or restrictions of family. The one dissenting voice came from a female attender, "Well, it is supposed to [benefit me]. We'll have to wait and see if it comes." Unfortunately, she did not elaborate on this statement.

Comparison with Findings from Dementia Care Mapping (DCM)

The evaluation was also able to put the responses of the interviewees in some context through the DCM exercise (Kitwood and Bredin 1992), which was carried out to supplement the interviews. Essentially, DCM attempts to measure the extent to which the individual with dementia maintains a sense of well-being while in a formal care setting (in this case, day care). One of the statistics that the DCM tool produced at that time was an "average individual care value" (now renamed "individual well/ill-being value") for each client being observed. This value was averaged from care values assessed for these individuals over a large number of five-minute time periods. These individual averages were classified as "low," "medium," or "high" according to the respective DCM categories of "fair," "good," and finally "very good" combined with "excellent." Those members of the day center who declined to be interviewed were included in the mapping exercise, although three of the interviewees were not present during the map-

Table 10.2. Comparison of Interview Responses with
Dementia Care Mapping Scores ($N = 9$)

	DCM Score (Average Individual Care Value)		
Interview Responses	Low	Medium	High
Positive	0	0	5
Negative	0	1	0
Refused	1	2	0

ping. These three all responded positively to the question about benefiting from attending the day center.

Table 10.2 shows that those who did not score highly in the mapping exercise either declined to take part in the interviews or did not feel that they benefited from day care. At the same time, those who scored well in the mapping all felt that they benefited from day care. This indicates that perhaps it ought not to be assumed that those who refused to be interviewed would have given similar answers to those who were interviewed. Were those who declined to be interviewed commenting on the service by their refusal to take part? In DCM work, it is often the people who have the lowest care value scores with whom workers have greatest difficulty communicating. Therefore, they are left alone and not engaged with or included in activities, with the result they experience less stimulation than the others. Fortunately, the DCM tool is one of "developmental evaluation." It allows the mapper to address such issues when feedback is given to workers. The feedback session then usually involves developing strategies to increase the inclusion and involvement of those with lower care value scores.

How Would Members Change the Center?

For a variety of reasons, it can be difficult to get users of community care services to suggest changes to the service they receive. In this instance, this task was approached in three different ways. Members were asked directly if there were any improvements or changes that they would make; they were also asked if there was anything they would like to do instead of attending the center; and finally they were asked whether they had any advice for the workers.

Generally these questions provoked similar positive responses to those about the benefits of attending. Seven people expressed a general contentment with the center and said they had no wish to do anything else instead. One of these elaborated on this, saying that he preferred the center to other centers or clubs because "the other clubs, they're just sitting." This attender was implying that nothing happened in the other clubs that he attended.

The issue of free choice, both in attending the center and in participating in the activities program, was raised as a result of these questions. Two people mentioned how much they appreciated not being forced to attend the center or to participate in specific activities, saying "The ones that's in here, they are all helpful and if there's something you can't do, they don't force you" and "I think to me it's good that you people . . . you've not forced me to come . . . but realized that I needed this place." Similarly, in the reminiscence evaluation referred to earlier a woman at the day center in the south of Edinburgh talked about how much she appreciated being "asked" to join the reminiscence group.

Most of the advice that members said they would offer to workers was along the lines of "Keep up the good work." One member, referring to how much she enjoyed the various activities, also mentioned her desire to be allowed to help with the jobs at the center (e.g., drying the dishes): "If you don't mind, I want to help because I feel I must be doing something." This was a particularly striking comment, as the center did miss opportunities to involve the members in activities of daily living, such as setting or clearing tables. This can sometimes be the case when volunteer helpers are involved, as it can be difficult to instill in them concepts of "doing with" rather than "doing for."

One suggestion that was not directly made by any interviewee but arose through the process of these interviews was the option of formal one-to-one time to support the emotional needs of the members. During the course of the interviews several members talked to the interviewer about other, personal things in their lives. This may have been prompted by the intimate one-to-one atmosphere induced by the interview process. A few of those interviewed shed tears and seemed to feel better after the chat that accompanied the interview itself. The provision of a simple, unobtrusive way to facilitate this sort of exchange was one of the recommendations of the final

evaluation report. It was felt that this would be valued as it might open people up to deep sharing and emotional expression. The impression given to
the interviewer was that many members would not ask for "counseling" as
such but would appreciate the opportunity to share their concerns informally.

The Befriending Service

A befriending program traditionally matches up a user with an individual
volunteer based on some common background or particular interests expressed by the user. In Britain such programs are becoming more common,
especially as government policy places more emphasis on continuing to
care for people in the community and on such community services being
driven by what individuals need (Dean and Goodlad 1998).

This befriending program is unusual in that it was established exclusively for people with dementia. The Scottish Befriending Development
Forum reports that it is the only such program among ninety-plus member
programs. The program has been in operation since 1994, and during the
evaluation it received its hundredth referral. The program is run by a voluntary management committee made up of former caregivers, representa-
tives from the social work department, and from Alzheimer Scotland Action on Dementia. There is a part-time paid coordinator, and there are
twenty to thirty friendships at any one time. The program covers a predominantly rural area containing one small town and some large villages.

Two major challenges face such a befriending program. First, it is difficult to recruit and match up befrienders over such a large rural area; in particular, it can be difficult to recruit male volunteers. Feedback to befrienders from service users (or, more accurately, the lack of it) is the second
challenge facing such programs. Often those being befriended may not be
able to communicate to the befriender what they did together the previous
week. Thus, volunteers' sense of contribution may be undermined. Two examples from the befriender program are presented below, followed by the
evaluation findings.

Case Examples

Jenny lives on her own. She is 85 years old and has mild dementia. Her
physical health is very good. She previously did a lot of entertaining and

socializing; these are the things that are most important and most familiar to her. For Jenny, the befriending relationship is about her hosting the befriender for morning coffee. The befriender visits every Friday morning. Jenny will lay out an elegant tray of tea or coffee and biscuits for her visitor. Their conversation covers many topics, and they talk about the past in a general way, reminiscing about countries visited and interesting people encountered. Jenny was keen to emphasize that they do not gossip. The visits seem to echo familiar occasions for Jenny; she was accustomed to such visits and consequently felt at ease during them. At the same time, the befriender accepted her role as guest, so Jenny poured the tea, found the sugar, and so on.

George's relationship with his befriender revolved around walking. Walking—indeed, exercise generally—had always been an important part of George's life, as he had been a professional sportsman. However, his wife could not go on walks with him due to the deterioration in her own physical health. George was 69 years old and had moderate dementia. He still retained his athletic appearance from his sporting days. George's befriender was a retired outdoor-pursuits leader from the nearby village. Together they walked through the forest beside George's home, along with the befriender's two dogs. The walks gave George many positive experiences. George and his befriender jointly gave directions to other walkers they met ("we helped them," George commented during his interview); George called the befriender's dogs by clapping his hands. George seemed to have gained much from the social nature of the walk and the encounter with other people along the route. The walks had a comradely nature, as George advised the befriender on the best ground to walk on. Also, the links with his sports training seemed important for George. Without a befriender, George might have been denied access to such experiences and feelings.

The Sample

I was responsible for the interviews in this evaluation. Unlike in the previous day care evaluation, there was not a key individual who was familiar with the service users since befriending is by nature a more private activity. Ten befriendees were selected randomly for interview from the list of all current befriendees. Eventually six of these were interviewed by me. Two of the "refusals" were initiated by the persons' befrienders. In the first instance this was because the user had a severe hearing impairment and became very agitated when any new person entered her house. In the second instance the befriender thought that the person would have no recollection of the befriending visits. This was also the reason one woman vetoed her husband's being interviewed. The final "refusal" raised an interesting issue: the relative reported that her mother became quite distressed at the thought that she was being *befriended*.

Four of the six interviewees were female. Both of the men who were befriended regularly left their house as part of the visit, whereas this was the case for only two of the women, though not as frequently as for the men. Half of those interviewed were 65 to 70 years old, while the remainder were in their mid-eighties. Two interviewees were in the mild stages of dementia, and four were described as moderate. There was a broader range of social classes in this group than in the day care group, with one middle- to upper-class woman, as well as a teacher and a nurse. One woman had been receiving her weekly befriending visits since the scheme started, more than three years previously. The majority had been taking part from one to two years.

Needs

Only four of the six users who were interviewed articulated needs. Two interviewees found it difficult to think of their needs; for example, one said, "I can't say. What would I need?" The remainder spoke of things they were *not* able to do or other restrictions, a sense of things being missing until the befriender came. "There was a time when I was going out. I'm not part of the world now," said one woman, who seemed to be talking about a dislocation from society. She also felt that she could not call on her family, or perhaps she did not want to: "I have got my own, but they can't always be at your beck and call as it were." Thus, her need seemed to be someone to call on besides her immediate family. This recalls the comment made by one of the male interviewees in the other evaluation that an advantage of day care was that it gave him and his family time apart.

The remaining three users spoke of varying needs for occupation. "I wasn't lonely. . . . I'm here and I have nothing to do," said one woman, who went on to say that she likes people—"I like people. I always have"—perhaps indicating that having company was a way to have "something to do." Another user spoke of his need for company in a more qualified way. "Lots of things I'll not get to do so I can scrub them out. . . . I can blether away, but I'm a wee bit wary." This man seems to be referring to things that he is no longer allowed to do because of his dementia. The second sentence seems to indicate that he enjoys talking but that he is apprehensive, perhaps because he recognizes his failing abilities due to his illness. Hence the need to be with someone that he feels he can trust.

For the final user, the professional sportsman, George, referred to earlier, it was a more specific need: for exercise. "The nights weren't too good before [the befriender] came, I was out on my own walking myself. . . . I don't do any exercise at all in the house." The first half of his sentence is probably a reference to what others might refer to as wandering.

Benefits from the Friendship

All six interviewees talked about beneficial aspects of "company." Their comments ranged from "It was company. . . . We talked away at one another" to "You've got someone who's interested in your well-being, it gives you a wee boost." One interviewee, Jenny, attached much importance to the nature of the conversations she had with her befriender: "Not much gossip, that's me. . . . [We] speak intelligently about intelligent things." Some people had greater recollection of what they did during their time with their befriender than others had. Also, some were able to recollect more if the interview took place soon after the befriender's visit.

Four interviewees noted that the befriender helped them to get out of the house, either for a walk or for a drive in the car. Another specifically mentioned that the befriender massaged her arm during visits. Two interviewees talked in extensive detail about what they got from the relationship. One female user replied: "They have time to listen to all your wee troubles. . . . You feel they are interested and want to listen. . . . She takes me out nice little runs . . . have a seat and a talk, and also the scenery is so lovely—it really is a treat to go—it is so nice. . . . She brings me wee titbits [food] and I enjoy them. . . . She has been my life line definitely—just the feeling that she is there even." This quotation reveals someone made to feel special through the relationship, both in material terms and in terms of emotional support. This woman, who certainly saw herself as a service recipient, described the overall program thus: "When I need help to feel alright, this is where I see the befrienders." She emphasizes here the therapeutic and supportive benefits of having a befriender.

A male interviewee who spoke more extensively said: "He [the befriender] just puts you at your ease. . . . He has got a knack for it, and that sort of helps you a bit. . . . He kind of tries . . . if he is there, you are alright; when he goes away you can do the opposite. Put it this way: I'm not very good—if he came in here just now, he would come in and say something . . . that's it . . . he just puts you at your ease. . . . We've just got to get together and try and do it. . . . You don't need to go places, but it's nice to get a bit of fresh air. . . . It gets me out of the house; . . . to get me to be the same."

This is the user who spoke earlier about "being wary." Here he seems to be acknowledging the ways his befriender helps him in social occasions, as well as welcoming the opportunities to get out and enjoy the fresh air. The phrase "get me to be the same" is a fascinating one, as it is open to various interpretations. Is the individual with dementia saying that he should be the same as the befriender, as everyone else, or as he was before his dementia? This was the only individual who was also interviewed in the earlier day care study, where he used the expression "making the best of it," which suggests that the third explanation—getting him to be the same as he was—is the most plausible.

A key factor in the responses was the emphasis on the relationships being two-way. In three of the interviews, direct and indirect references were made to the contribution of the person being befriended. One person talked about being an independent woman and not liking to be dependent. The befriending relationship seemed to appeal to her sense of remaining in control; it was a shared experience. She was not, for example, going to day care to be looked after. Indeed, when this woman commented on the program as a whole, she reflected: "Good that it happens. Some people [are] too shy or too withdrawn to get company." Thus, she viewed the program almost as an introduction agency, certainly not something that was being "done" to her. Her viewpoint is further reinforced by the befriender's comments when asked about what she got out of the befriending relationship. The volunteer stated that it was the best conversation that she had all week!

In the other two cases in which the users spoke of a two-way relationship, they talked about things that the *befriender* got out of the relationship or that they had given to the befriender. For one, it was the simple fact that they both watched a television program that was a favorite of the befriender. For the other, George, it was that he had introduced the befriender to a new place to go walking. "He just knows it since he came up with me." Irrespective of the accuracy of these comments, they do point up a need for the person receiving the service to have a sense of "contribution" to the relationship.

Lessons Learned

Ethical and Practical Considerations in Interviewing People with Dementia

In interviewing potentially vulnerable service users about services, the most important balance to achieve is that between intrusion and data collection (McConkey 1996). Those carrying out such work should be prepared to postpone the interview if necessary. The data collection ought to remain secondary to the well-being of the individual with dementia. Therefore, any sign of distress should be a signal to the interviewer to consider postponing the interview. The interviewer may need to offer high levels of reassurance and support to users who cannot remember words or have difficulties in expressing themselves. Relationship building is more important than asking questions. On one occasion I left an interviewee's house knowing very little about her views on the service but a considerable amount about her life story: how she met her husband, where she worked during the war, where her granddaughter had gone on holiday. I did not consider this interview a failure.

The ethos of avoiding intrusion can be supported in practice, first by serious consideration of the consent issue. Both the letter and the spirit of consent need to be observed. Although the individual with dementia may have given formal consent, perhaps in the way that it can be hard for some older people to say "no," it may become clear once the interview starts that he or she is unhappy. Applying the spirit of consent here, the interviewer might read the nonverbal communication as a withdrawal of consent.

There are a number of practical decisions to make, such as who might conduct the interviews and where these can take place. In selecting an interviewer a balance must be struck between independence and familiarity. The former is more conducive to receiving critical opinions, while the latter can be especially important for ensuring that the individual feels secure and comfortable. Whoever is chosen, it must be someone with an understanding of dementia, someone who will not pursue answers to questions when the individual with dementia is obviously distressed, someone who will not "correct" the individual. The ideal environment is not threatening to the person, is free of distractions, and has some connection to the subject of the evaluation (sometimes called *immediacy*). In the reminiscence-program evaluation some of the interviews had to take place away from the place where the reminiscence session had taken place. Two of the three interviewees for whom this was the case specifically stated that they could not remember details. At the same time, it can be difficult to retain immediacy and avoid distractions. A final factor is having a venue that allows the person to leave if he or she needs to (i.e., an open door). Table 10.3 lists other key issues that need to be considered.

Final Thoughts on Interviewing People with Dementia

Before getting started with the interviews, it is prudent to anticipate certain situations that might arise. In the day care evaluation many of the day-center members told the interviewer that they welcomed the opportunity for one-to-one time with her. The project agreed to try to make available such more intimate opportunities. Similarly, the external evaluator may be asked by the person or the family caregiver about additional services. Are there channels of communication to refer such issues back to the appropriate people? Additionally, for those situations in which the interviews will take place at the home of the individual with dementia, interviewers need to think about the involvement that the family caregiver will want or will have. On one occasion, in particular, the family caregiver (spouse) frequently wanted to make her comments about the service in question during the interview with the service user. She may have been offering her own perspective, or she may have been giving her interpretation of her husband's perspective. Has the evaluation made provision to ask family caregivers for their views separately? If so, this could be helpful in explaining to family caregivers why the interview in question is purely about the individual with dementia.

Along with the actual interviewing of service users, it is necessary to reflect on other ways to "hear the user's perspective." It was shown earlier how the Dementia Care Mapping method was used as an additional way to understand the perspective of the person with dementia at the day center.

Table 10.3. Issues to Consider in Interviewing People with Dementia

Word or phrase to use to describe the service being evaluated	Users may refer to the service by a variety of different names. For example, it may be the name of the building or the day of the week that the day care takes place. Many of the people that were interviewed for the befriending evaluation were not aware that they were part of a befriending program; for one woman this information caused her distress. Some identified the service simply in terms of the person who befriended them.
Prompts or cues for the person with dementia	This applies especially to interviews taking place away from the subject being evaluated, with a consequent loss of immediacy. Photographs from day care have proved useful as a memory aid.
Preferred time of day	Knowledge of when the individual functions best can help to ensure greater participation. Also, the interview time should not disrupt any routines.
Information from other sources	There may be factual information that can be collected from, for example, attendance records, which will obviate the need to gather such information from the individual with dementia. In the befriending study the befriender could specify the different types of outing that he or she shared with the individual with dementia so that the user would not have to recall such details. Essentially these two studies have sought the users' *views* (i.e., their opinions, not their recall of factual information).
Useful advance information	What can be found out about the service user's use of the project in advance to help the interviewer? For example, knowing something about the things that a befriender and befriendee do together may help you to interpret a tangential reference in the interview.
Pilot the instrument	In the befriending interviews less than 50 percent of the questions on the original schedule were used eventually.
Recording method	A tape recorder is ideal, as it allows the interaction to be natural and the interviewer to be more directly responsive. Permission should be sought. One befriendee, Jenny, refused, arguing that the subsequent transcription would highlight her "poor grammar." If the interviewer has to write during the interview, he or she should schedule free time immediately after each interview for expanding the notes.

The other main alternative to hearing the user's views is to use a proxy. The proxy view may be useful in supplementing the factual information gathered. However, the day care study also illustrated how family caregivers, when serving as proxies, can miss aspects of the viewpoint of the individual with dementia. None of the family caregivers identified "enjoyment" as a reason why the relative attended day care, whereas four out of nine users did.

Clinical Considerations

The material referred to in this chapter confirms that individuals with dementia can comment on community services. The quotations should show practitioners that individuals with dementia are not passive recipients of care; they are experiencing it and have views on it. At the same time, the limitations of these studies must also be acknowledged. Both of the main evaluations took place in well-run services. Also, a certain amount of interpretation was necessary. Nevertheless, specific points can be drawn from the comments in the two main evaluations and from the subsidiary sources.

• *People with dementia can reflect at length on their need for support despite their illness.* In these studies, what allowed people to express their needs was a combination of making a generous amount of time available, offering individual attention, and having a sympathetic listener. Often it can seem more convenient for the staff to assume that individuals with dementia have little or no insight. Insight implies some understanding of the situation, and this in turn entails the capacity to make choices. If the person has little insight, then the staff might feel that they can get by with offering limited choices. As with all disabilities, the maintenance of remaining skills is important. This involves recognizing people with dementia as individuals and not grouping everyone together under the dementia banner.
• *Some people with dementia welcome being among people who are in similar situations.* One can only speculate on the importance for people with dementia to recognize that they are not alone, that others are having similar experiences. Staff can sometimes miss out on the conversations that service recipients have among themselves, where, certainly in the early

stages of dementia, there is the potential for peer support. Such potential should be encouraged by staff. Witness too the rise in formal support
groups for people in the early stages of dementia.

• *Interviewees welcomed the opportunity to socialize in an inviting unstructured environment that lessened their social isolation.* Workers in
community projects may underestimate the benefits they provide simply through offering a place where people can meet others. The activities for individuals with dementia in the day care setting that gained
most uniform acclaim were those more normal activities, for example,
chatting, singing, and reminiscing. Commentators in dementia care
speak of a decreasing social circle for both individuals with dementia and
their family caregivers as many friends and family "cope" with the problem through avoidance of contact. Transport, a comfortable environment, refreshments, and time for normal socializing behavior all contribute to an attractive setting for mixing with others.

• *The interviewees from the day care setting liked being able to decide for themselves whether to take part in activities programs.* The *option* to be a specta-
tor at a given activity is often ignored in day care settings. Many people
previously may have taken more pleasure from observation than from
participation. Also, forced participation in a particular activity may
highlight the things that the person can no longer achieve.

• *While interviewees talked about the need to be doing or helping, allied to this
was a need to do the thing "right."* What measure of success do staff have
for tasks that members may carry out at day care? Compensating for disability is one criterion. However, where do the individual's own standards for achievement fit in? Allowance must be made for *insight* from
the individual with dementia that he or she may not be carrying out a
particular activity the way he or she would like, that is, according to his
or her internal standards.

• *Some interviewees were conscious of the positive role that community services could play in providing respite for their family caregiver.* Again, this
challenges practitioners on their understanding of the insight that individuals with dementia might have into both their situation and that of
the person(s) looking after them. In another day care project with which
I am involved, some members have commented on their spouse being
left at home while they have an opportunity to get out—to the day center. Such observations were partly responsible for the subsequent estab-

lishment of a monthly "companions club," where members and their spouses' socializing together was supported.

• *Many service users with dementia do not desire to be purely recipients, and this seemed more marked in the one-to-one relationships of the befriending service.* All of us, persons with dementia included, can derive positive feelings from doing things for others, from being the giver or helper in a relationship. Individuals with dementia do not want simply to have things done for them. How can we promote opportunities for individuals with dementia to be givers? We must begin by recognizing the individuality of the person with the illness. Life-story work can be an important tool in developing this recognition (Murphy and Moyes 1997). Life-story work allows for the recording of individuals' likes and dislikes, past history, and particular skills and talents. For example, someone who had been a florist may still be able to direct staff in arranging flowers for a display even though her disabilities may prevent her from making up the display herself. Life-story work thereby points to ways that people with dementia themselves can "give." Allied to recognizing this individuality is building on their remaining skills.

Conclusion

Acknowledging that hearing the users' voice can be done within services does place an onus on staff working with individuals with dementia to be *open* to hearing these views (Murphy 1999). Staff also need to recognize the individuality of the people they work with. This could form part of the staff induction training. Staff can support one another in this process, for example, by sharing strategies that have proved successful in helping an individual to communicate. Ultimately this should make staff's work easier, although paradoxically more difficult in that one must discard the preconception of dealing with a homogeneous group. For all of us working in the field of dementia care, though, listening to the views of users entails an implicit commitment to take action and responsibility to provide more person-centered care.

REFERENCES

Archibald, C., and C. Murphy. 1995. *Not "them and us"—simply us!* Stirling, Scotland: Dementia Services Development Centre.

Dean, J., and R. Goodlad. 1998. *Supporting community participation? The role and impact of befriending.* Brighton: England: Pavilion.

Kitwood, T., and K. Bredin. 1992. A new approach to the evaluation of dementia care. *Journal of Advanced Health Nursing Care* 1 (5): 41–60.

McConkey, R, ed. 1996. *Innovations in evaluating services for people with intellectual disabilities.* Chorley, England: Lisieux Hall.

Murphy, C. 1999. Commentary. *International Journal of Geriatric Psychiatry* 14:131–32.

Murphy, C., and M. Moyes. 1997. Life story work. In *State of the art in dementia care*, ed. M. Marshall, 149–53. London: Centre for Policy on Ageing.

11

Volunteerism

Contributions by Persons with Alzheimer's Disease

JANE STANSELL

Volunteering makes me aware that I can still help others, despite what I have.
It keeps Alzheimer's from taking over our lives.
—Annette, a 72-year-old retired real-estate agent

Persons with AD are often described by professionals and the public in terms of their deficits and need for care rather than in terms of their abilities and skills. Many of these widely held negative perceptions of persons with AD cause distress for those with the illness. Being a burden to others is a frequently cited concern of older people, especially people in the early stages of AD. Perhaps because so much research and public discussion about caregiving has focused on the burden and stress experienced, it has become generally accepted that persons with AD are a burden to their families and that the cost of their care is a burden to society. This belief of the general public is also held by persons with AD, who often tell clinicians that they wish they could "ease the burden" for their spouses or children. They seem to have accepted the notion that since they have AD, they are, or will be, a burden to their families. Possibly the best-known expression of this feeling can be found in former President Ronald Reagan's "Open Letter to the American People," published in newspapers across the country in November 1994, in which he expressed concern about the difficulty his illness will cause for his wife, Nancy.

Despite these sincere concerns about being a burden as the disease pro-

gresses, persons with AD do not define themselves by their illness; they normalize the symptoms they experience and express the desire to continue
their lives as usual. Indeed, most persons with AD continue their usual activities until the symptoms of the illness interfere with their ability to participate in their customary ways. Among the activities they continue with
are volunteering and helping others, informally or in organized programs.

Volunteerism is an important part of the lives of many people, and the
desire to help others in this way does not diminish with the diagnosis of
AD. As one person with AD said, "It is a great feeling to be able to help somebody else, despite what we have." Having the opportunity to provide real
assistance to others promotes feelings of usefulness instead of feelings of
uselessness and burdensomeness. The personal satisfaction inherent in volunteerism is bolstered by the public recognition of one's contributions by
community agencies. In addition, volunteerism provides the opportunity
to be not only productive but part of the normal life of a community. This
focus on abilities and contributions, rather than on one's disease and limitations, also promotes a feeling of wellness rather than one of illness for a
person with AD.

However, for many persons with AD independent volunteer activities
are not possible. The symptoms of the illness make it difficult to make the
necessary contacts and the arrangements to get to the volunteer location.
Therefore, structuring opportunities for persons with AD to continue or re-
new life patterns of volunteerism should be an integral component of any
program for them, especially early in the illness, when they still retain many
skills.

This chapter focuses on the ability of persons with AD to make real and
needed contributions in their communities. After an overview of volunteerism and the elderly, I describe a program that provides volunteer opportunities for persons with AD, followed by a description of the reactions
of the group's participants and a discussion of lessons learned.

Volunteerism and Older Adults

Scholars and researchers have recognized that volunteering can serve a
central purpose in one's life. Victor Frankl (1984) contends that "man's
search for meaning is the primary motivation in his life," that a person's
values and ideals are a driving force in his or her life (105). While volun-

teerism may not in itself provide a purpose or meaning in a person's life, it can be a way for people to act on the values and ideals that are meaningful to them (Crist-Houran 1996). Volunteering has been found to provide opportunities to act on one's beliefs about the importance of helping others, to learn about one's self and the world in which one lives, and to feel useful and good about oneself (Okum, Barr, and Herzog 1998).

The abundant literature on volunteerism by older people shows that participating in this type of activity benefits them. Weinstein and Xie (1995) found that retirees who volunteered more than ten hours per week scored significantly higher on a Purpose for Life Test than those who volunteered fewer than ten hours per week. According to Herzog and House (1991), "The most useful strategy for facilitating health and well-being among older people is to provide opportunities for productive involvement that permit them to tailor their participation according to their existing health limitations" (54). Brim (1988) contended that the processes that underlie the maintenance of feelings of usefulness and well-being require behaviors and activities that permit older people to continue viewing themselves as successful in their daily endeavors. A study of Senior Volunteers by Marriot's Senior Living Services found that while the main reason for volunteering was to help others (83%), feeling useful or productive was the second most frequently given reason (65%) (Marriot Senior Living Services 1991). Volunteerism is also a continuation of life interests for many people; in 1990, 41 percent of all people over the age of 65 worked as volunteers for a wide variety of organizations (Chambre 1993).

Interestingly, Richardson and Kilty (1991) found that volunteering can help persons adjust to critical life events and can mitigate some of the stresses related to retirement and widowhood. Even more importantly, volunteerism has been found to validate the volunteer's perception that he or she is a competent person (Herzog et al. 1998). A meta-analysis of thirty-seven independent studies about older volunteers confirmed the finding of earlier studies that the volunteer's sense of well-being was significantly enhanced by the volunteer experience. In fact, 70 percent of the people in these studies reported enjoying a "greater quality of life" than the average nonvolunteer (Wheeler, Gorey, and Greenblatt 1998). However, it has been found that the perception of poor health often acts as a barrier to volunteering and that there is a strong relationship between perceived good health and volunteering (Warburton, Le Srocque, and Rosenman 1998).

Volunteerism and the Person with AD

Given the many potential benefits of volunteering for people of all ages, with and without health problems, it seems reasonable there are benefits to be derived for persons with AD, especially those in the early stages of the illness. According to Frankl (1984), what matters is "not the meaning of life in general, but rather the meaning of a person's life at a given moment" (113). Since Kitwood (1997) contends that a primary focus of care for the person with AD should be helping the person maintain a relative sense of well-being, volunteer activities seem to be a natural fit for a person with early-stage AD.

However, the current literature on volunteerism by persons with AD is limited essentially to their participation in drug or research studies (Rasmusson et al. 1998; Smith et al. 1998) The number of persons with AD involved in these and similar research projects suggests that they are often willing volunteers. However, their eagerness to participate as volunteers is often surprising, even to experienced professionals. A physician who had worked with persons with AD for many years and supported the development of early-stage support groups was invited by one such group to talk about the illness and research progress. Even this experienced clinician was surprised by the extent of the group's generativity concerns. They expressed concerns about heredity risk factors and whether their children and grandchildren were likely to get AD, and they wanted to know if they could help in the research process. As one man put it, "It's good to know that so much is being done. Is there any way we can help?" Another person with AD said, "I wish I didn't have this, but since I do, can't you use me as a guinea pig? Maybe it will help my children." A woman whose physician had encouraged her to join a support group said, "I want to do anything I can to help them find out what causes this, but I am not interested in just talking about the disease."

The eagerness of this group of people to volunteer for research projects, the many positive effects of volunteering, and the requests of people in support groups for some sort of ongoing activities raised the question whether people in the early stages of AD could be successful volunteers for community organizations? Since a loss of purpose and social connections are not inevitably part of the illness, the leadership and staff of an adult day center in Chicago decided to develop a program that would provide both social connections and the opportunity for volunteerism. People such as Josephine, introduced below, were our motivation.

Josephine: A Case Example of the Need for a Volunteer Program

Josephine has six children and had been married for forty-five years when her husband died. She described her husband as a person who was not easy to get along with, especially when he drank. Joesphine had worked during most of her married life and retired after working in a factory for twenty years. After retirement she stayed busy with volunteer work and family activities. Josephine volunteered at a local hospital and at a facility for developmentally delayed children. She was devoted to working with these children and would arrange all her other activities in order to be available to spend time at this facility. Twice a week she took two buses from her home to the facility and spent the day working with the toddlers. Then in 1994 she began experiencing significant problems remembering things. She gradually cut back on many of her usual activities but continued her volunteer work with the children. After she took the wrong bus several times and got lost, her family, who worked full-time and were unable to arrange transportation for her, insisted that she stop going to the facility out of concern for her safety. She became depressed, lost weight, stayed in her apartment all the time, and even began to withdraw from family activities. Her family physician prescribed an antidepressant, and her weight stabilized, but her usual active demeanor did not return. In an early-stage support group she often talked about feeling useless because she could not continue her volunteer activities.

Josephine's experience was not unusual. Many people in early-stage support groups in the Chicago metropolitan area expressed a yearning to maintain connections to the community. This was especially true for those whose driving had been curtailed or limited to the immediate neighborhood. Feelings of isolation and uselessness were common.

The Program

Program Philosophy

Compensating for people's losses so that they can continue to use their retained skills is a fundamental responsibility of those who care for persons with AD (Fazio, Seman, and Stansell 1999). Identification of losses and especially barriers to using retained skills is an obvious first step. These limitations are usually very subtle early in the illness but can be discerned in a careful assessment. There is usually some impairment of executive skills—the ability to plan, initiate, and sequence. Most people early in the illness experience memory loss and forget appointments or how to get to a specific location, whether driving or using public transportation. Impairment of one's sense of time and the ability to maintain a schedule of activities is another common experience of people early in the illness. Therefore, it seemed clear that a program to facilitate volunteer activities in the community had to be designed to accommodate these symptoms of the illness and would require much more than simply connecting an interested person with a community agency in need of assistance. A volunteer program for people in the early stages would have to compensate for the volunteer's impairments without calling attention to them.

Program Description

Thus, in 1996 a program was developed in Chicago to assist people in the early stages of AD or related dementias to actively participate in the community and receive the emotional support they needed to cope with the symptoms of their illness. The program had two basic components, social and support activities and volunteer services at community agencies. Since it was based on the premise that knowledgeable staff with considerable expertise would be needed to make the adaptations in the community to compensate for the participant's impairments, thoughtful attention was given to the skills and abilities staff would need. Professional staff who were knowledgeable about the abilities and deficits of persons with AD, about individual and group dynamics, and about available community organizations were essential to the success of the program.

Among the needs expressed by people in the AD support group were getting together "frequently" and to do things "regularly," "not just occassionally." It was decided to try to provide a full day's activities twice weekly during the pilot phase of the program. While some people expressed a desire for a daily program, the twice-a-week program seemed to be a good fit for the majority of people and their families.

Recruiting participants for the program did not go as quickly as anticipated. Admission criteria, developed during the planning process for the program, included a diagnosis of early-stage AD, consistent aware-ness of the diagnosis, ability to participate in activities (including physical strength and stamina), and independence in activities of daily living. In as-sessing the participants in the early-stage support groups of the local chap-ter of the Alzheimer's Association, it quickly became apparent that many were no longer in the early stages of the illness. We linked these people with services appropriate to their needs and abilities and began to recruit people more intensively from the dementia diagnostic centers.

Since most people in the early stages of the illness wanted to continue with their own life patterns as long as possible, many did not want to join any group until they absolutely could not continue to do things indepen-dently. "I'm not ready to do this yet" is sometimes how people describe their need to continue their activities independently. A minister in the early stages of the illness was very articulate in his explanation of the need to continue working for his church rather than joining the group. "I feel like I have the sword of Damocles hanging over my head and I need to work hard to make as many contributions [to the church] as I can while I am still able. I was brought up to think about others first, and I feel there is still a lot I can do for oth-ers before I get too sick."

We found that the program was wanted and needed by people who could not continue their usual activities in the community on their own but did not yet need or want the structured environment of an adult day program. Although the average program census built up slowly, the average atten-dance is now about ten people per day with scores ranging from 16 to 28 on the Mini-Mental State Examination, or an average score of 21. The pro-gram seems to attract more women than men and more Caucasians than minorities. Most participants have a high-school education, although some have college degrees. Most of the participants have worked outside the home in a wide range of positions, from factory worker to professional. Al-though most of the women in the group worked outside the home at some point in their lives, many did not do so when their children were young. The average length of stay in the program is about two years.

Participants in the group were not able to independently offer sugges-tions about the kinds activities that interested them and needed suggested alternatives from which to choose. In the pilot phase of this program it was found that some organizations were unwilling to have persons with AD serve as volunteers. It seems that some people do not perceive AD as a progressive degenerative disease but rather as a disabling disease that renders a person incompetent and incontinent. Several organizations somewhat reluctantly agreed to participate and did not seem to have very high expectations of the volunteers or their abilities (Swanson, Levi, and Mantano 1999). It was often necessary to make personal visits to the prospective volunteer site in order to educate the agency staff about the abilities of persons with AD, as well as to assure the agency that the volunteers would always be accompanied by two staff members, who would be responsible for them, before an agency would agree.

The group volunteered for a wide variety of activities in a wide variety of settings. They worked at a natural-science museum, preparing materials for a children's program; provided activities for children at a shelter for abused women and their children, in a homeless shelter, and at a school for emotionally disturbed children; sorted clothes at a Salvation Army resale shop; helped first graders with reading activities in a public school; and helped with mailings for the Red Cross, the local chapter of the Alzheimer's Association, and the Chicago Department on Aging. These organizations and many others have been, and continue to be, active partners in this program.

After witnessing some of the volunteers' abilities and the responsiveness of the program staff both to the participants and to the agency, agencies' expectations and perceptions of the group began to change. We now receive calls from community agencies asking for our volunteer participants to assist with special projects or to increase the amount of time they presently give. One of the most positive outcomes of the program has been the increasingly positive responses of community organizations to the program participants and to persons with AD. The Salvation Army presented the group members with achievement awards for their work at the resale shop. The director of the Illinois Department on Aging presented each member of the group with a certificate of appreciation from the governor for the group's work helping first graders develop their reading skills.

While these achievements are a real testament to the many abilities of the group members, considerable support is needed from the staff, family, and friends to enable the participants to be so successful in these volunteer endeavors. Some sort of personal support system needs to be in place to compensate for the person's deficits and make participation in the group's activities possible. Family members, friends, or staff in assisted living facilities often need to provide reminders about scheduled volunteer times. Even when people are still driving, it is usually only within their own neighborhood, so help is needed to get the person to and from the group's meeting place.

The group does not simply become part of an organization's existing volunteer programs; rather, it works on specific projects or activities for the organization. While input of group members is an essential component of the planning process, the staff are responsible for contacting organizations, determining the appropriateness of the location and activity for the participants, and making the specific arrangements. They organize the task in a way that will provide a successful experience for everyone, breaking the task into manageable bits that fit the retained skills of each member of the group.

Limitations to Program Participation

Although the program is designed specifically for people with early-stage AD, there are limitations to participation.

- While a goal of the program is to compensate for people's losses so they can use their retained skills, we have found that not all the symptoms people may experience early in the illness can be accommodated in a volunteer program. A relatively rare but very difficult symptom to accommodate is difficulty with spatial relationships and fine motor coordination.
- A person's physical strength, stamina, and dexterity may not be sufficient to permit full participation in volunteer activities. Since volunteering is done in a variety of community organizations, people have to be able to negotiate in a range of different environments, including those with steps and uneven surfaces.
- Safety issues, especially getting lost, are a serious concern for all programs for persons with AD, even in the early stages of the illness. Since this is a concern of most group members, there is a vigilance on the part of both staff and participants "to keep an eye on" one another, and all participants in the program are required to wear an identification bracelet, like the Alzheimer's Association's "Safe Return" bracelets.

• Since the ratio of staff to participants for this group is potentially 1 to 7, it is not possible for the staff member to be with each person in the group at all times. Although independence is supported and encouraged, the participants have to be willing and able to stay with the group.

• Transitions from the program are often difficult for everyone involved—the person, the family, other members of the group, and staff. It calls attention to and challenges acceptance of the progressive nature of the illness and the feelings it raises for everyone. It has sometimes been helpful to the person and his or her family that the early-stage program is part of a larger adult day service program, so that the transition from the volunteer component is less painful than it might otherwise be. Focusing on the functional ability and comfort level of the person with AD seems to help many people through the transition.

• While this program focuses on volunteer work, the level of organization and support necessary to make it possible clearly has a financial component. Funding, which can be a major barrier to the development of a new program, has not been a significant problem for this particular program because the pilot project was funded by two local foundations. When it became clear that it was a viable program for some people in the early stages of AD, other funding options were explored. When the grant funding ended, a fee was established to cover the cost of the program. Since it is the policy of the organization to provide needed care regardless of a person's ability to pay for services, a sliding fee scale was made available. In addition, every effort is made to utilize all financial-assistance programs available to the participants, such as a state-administered Medicaid waiver program.

The Response of the Volunteers

From the inception of the project the opportunity to learn from the participants in the group was recognized. While this was not a research study, a qualitative-like approach was used to gather and analyze information shared by group members. Discussions in the morning support group were taped. Staff also noted comments and discussions at lunch that were particularly pertinent. In this way, we were able to identify five common themes in the group members feelings about their volunteer work: being who I am, helping others, providing meaning, feeling competent, and maintaining a sense of well-being.

Being Who I Am

A common theme among many people early in the illness is the need, in the words of one participant, to "keep on being who I am, doing what interests me." In this group of persons with AD who are currently actively in engaged in volunteer activities, the members have a history of volunteering throughout their lives. They participated in a wide variety of children's activities, both when their own children were small and after they retired—as girl scout leaders, as den mother, as room mothers at school, and working with developmentally challenged children. Several were involved in church and temple activities—as Sunday school teachers, as choir members, leading Bible study, helping with church dinners, baby-sitting, cleaning the church, and participating in volunteer activities in the community as a part of a church group. People were also involved in other volunteer activities in the community—as members of the League of Women Voters, as symphony ushers, as volunteers with Marines in annual "Toys for Tots" drive, and teaching skills like crocheting at the community center. In addition to formal volunteer activities, there were examples of informal volunteering—helping neighbors, caring for children of friends, or taking an older person shopping. They describe their past volunteer experiences as important ones in their lives. Elaine was described by her son as a "professional Mom," focusing most of her time and energy on her children and helping with many of their activities. After her own children left home, she worked in a local school as the administrative assistant to the principal.

Elaine, who is 73, has fond memories of teaching Sunday school: "I loved working with the children and helping them. It was a very precious part of my life."

Marie K., 76, had a difficult marital relationship with a husband who was "an alcoholic and not emotionally available," according to her daughter. Marie was a girl scout leader when she was not working outside of the home. Later she worked as a receptionist and was active in her church's social activities. After she retired, she volunteered at the senior center. Marie tells about how much she "loved teaching crocheting at the center. Everyone was different and did things differently. I learned so much about the people I was teaching."

Helping Others

For many people, helping others is an important part of their lives, and this is especially true of the members of this group. Annette, a former real-estate broker, was active in her synagogue. She believes that "helping others is something that comes naturally. I think there is something missing in people who don't want to help someone less fortunate. I feel sorry for people who are so self-centered that they won't make time to help others. It's natural to want to help make someone's life a little better. Because of Alzheimer's I don't always remember what we do, but I know that we always do good things for others. That's important, to know that you help others, even when you don't remember the specifics."

Elaine has focused much of her time and energy throughout her life on children. "The children feel good when we come. It's a good feeling that we can make a difference in their lives. Letting them know we care about them is important. Giving them the attention they need and should be getting is very important for them to grow up to be happy and lead useful lives. The volunteer work lets us keep on doing things for children."

Meaning

Volunteering has provided the group members with a means of renewing a sense of purpose and meaning in their lives. For Annette, volunteer work "makes me aware that I can still help others despite what I have. It keeps Alzheimer's from taking over our lives." Sylvia, aged 80, never worked outside the home but had a very active social life that included a number of volunteer activities. She talks about the boredom she experienced when she could no longer drive and before she joined the group. "I'm not happy staying at home and doing nothing. I use to go, go, go. I was always doing something for someone or going somewhere with my friends . . . but now I don't initiate things. I was just sitting at home doing nothing until I joined the group. Now I get out and do things . . . I'm not so bored and I feel good about being able to help out."

Agnes, aged 81, also had a very active social life that included volunteer work. After her husband died, she traveled extensively with a senior group and volunteered at the Salvation Army and a church. She too talks about "feeling isolated and useless" prior to becoming a part of the group. "At least we aren't sitting at home twiddling our thumbs . . . we are doing something important for the kids. That makes me feel useful again." Annie, 86, is a plain-spoken woman with little formal education but great wisdom who talks about good and bad in very fundamental ways. For her, "it's good to get out and do things for other people, especially those little ones at the shelter."

Feeling Competent

The impairments that result from AD challenge the person with the illness in many ways, including challenges to their confidence in their own abilities. Volunteering and receiving public acknowledgment of their contributions seems to help people to focus on their abilities rather than on their losses. According to Marie, "When we are volunteering, I feel like we are still a part of the normal world. I like feeling normal, not like we are sick."

Lucille, who is 86, only completed grade school. She worked at a drugstore, first as a cashier and then as a bookkeeper. After retirement she volunteered at her church's grade school as a "lunch mother." She was always pleased with her accomplishments and wanted to share these with others. "Wait till I tell my daughter what we did today!" was a frequent comment as she was about to leave for home. She was particularly excited about the public recognition the group received; it validated her sense of competence. "Some people think we can't do anything just because we forget some things. I like people to know that we can still do things . . . now other people know we can still do things even if we do have Alzheimer's disease! We got our awards, and it's something you can have and show people. They announced my award at my Bingo Club, and everybody congratulated me. I was so proud. No one there ever got an award from the Governor!"

A Sense of Well-being

Kitwood (1997) contends that persons with AD can maintain a relative sense of well-being if people around them are supportive. It is not uncommon for people to be somewhat depressed and/or withdrawn when they join the group. Annette, who seemed more depressed than most people when she joined the group, says that she became despondent after she was diagnosed. Giving up her work as a real-estate broker, which she loved, was very traumatic for her. "I used to get so sad and really despondent because I thought if I couldn't work, I was useless. I was afraid my friends would think I was crazy, so I didn't want to tell anyone I had Alzheimer's. I just cried a lot and wished this would go away. I still wish that, or at least they would find a cure. Now I know I can still do things for others . . . still have fun with my new friends and some of my old friends. Just because I can't work doesn't mean I can't do anything! I am a lot happier now!"

Angel, who is 66, was born in Puerto Rico, moved to Chicago as a young man, and worked at the post office for thirty-three years. "Sometimes this thing, the Alzheimer's, makes me feel so stupid and I get to feeling really sorry for myself. But when we are together and work with the children, I feel good, not stupid. I feel normal."

Marie S., 85, was a tiny woman who had worked as a riveter in a factory during the war. After retiring, she had remained active by doing volunteer work at church and helping to care for her great-grandchildren. She believed that "you have to keep busy. It keeps your troubles off your mind. This keeps me busy, and I feel happy when I am doing something for others."

The social interaction and support of the group seems to complement the volunteer work in helping people maintain a sense of well-being. According to Annie, "It's good working together with each other. You don't have to worry about making a mistake, and it's good being together. Helping those in need makes us feel good."

THESE FEW COMMENTS ARE REPRESENTATIVE of those made by participants in the program and help us better understand what is important to them. Their reasons for volunteering are multidimensional, related to long-held values and life patterns. For the participants of this group, the opportunity to see themselves in a helping role bolstered their feelings of competence and supported normalization of their illness. These people do not define themselves by their illness and are pleased with the opportunity to enable others to see them as people with abilities.

Lessons Learned

From our experience of running the volunteer project we learned some valuable lessons.

• All abilities are not lost due to the disease process. Especially early in the illness, persons with AD have a great diversity of life skills and abilities that can be used to help others.

• Persons with AD do not define themselves by their illness but normalize the illness and want to continue doing things that are important to them.

• Professionals who think of persons with AD in terms of loss rather than ability are likely to limit opportunities for people to continue to be contributing members of the community.

• We are just beginning to learn about the needs and experiences of people in the early stages of AD. A variety of programs are needed so that everyone can continue "being who they are." This program is not for everyone. Not everyone is interested in volunteering. As Harry stated so eloquently, "I'm looking for someone to help me, not the other way around. How many 90-year-olds do you see working?" Not every person with AD is a "group" person, just as not every woman with breast cancer joins a support group. Some people are not "ready yet" and want to continue doing things independently as long as they can.

• As more is learned about the experiences of people in the early stages of the illness, it is clear that more needs to be learned about the kinds of adaptations that are needed to help people do the things that are important to them. Nick said that "What bothers me the most is that I can't spin like I use to when I dance," a reminder that not only the loss of memory is frustrating.

• Given common myths about persons with AD, some reluctance from community groups should be expected. Contact a few community organizations, preferably ones with which staff members are familiar, learn what kind of help they need, and assess their willingness to have persons with AD as volunteers. Visit the organizations to assess the appropriateness of the locations and projects for the group members. Take a group member along, if possible, so that the agency staff can see that people with AD have skills and abilities.

• Establish clear admission and discharge criteria for programs that are based on functional abilities, not just a diagnosis. Sometimes physicians tell family members that a person is in the early stages of the illness as long as the person is continent. Transitions from the program are often difficult for everyone—the person with AD, family members, staff, and other group members. It is somewhat helpful if the volunteer program is a part of a larger adult day services program so that people are familiar with the place and the staff.

• Staff with expertise, knowledge, and judgment are essential to the success of the program. The staff must have exceptional verbal and non-verbal communication skills, the capacity to respond to changing situations without becoming flustered, and the ability to transport the group to the volunteer locations. They have to be able not only to match the person to an appropriate task but also to monitor the flow of the work and make subtle adjustments or adaptations to ensure success in each activity for each person. A high level of vigilance is clearly required, but this must be subtle and not perceived as controlling or demeaning. The relationship between staff and participants is much more collegial than directive. Staff do not simply set up activities and facilitate when necessary; they are active participants in the work of the day and part of the social fabric of the group.

• As with any new program, especially one without clear guidelines to follow, there are the customary two steps forward and one back as the program is developed and adapted to make it better fit the participants. It is an untidy process that requires perseverance, optimism, and a willingness to make changes based on what is learned from experience, and from the ideas and feelings of those involved.

Conclusion

This chapter describes an innovative program for persons with AD that grew out of the comments of support group members. It has been successful in meeting the goals of providing social support and activities, as well as opportunities for volunteerism. Volunteerism is not just a means of staying busy or using retained skills and abilities. It is also an opportunity for persons with AD to act on and connect to lifelong beliefs and values and to help others. In addition, it seems to provide meaning and to promote feelings of competence and well-being in persons with AD. The program does not meet everyone's needs, and it is not of interest to everyone in the early stages of AD. However, most importantly, such a program shows that persons with AD can be contributing members of society, not burdens.

What is more, their ability to make real and significant contributions can also change the perception of others about persons with AD.

REFERENCES

Brim, O. G. 1988. Losing and winning. *Psychology Today*, September, 48–52.

Chambre, S. M. 1993. Volunteerism by elders: Past trends and future prospects. *Gerontologist* 33:221–28.

Crist-Houran, M. 1996. Efficacy of volunteerism for role-loss depression: A complement to Weinstein, et al. *Psychological Reports* 79:736–38.

Fazio, S., D. Seman, and J. Stansell. 1999. *Rethinking Alzheimer's care*. Baltimore: Health Professions Press.

Frankl, V. E. 1984. *Man's search for meaning*. New York: Simon & Schuster.

Herzog, A. R., M. M. Franks, H. R. Marcus, and D. Holmberg. 1998. Activities and well-being in older age: Effects of self concept and educational attainment. *Psychology and Aging* 13:179–85.

Herzog, R., and J. House. 1991. Productive activities and aging well. *Generations* 15:49–54.

Kitwood, T. 1997. *Dementia reconsidered*. Philadelphia: Open Univ. Press.

Marriot Senior Living Services. 1991. *Marriot Senior Volunteerism Study*. Washington, D.C.

Okum, M. A., A. Barr, and A. Herzog. 1998. Motivation to volunteer by older adults: A test of completing measurement models. *Psychology and Aging* 13:608–21.

Rasmusson, D., A. Zonderman, C. Kawas, and S. Resnick. 1998. Effects of age and dementia on the trail making test. *Clinical Neuropsychologist* 12 (May): 169–78.

Richardson, V., and K. M. Kilty. 1991. Adjustment to retirement: Continuity vs discontinuity. *International Journal of Aging and Human Development* 33 (2): 151–69.

Smith, A., E. King, N. Hindley, L. Barnetson, J. Barton, and K. Jobst. 1998. The experience of research participation and the value of diagnosis in dementia. *Journal of Mental Health (UK)* 7 (3): 309–21.

Swanson, N., G. Levi, and T. Mantano. 1999. Volunteer program gives pride to people with dementia. *Rush Alzheimer's Disease Center News*, spring.

Warburton, J., R. Le Srocque, and L. Rosenman. 1998. Older people—the reserve army of volunteers? An analysis of volunteerism among older Australians. *International Journal of Aging and Human Development* 46:229–45.

Weinstein, L., and X. Xie. 1995. Purpose in life, boredom, and volunteerism in a group of elderly retirees. *Psychological Reports* 76:482.

Wheeler, J., K. Gorey, and B. Greenblatt. 1998. The beneficial effects of volunteering for older volunteers and the people they serve: A meta-analysis. *International Journal of Aging and Human Development* 4:69–79.

12

The Experience of Support Groups for Persons with Early-Stage Alzheimer's Disease & Their Families

ROBYN YALE AND LISA SNYDER

It helps to know you aren't alone—listening to how others deal with similar problems. . . . It makes me feel much better to know that there are people like me.
—Stan, a 74-year-old retired mail carrier

In the 1990s there was a significant shift in professionals' awareness and response to the social and mental health needs of persons with AD. These needs had been overlooked largely because of the mistaken belief that invariably persons with AD had limited insight into their symptoms and that little could be done to treat their condition (Goldstein et al. 1991). Even those diagnosed in the early stages of AD are often sent home with no information about the disease and few, if any, resources. With the advent of earlier and more accurate diagnosis this gap in service and treatment has become very apparent. A movement is now under way to establish supportive services earlier in the course of the disease, including a range of programs that never before existed. A cornerstone for this new foundation is support groups for persons with early-stage AD to help them understand, accept, and adjust to their condition (Yale 1995). This chapter explores the development and benefits of support groups, discusses types of models, and identifies recurrent themes in the group process, group discussion content, and participants' reactions.

Although some persons with AD deny memory or functional problems, many others are able to express their feelings and concerns about having the illness. Keady and Gilliard (1999) detail a process of transition in which individuals may move from awareness that something is wrong, through a period of secrecy, to the point of wanting to make sense of the symptoms they are experiencing. As one newly diagnosed woman stated, "The main issue is to help people to be open about Alzheimer's—not to privatize it, especially within the family. Very often the tendency with something like this is to hold it in and suffer with it. But it isn't necessary to suffer alone. People with Alzheimer's are curious about what all of this is going to mean to their lives, and if they can get some sense of this through a support group, then they can move into this process more at ease. That's very important" (Snyder 1999, 127–28).

Reported Benefits of Participating in Early-Stage Support Groups

Therapeutic Benefits for the Participant with AD

In her early work developing support groups for persons with AD, Yale (1989) notes the therapeutic potential of the group process to decrease feelings of isolation, facilitate grief work, and provide for the exchange of information and resources. Drawing on the work of the psychiatrist Irving Yalom (1985), she confirmed the "curative factors" of support groups for participants with early-stage disease. The instillation of hope, interpersonal learning, socialization, catharsis, universality, and altruism are attributable to support groups for persons with AD. In her research into how participants with early-stage AD respond to the support group experience, Yale (1995) observed that participants bonded and became self-disclosing early in the group process; they were able to share information and express feelings with one another with remarkable candor. LaBarge and Trtanj (1995) confirmed the ability of group participants to bond through verbal and nonverbal communication (compassionate use of touch) and to gain a sense of comfort and decreased isolation from hearing the experiences of others. Snyder et al. (1995) also validated the presence of group cohesiveness and self-disclosure in their supportive seminar groups for persons with mild AD. Participants freely initiated conversations, and the more vocal participants elicited sharing from the quieter members. Morhardt and Johnson (1998) observed a strong sense of group cohesion and camaraderie in their support group. Group members looked forward to seeing one another, expressed enjoyment and humor when together, and asked about those who were absent from a group session.

In an analysis of communication and the group process for persons in early-stage AD, Goldfein, Stilwell, and Kahn (1995) noted a wide range of speech acts by participants, including affective, informational, empathetic, altruistic, and humorous statements. Topics were generated by the group and included an array of emotionally and informationally based themes pertaining to the disease, as well as discussion of issues related to group structure and extraneous topics pertinent to their lives. Although language ability varied among participants, group communication was effective; facilitators or less impaired participants compensated for others' language difficulties. Goldfein and her colleagues also confirmed that many of Yalom's curative factors were evidenced throughout the group process.

Although the support groups referred to above have been conducted with persons with mild impairment, persons with moderate impairment may also benefit from the group process. Shoham and Neuschatz (1985) led groups for persons with AD and reported that the use of structured topics in sessions helped to keep participants focused and on track. Individuals seemed better able to organize their thoughts and to make more appropriate comments. David (1991) led a small support group for moderately impaired persons with AD twice a week. Although the participants' insight, abstract thought processes, and attention spans were limited by the disease, they developed strong interpersonal relationships. They generated topics such as memory loss, aging, illness, and adjusting to word-finding problems. Although they did not always remember that they had been diagnosed with AD, they were comfortable enough with one another to share difficult feelings about their symptoms. They were able to compensate for one another's disabilities through assistance with word finding, patience with perseveration, and the effective use of humor.

Therapeutic Benefits of Family Involvement

Cohen (1991) suggested that interactions can be much more positive when those diagnosed and their caregivers recognize each other's reactions to the disease. Many caregivers with early-stage loved ones do express a need to develop empathy for their relatives' viewpoint in order to better understand their own changing roles and responsibilities (Kuhn 1998; Yale 1995). A growing body of literature describes experiences with conjoint support groups made up of persons with AD and their significant others that work toward these goals. Both partners attend sessions together, or more commonly, they attend separate group meetings concurrently and then reconvene for a final, conjoint discussion period. In their experience leading concurrent groups McAfee et al. (1989) noted that family members expressed a feeling of empowerment as a result of their loved one's being included in important discussions of family matters. Diagnosed participants commented that the discussions helped them better understand the disease, and some expressed increased understanding or concern about issues facing their caregivers. McAfee et al. did not observe any negative outcomes of this conjoint process and concluded that conjoint groups may help preserve the dignity and self-esteem of families as a whole. Yale (1995) found that individuals with AD and their family members felt that they were coping as a team, pulling together to face the challenges, and learning to better understand and tolerate each other through the support groups. Caregivers felt that the support group experience helped their loved ones by "normalizing" their experience, improving their mood, decreasing their isolation, and adding organization to their lives. Participants seemed to be more open emotionally and to have an enhanced understanding of their own personal behavior.

Khurana (1996) and Snyder et al. (1995) also stated that in their experience facilitating concurrent groups, both groups gained understanding of the disease and each developed empathy toward the other's circumstances. Individuals and families often formed social bonds outside of the sessions. Nemeroff and Genier (1999) described instances when topics that originated in the session for diagnosed participants were then brought (with permission) to the conjoint group so that a more open dialogue could be established between those diagnosed and their caregivers. Two caregivers commented on the value of their loved one's involvement, stating that they would not have joined a support group without their spouse's participation.

A final report issued by the Alzheimer's Association of South Australia (1999) also addresses the value of concurrent group education and support for people with early-stage dementia and their caregivers. Results of group evaluations strongly suggest that the most helpful aspect of the concurrent six-week support groups was meeting with others in a similar situation.

Both diagnosed participants and their caregivers felt less alone in dealing with the disease and were afforded an opportunity for mutual support and information sharing. Although some participants had already felt comfortable talking about dementia with family members, for others the group helped to increase communication between them and their families. In a research study comparing four early-stage program interventions, Quayhagen et al. (2000) found that 50 percent of the caregivers who participated in a dual supportive seminar group documented enhanced communication and interaction with their loved ones.

Although qualitative, survey, and anecdotal documentation attest to the value of support groups for persons with early-stage AD and their caregivers, statistically significant quantitative findings have been much more difficult to obtain. Researchers report small sample sizes and insensitive outcome measures as primary obstacles to significant findings (Fine et al. 1995; McAfee et al. 1989; Morhardt and Johnson 1998; Quayhagen et al. 2000; Yale 1995). Clinicians and researchers must work together to construct or employ measures that more effectively target qualitatively defined outcomes.

Support Group Models and Participant Criteria

Many administrative matters must be considered when developing support groups for persons with AD. These include securing professionally trained facilitators, recruiting group participants from the community, prescreening and selecting group participants, establishing a group model or structure, and working with sponsoring organizations to secure support or necessary funding. Yale (1995) elaborated on these issues and outlined a model that has been refined and widely replicated nationally and internationally. Designed for early-stage individuals, the group format has evolved to include the addition of a concurrent support group for family members. In one such format the groups meet for ninety minutes once a week for eight consecutive weeks, with two-week breaks between series. The two groups meet together for the first half of the first meeting for orientation and introductions and for the last half of the eighth meeting for final interactions and evaluations. Otherwise, the groups meet in separate rooms, but at the same time. Meetings involve discussion and support, with topics generated by participants or initiated by the facilitator. Participants can repeat the eight-week series as long as they are able. Although this format is often used as a long-term model, at some sites the program is limited (e.g., a one-time six- or ten-week series) and monthly "graduate groups" are offered for those who want more ongoing support or continued social interaction.

In another variation of the format, Snyder et al. (1993) developed an eight-week educational group for individuals with early-stage AD and their caregivers. The weekly structured topics incorporate handouts for both those diagnosed and their families to facilitate learning and to provide references for enhanced communication between family members during the time between group meetings. Participants with AD and their family members meet in separate groups for the first hour. Each group discusses the same topic (e.g., coping with memory problems, the impact of the disease on social and family relationships, disclosing the diagnosis, health and stress management), and then the two groups meet together as a whole for the last half hour to share experiences from their separate groups. Although confidentiality is honored in both groups, the combined half-hour allows for voluntary sharing about the weekly topic and can facilitate more open communication between participants with AD and their family members.

Long-term, open-ended support groups typically do not utilize structured topics and do not always offer a formal support group component for caregivers. These groups usually meet weekly and enroll participants or help them move on from the group as needed. Support group discussions are influenced by the needs and concerns of the participants. Clinical experience has shown that groups cover similar topics regardless of whether they are initiated by facilitators or participants. Snyder and colleagues currently facilitate a long-term group in which caregivers meet informally without a facilitator while their diagnosed relatives participate in the group. These family members initiate and organize monthly social outings for the group as a whole as a way of further facilitating a sense of community.

Although support group formats vary, it is necessary to establish participant criteria consistent with mild impairment. Criteria based on the functional, cognitive, and social abilities necessary to participate in an interactive group process are common to most group models and usually include

• a complete medical workup resulting in a diagnosis of AD or a related disorder;

- the participant's having been informed of the diagnosis;
- acknowledgment of memory loss and some degree of recognition that it may result from AD or a related disorder;
- an interest or willingness to try participating in a support group (as opposed to caregiver insistence);
- the ability to converse adequately to convey and comprehend a verbal message;
- the ability to sit for the duration of the group session without problematic restlessness, agitation, or other disruptive behaviors;
- sufficient hearing to understand the group discussion;
- being free of functional impairments requiring staff assistance or supervision (i.e., assistance with toileting or with eating snacks in group);
- being free of psychiatric disabilities that would negatively affect participation in the group process (i.e., significant paranoia, delusions, hallucinations, or substance abuse); and
- transportation to and from group meetings.

Screening interviews, which are conducted in person, give facilitators an opportunity to assess each person's abilities, insight, communication skills, and receptivity to the group process. Yale (1995) developed extensive screening tools that have been duplicated and modified successfully by many group facilitators. Sensitive and thorough screening increases the likelihood of a successful group experience.

Support Group Content

Group Themes and Interactions

In her study exploring the responses of people with early-stage AD to a support group Yale (1995) noted recurrent themes in group discussion content. These themes included AD and the diagnostic process; current research; awareness of the stigma attached to the diagnosis of AD; relationships with family and friends; changes in lifestyle and abilities; keeping life full and meaningful for as long as possible; and preparing for the future. A variety of feelings and experiences were expressed in support group interactions, including self-concept and AD. One support group participant stated, "I hope we're not going to discuss the past much, because I'm no longer the person that I was then." To which another replied, "Well, I'd rather discuss the past than the present because I can remember it much better." The group process enabled persons to integrate the past, the present, and the future and how they saw themselves at these varying points in time.

Participant dialogue also reflected struggles to accept and cope with the disease. One person spoke about the loss of autonomy: "It's hard to start depending on others—I've coped with responsibility since I was 4 years-old." Another expressed concerns about the future and said, "My grandchild worries that I will forget who she is." Feelings of both fear and resilience are evident in the question of one client, who asked, "Will I soon not be a person anymore?" Another answered, "No, you may have Alzheimer's, but that isn't all there is to you—we all have strengths and weaknesses." Dialogues developed that illustrated differing perspectives. When one participant stated, "I'm only 75, and I'm angry this is happening to me," another responded, "I'm 75, and I figure something's bound to happen to my health. At least Alzheimer's doesn't involve physical pain."

A powerful group process emerged as people shared their knowledge, feelings, and experiences with one another. One participant brought up the sensitive issue of driving, saying, "There are laws against driving when you have Alzheimer's." Safety concerns were also discussed. Yale noted that the cohesiveness and camaraderie as people with AD reach out to and support one another is significant and incorporates sensitivity, humor, and tolerance.

LaBarge and Trtanj (1995) also defined general categories that were discussed by participants in their support group for persons with early-stage AD. The five categories include subjective descriptions of difficulties with disease symptoms; questions about AD and responses to the diagnosis; coping mechanisms; responses of others to their altered abilities; and responses of participants in the group. Participants expressed feelings, including panic and loss, and group members offered one another both empathy and pragmatic support. Group members listed practical strategies for coping with the disease and also discussed the benefits of a positive attitude. And as many facilitators of support groups for persons with AD have emphasized, a sense of humor was an important strength that emerged repeatedly in group interactions.

Morhardt and Johnson (1998) confirmed that participants in their support group established an easy rapport with one another and that most were willing and able to discuss the impact of the illness on their lives. The themes were consistent with those previously noted, and many participants were able to identify specific problem areas. One acknowledged, "I've recognized the change; I'm not doing everything I did before. It would be embarrassing. When it comes to vocabulary, it used to be outstanding. Now it's not. I can't remember names of people I know very well." Reactions to the illness ranged from acceptance to despair. One participant reflected, "It's not really bothering me. . . . My memory problems are not overwhelming, just more of a nuisance." Others, however, expressed much greater distress. One participant lamented, "This has me very disturbed and depressed . . . I feel worse. I'm grateful we all understand each other here, and I feel comfortable saying what I just did. My concerns are very great. It weighs very heavy and I don't want to go through it."

Participants' feelings about admitting their diagnosis to others varied. One woman asked the other members of her group, "Don't you feel ashamed sometimes? I feel ashamed sometimes when I can't remember stuff." A male participant responded, "When I'm shopping and I get all screwed up, I just tell people I have something wrong with my brain and ask them to help, and they do. The salvation is in being honest and open." Many in the group discussed the importance of humor and hope. "We are still looking for the wonderful piece of medication that will do the job," one man said, "but in the meantime, we need to learn some new songs and some new jokes."

Participants' Reactions to the Support Group Experience

Many facilitators report that participants with AD frequently mention the value of the support group experience. In their qualitative analysis of support group content Snyder et al. (1995) noted that participants' statements that convey feelings of gratification and belonging often stem from references to the group. One man commented that "if you lost your memory fifty years ago, they put you off in a closet somewhere. They never had classes like this." Another participant spoke about the experience of camaraderie generated by group participation and said, "With this group, you're all in the same category, so it feels more open."

Some individuals report feeling less depressed as a result of the support group experience. "The big thing for me," one man said, "was the fear of not knowing what was going to happen, the fright of mental confusion, the fright of what you hear about it [AD], the frightening effect it has on your spouse and children. But learning more about it has helped. Groups like this are survival. . . . I'm having less trouble crying and being depressed, which is really great. Problems aren't as drastic as they used to be." For others the primary benefit of the group was sharing and learning from other participants. One man with early-onset dementia said that what he liked best was "the interaction—being here talking to everybody and being able to express myself without being criticized. We learn from each other. Everyone has so much wisdom. We also get lots of laughs in this group." Some specifically value the educational components of their group experience. One participant stated, "I like the exchange of information about medicines and treatments." Support groups also establish a feeling of community for participants. One woman put it simply: "I'm not alone" (San Diego Chapter, Alzheimer's Association, 2000).

Lessons Learned

Although there are many similarities between facilitating groups for people with early-stage AD and facilitating other support groups, special skills are required of facilitators who manage the unique and challenging group dynamics of this population. Yale (1995) elaborated on the following issues that warrant particular attention when developing an early-stage support group.

Facilitator Credentials

Although caregiver support groups can be well led by volunteer laypersons, support groups for persons with AD need well-trained professional facilitators. Facilitators should have a clinical license (or supervision available) and a background in dementia care, group work, and mental health. Orientation and ongoing training and support should be available to facilitators, including established protocol, guidelines, and techniques so that each one does not have to "reinvent the wheel."

Cultural Considerations

There are cultural differences to consider when offering Alzheimer's support groups to different populations, including variations in openness about feelings and norms about accepting help from outside the family (Yeo and Gallagher-Thompson 1996). We have experienced successful early-stage groups with members from varied cultural backgrounds and age groups. Some potential participants, however, may not have come forward for reasons of language, location, or other barriers to participation. It is important to do outreach to minority communities to determine their receptivity to the support group experience or to modify the format or structure as needed to accommodate differing views or values.

Maintaining a Delicate Balance

It is a compelling and delicate clinical challenge for the facilitator to acknowledge both the positive and the negative aspects of AD. It is important to address feelings of grief, loss, fear, and frustration while also embracing the opportunities, capabilities, and joy that can exist in the present. This integration is an important part of the group dynamic, and the facilitator must monitor this process.

Fluctuations in Denial

There are many reasons for denial. Some persons with AD forget that they have been diagnosed with the disease. For others denial serves as a defense against shock and loss and may result from the disparity between one's relatively minor symptoms and the prevailing images of persons with severe symptoms. Some individuals remain staunchly and adamantly in denial; others fluctuate or work through it over time. Some will more readily acknowledge the widely accepted condition of "memory problems" than they will the specific diagnosis of AD. Facilitators can express empathy that one of the challenges of memory problems is that sometimes people forget that they have one. It is helpful to ask others in the group whether they also have times when they are unaware of any problems. The support group models described here are intended for those persons with AD who are at least intermittently able to acknowledge the diagnosis and want to meet with others to discuss its impact.

Memory Impairment

If members occasionally repeat themselves, this may allow others to see that it is safe to repeat or ask the same question. The facilitator must stay structured in the group process and move forward with the material to avoid tangential or repetitive remarks. Forgetting the subject, one's train of thought, or the right word to finish a sentence would be disruptive in any other support group, but in a support group for persons with early-stage AD it becomes part of group process. The facilitator can respond by saying, "It's okay that you've forgotten—that's what we're here to talk about. Does that ever happen to anyone else in everyday life? If so, how do you handle it?"

Some participants may perseverate on a topic or statement. The facilitator can gently let the participant know that he or she has said the same thing a few times and comment, "This must be very important to you." It may be possible to derive something different each time the comment is made (i.e., the content, the feeling, or a particular way in which it might be integrated into other group-session content).

Communication Difficulties

Communication difficulties include problems with aphasia, word finding, and sentence completion. It is helpful for facilitators to avoid run-on sentences or raising many questions and points all at once. Allow silence or extra time for participants to find their words. Ask permission to help them find a word or paraphrase a thought. It is helpful to respond to the *feeling* if the content is unclear.

Agitation

Persons with AD can express a great deal through body language or the tone of their voice. Body language may be restless or the tone of voice may be challenging or argumentative. The facilitator can address the feeling and validate it (e.g., "You seem frustrated") and provide reassurance. Physical agitation may also indicate a need to use a restroom. Offer to take a brief break with the member if possible and take him or her to the restroom or to get a drink. Intense topics can be diffused by addressing the feeling and then asking others if they ever feel the same way. If agitation about a certain topic persists, change the topic.

Family Dynamics

Facilitating a concurrent support group for family members of persons with early-stage AD is similar to facilitating other caregiver support groups, but the themes and interactions may differ. The unique issues of caring for someone in the early stages of AD, including an emphasis on involving the person with AD in problem solving, planning, and decision making, must be addressed. Caregivers need assistance in processing current changes and acknowledging the future course of the disease. A positive attitude about their loved one's present capabilities allows them to focus on the beginning of the illness rather than being overwhelmed by a focus on the concerns of later stages.

Family members often wonder what occurs in their loved one's group. As with any other support group, confidentiality applies, but facilitators can summarize what is being discussed and how group members are doing. Some participants with AD are able to tell their families what issues arise in the group, but others are unable or may choose not to. It is clear that participants with AD experience the group "in the moment" even if they cannot articulate everything about it. They often sit in the same seats, greet one another by name, reveal things about themselves and respond to one another, and say how much they appreciate being there.

Moving On

Due to the progressive nature of the disease, participants with AD must eventually leave the support group. This often poses considerable challenges for the participant, family members, and the facilitator. Time-limited support groups have a built-in end point. For those in long-term groups, however, the transition process is more delicate and involves ongoing evaluation on a case-by-case basis. The criteria and process for moving on should be mentioned at enrollment so that both the participant and the caregiver are aware of these guidelines. Snyder and colleagues developed the following criteria to determine when a participant is no longer able to participate effectively in the support group and needs to move into other programs in the community:

VERBALIZATION OR COMMUNICATION
• Contributions lacking in substance necessary to facilitate conversation or inability to initiate or demonstrate engaged participation in the group process
• Consistently inappropriate, tangential, or disruptive to topic continuity—inability to keep track of conversation
• Persistent expressions of denial or persistent minimization of problems associated with AD
• Aphasia resulting in inability to adequately comprehend or communicate through verbal or nonverbal means

BEHAVIORAL OR FUNCTIONAL
• Psychiatric disturbance (delusions, hallucinations, paranoia)
• Disruptive impatience or agitation with the group process or with other group members—low frustration tolerance
• Significant functional problems requiring staff or caregiver assistance (e.g., toileting, inability to eat a snack in group)
• Persistent falling asleep
• Hearing loss not adequately corrected
• Persistent irregular attendance, including late arrival and pickup, that is disruptive to the group process or staff schedules

Transitions to different levels of care are inherent in the progressive nature of AD, and professionals must work to help individuals and families grieve and reconcile these ongoing losses. Some participants accept the need to move on and show considerable generosity in giving up their seat to someone else who needs a chance to benefit from the program. Others may feel abandoned or rejected, and the facilitator will need to give considerable attention to these concerns. The participant may choose to come to the group for a final closing meeting. Others choose not to, and the transition is processed by the remaining group members. Group members may want to share concerns over their peer's absence and the progression of the disease. As one participant with AD stated, "It hurts me to see some people in the group who I know and care about go down faster than it seems they should. It's sad. But I'm there. I'm a part of the group, and that's it" (Snyder 1999, 128). Others may express anxiety about when they will have to leave the group.

In long-term groups it is not uncommon for participants to reflect on past group members long after they have moved on. Training, ongoing supervision, and peer support for facilitators are necessary to enable them to work through their own grief in observing participants decline during the support group experience.

The lack of programs to refer people to as a "next step" is also an obstacle when asking people to leave the support group. A few regions have experimented with offering second and third levels of early-stage programs to accommodate gradual cognitive decline and encourage families to transition to concurrent support groups. Families generally develop close bonds in support groups, and it is frequently difficult for them to move on when it is time for their loved one to leave the group. Although transitions between levels of care are anticipated, they still signify milestones in a progressive disease, and families may need supplemental services, such as counseling, for additional emotional support.

Conclusion

Support groups and other programs for individuals with AD and their families provide a new starting point on the continuum of dementia care. Many people with AD are willing, able, and relieved to discuss their condition when given the opportunity, countering biases that have traditionally dehumanized them. What began as pilot projects for persons with early-stage AD in a few regions in the mid-1980s has grown substantially in scope and scale, but early-stage support groups and services still are not universally available. Many regions in the United States and other countries do not have these programs. According to Keady and Gilliard (1999), planning and coordination at the national level must include public-awareness campaigns, professional staff training, and clear objectives to identify and respond to the individualized experience of early dementia. While much new ground has been explored, there is much more to investigate and learn. We need more program development (to expand services and tailor them to the early stages); advances in research (to design outcome measurements sensitive to the experience of early-stage AD and program interventions); innovative educational materials (including new written materials for the public and professionals); and expanded outreach, advocacy, and policy specific to early-stage AD. An international network of professionals involved in early-stage AD programming and research has been developed to exchange information and experiences through a newsletter and clearinghouse (Gatz 1998; Yale 1996). Countries now represented include the United States, Canada, New Zealand, South Africa, the United Kingdom, and Australia.

Aside from taking direct action in one's own region, perhaps it is a global shift in attitude that will most effectively fuel the development of programs that acknowledge the emotional and interpersonal needs of persons with AD. The need for such services is eloquently stated by Philip Alderton (1999), newly diagnosed with Alzheimer's. He clearly reminds us of the compelling task before us: "I ask you [professionals] to please treat each Alzheimer's client as an individual. Help them maintain their inner self, their personality. . . . The recipient of knowledge and understanding about Alzheimer's is indeed a lucky person—[without it] life can become intolerable and very lonely. . . . Educate others and help to draw away the veil of secrecy people use to hide their loved ones. Perceptions of the illness vary and it may take another generation before genuine understanding of Alzheimer's becomes universal."

ACKNOWLEDGMENTS

This chapter is based in part on Yale 1995 and Yale 1999, adapted with permission. It was supported by a grant through the National Institute on Aging (AGO5131).

REFERENCES

Alderton, P. 1999. *Early stage dementia group: National training course.* Paper presented at the regional workshop of the Alzheimer's Association, Adelaide, South Australia, February.
Alzheimer's Association, South Australia. 1999. *Group education and support for people with early stage dementia and their carers: A final report.* Glenside.
Cohen, D. 1991. The subjective experience of Alzheimer's disease: The anatomy of an illness as perceived by patients and families. *American Journal of Alzheimer's Disease* 6 (May/June): 128–33.
Cohen, G. 1989. Psychodynamic perspectives in the clinical approach to brain disease in the elderly. In *Psychiatric consequences of brain disease in the elderly*, ed. D. K. Conn, A. Grek, and J. Sadavoy. New York: Plenum.
David, P. 1991. Effectiveness of group work with the cognitively impaired older adult.

American Journal of Alzheimer's Care and Related Disorders and Research 6 (4): 10–16.

Fine, E., D. B. Marin, L. Williams, R. Mohs, and K. L. Davis. 1995. *Alzheimer's patients support groups.* Poster displayed at scientific symposium, American Psychiatric Association, 148th annual meeting, Miami, Fla.

Gatz, I., 1998. Meet Robyn Yale, LCSW: A pioneer in early-stage care. In *Early Alzheimer's: An International Newsletter on Dementia*, ed. I. Gatz, 1 (1).

Goldfein, S., N. Stilwell, and R. Kahn. 1995. Communication deficits and group process in early Alzheimer's disease. Panel presentation at the annual meeting of the Gerontological Society of America, Los Angeles, November.

Goldstein, M. K., L. P. Gwyther, A. G. Lazarosf, and L. J. Thal. 1991. Managing early Alzheimer's disease. *Patient Care* 25:44–70.

Keady, J., and J. Gilliard. 1999. The early experience of Alzheimer's disease: Implications for partnership and practice. In *Dementia care: Developing partnerships in practice*, ed. T. Adams and C. Clarke, 227–56. London: Bailliere Tindall.

Kuhn, D. 1998. Caring for relatives with early stage Alzheimer's disease: An exploratory study. *American Journal of Alzheimer's Disease* 13 (July/August): 189–96.

Khurana, B. 1996. An early stage group: Reflections over time. In *International Forum on Early Dementia: Multidisciplinary Perspectives on the Early Stages of Alzheimer's Disease*, eds. R. Yale and L. Snyder, 2 (1): 3–11.

LaBarge, E., and F. Trtanj. 1995. A support group for people in the early stages of dementia of the Alzheimer's type. *Journal of Applied Gerontology* 14 (3): 289–301.

McAfee, M. E., P. A. Ruh, P. Bell, and D. Martichuski. 1989. Including persons with early stage Alzheimer's disease in support groups and strategy planning. *American Journal of Alzheimer's Care and Related Disorders and Research* 4 (6): 18–22.

Morhardt, D., and N. Johnson. 1998. *Effects of memory loss support groups for persons with early stage dementia and their families.* Paper presented at the annual meeting of the Gerontological Society of America, Philadelphia, November.

Nemeroff, T., and B. Genier. 1999. The evolution of an ongoing early stage support group. Paper presented at the annual Alzheimer's Disease Education Conference, Long Beach, July.

Quayhagen, M. P., M. Quayhagen, R. R. Corbeil, R. C. Hendrix, J. E. Jackson, L. Snyder, and D. Bower. 2000. Coping with dementia: Evaluation of four nonpharmacologic interventions. *International Psychogeriatrics* 12 (2): 249–65.

San Diego Chapter, Alzheimer's Association. 2000. What do we value about the support group? *San Diego Chapter, Alzheimer's Association Newsletter.* 21 (3): 8.

Shoham, H., and S. Neuschatz. 1985. Group therapy with senile patients. *Social Work* 30:69–72.

Snyder, L. 1999. *Speaking our minds: Personal reflections from individuals with Alzheimer's.* New York: W. H. Freeman.

Snyder, L., D. Bower, S. Arneson, S. Shepherd, and M. Quayhagen. 1993. *Coping with Alzheimer's disease and related disorders: An educational support group for early-stage individuals and their families*. San Diego: University of California, San Diego, Alzheimer's Disease Research Center.

Snyder, L., M. Quayhagen, S. Shepherd, and D. Bower. 1995. Supportive seminar groups: An intervention for early stage dementia patients. *Gerontologist* 35 (5): 691–95.

Yale, R. 1989. Support groups for newly-diagnosed Alzheimer's clients. *Clinical Gerontologist* 8 (3): 86–89.

———. 1995. *Developing support groups for individuals with early-stage Alzheimer's disease: Planning, implementation, and evaluation*. Baltimore: Health Professions Press.

———. 1996. Transition from publication to clearinghouse. In *International Forum on Early Dementia: Multidisciplinary Perspectives on the Early Stages of Alzheimer's Disease*, ed. R. Yale and L. Snyder, 2 (4): 1–3.

———. 1999. Support groups and other services for individuals with early stage Alzheimer's disease. *Generations: Journal of the American Society on Aging* 23 (3): 57–61.

Yalom, I. 1985. *The theory and practice of group psychotherapy*. New York: Basic Books.

Yeo, G., and D. Gallagher-Thompson, eds. 1996. *Ethnicity and the dementias*. Washington, D.C.: Taylor & Francis.

13

The Person with Dementia and Artwork
Art Therapy

KATHLEEN KAHN-DENIS

What should I call it [her painting]? . . . *"The Edge of the Forest."*
—Mrs. A., an 89-year-old special care unit resident

"The senses don't just make sense of life in bold or subtle acts of clarity, but they tear reality apart into vital morsels and reassemble them into meaningful patterns" (Ackerman 1990). Accordingly, people with or without dementia use color, line, and shape in a way that cannot be separated from their unique "selves." The personality will assert its sensual, meaningful patterns by arranging art materials in a manner that is unique to the creator. The use of visual elements like color and shape in art therapy sessions provides opportunities for personal expression, which is so essential to the formation of self-concept (Johnson, Lahey, and Shore 1992).

Art therapy helps persons preserve and maximize their sense of self. Essentially nonverbal, it can draw on the sensory, affective experience of the person and evoke reminiscence and self-expression, and it can create opportunities to relate to another person. This chapter features striking examples of the personhood of individuals with dementia repeatedly surfacing in their artwork at various stages of the disease. Behavioral and creative styles consistently emerge in their artwork. The three cases presented were facilitated in an adult day care center, on a dementia special care unit, and in a nursing home setting within a continuing care retirement community in Cleveland, Ohio.

Background on Art Therapy

In the United States the synergy between art and psychology became formally recognized as art therapy in the early 1940s. It is a beneficial activity that the person with AD can enjoy, and it can also strengthen coping skills, even when the dementia becomes severe (Wald 1986). One-on-one art therapy sessions are usually quiet, allowing inner feelings and emotions to surface, and the artwork produced in these sessions is often highly personal. Art therapy in a group context provides an opportunity for the person with dementia to differentiate his or her "self" from others and to interact with people with similar problems. However, the inclusion of art materials in an interactive process categorically distinguishes art therapy from other types of therapy involving personal expression, for example, music therapy.

Using art materials to create images involves the person (creator), the process (moving art materials around), the product (the end result), and sometimes a witness to the process (an art therapist). The art therapist can take advantage of the integrative role that art can play in preserving the personality of the person with dementia. Art therapy offers persons with dementia a vehicle for nonverbal expression when their ability to articulate feelings or to use language meaningfully dissipates. Artistic mediums can spark a symbolic language full of sensory exploration and stimulation. Metaphorical equivalents for feelings take shape on paper or canvas or clay, and surprising self-reflection occurs; or the person with dementia might spontaneously tell a story that was not accessible prior to involvement in the art activity. Finally, the art therapist who witnesses this process should become familiar with as many aspects of the person's manner and demeanor as possible in the hope of establishing an environment that promotes creativity and self-expression (McNiff 1992, 22). The importance of revealing oneself to others is crucial to maintaining a sense of identity. Although the task of making art can be elusive or difficult for the person with dementia, the art therapist can help him or her deal with obstacles by fostering a nonthreatening creative process. Lowenfeld (1975) described the act of creation as expressing one's importance through one's own means. The self is allowed to emerge in art. The individual's feelings, thoughts, and emotions at the time of creating are portrayed through defined lines shapes, colors, and textures.

Case Presentations

In the three cases discussed in this chapter artwork became a means of personal expression that brought complex rewards and a source of personal satisfaction. For Mrs. T., drawing and painting were a means for showing herself to others and expressing who she was as a whole person in spite of her deficits. She would reveal personal experiences from her past, and she shared her art with those in her present experience as a means for developing new, social relationships. Mrs. A.'s artwork reflects a dimension of her personality that remained untouched by her disease. Her images illustrated imagination and humor, and she revealed her desire to remain connected with other people by asking them (both staff and residents) what they thought of her artwork. Mrs. W. exhibited determination and a strong will throughout the eight years of the disease. She made images that would graphically portray her experience of being demented so that others could understand or relate to that experience.

Mrs. T.

Mrs. T. was an 82-year-old African American woman who had been diagnosed with early Alzheimer's disease and hypertension. She began participating in art therapy sessions at the adult day care center that she attended three times a week. Born in Mobile, Alabama, she had moved to the Midwest to be near the members of her immediate family who were responsible for her care. Mrs. T. was tall, slender, and elegant with a proud demeanor. She always arrived at the center impeccably dressed, adorned with jewelry. She was usually pleasant and sociable and often assumed the role of helper or volunteer at the center, offering her assistance to those around her. She did not consider herself artistic and often said that her brother was the artist in the family.

Mrs. T. completed her first painting during a group session in which the intent was simply to "play" with watercolor paint. Unlike the other participants in that session, Mrs. T. painted in an orderly fashion, arranging color and shape in a manner that was relaxing yet purposeful (see Fig. 13.1). She used bright red, yellow, and blue. She applied the paint in much the same ways that she would arrange a tray of cookies for a festive event. For many

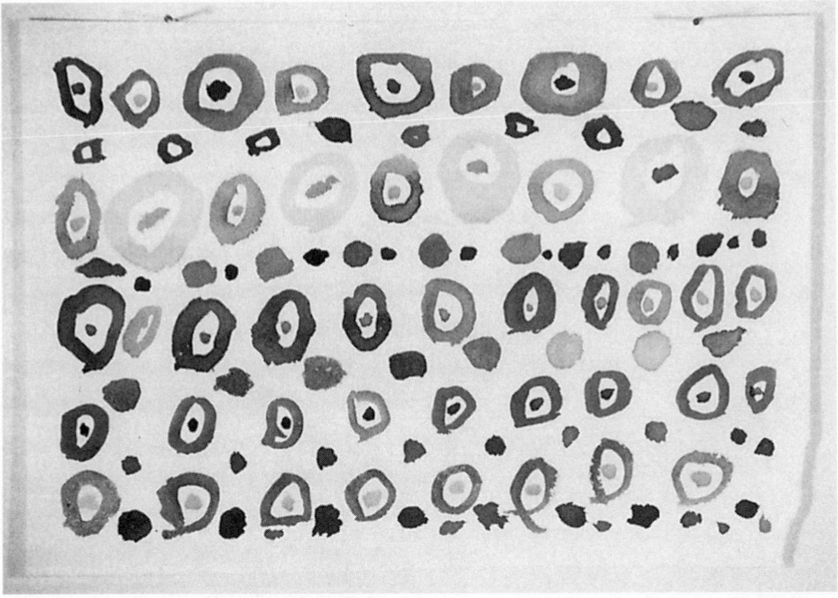

Fig. 13.1. Arranging primary colors

years she had been the head cook and baker for the Women's National Democratic Club, and she proudly spoke of those days in her life. She had the same concern for aesthetics in her artwork that she had shown in her culinary activities (see Fig. 13.2).

One year after her initial painting, Mrs. T. attempted a self-portrait (Fig. 13.3) with the assistance of an art therapist. Note the same attention to adornment in the dress as evidenced in her earlier painting. The painting had a decorative, creative style that was reminiscent of her earlier work. While painting, Mrs. T. would often stop and offer a recipe to whomever she was with at the time. Her "Seafood Bake" recipe became quite famous at the center, and again she would speak fondly of her days as a prominent hostess. At other times, however, she would speak about aspects of her life that had not been as pleasant. She would begin by describing the loss of the grandmother who had raised her and being "taken in and raised by a white family," who "saw that I got an education." The self-portrait shown in Figure 13.3, done at age 83, illustrates her desire to maintain a neat and proud appearance. She drew the portrait in an orderly manner, completing each

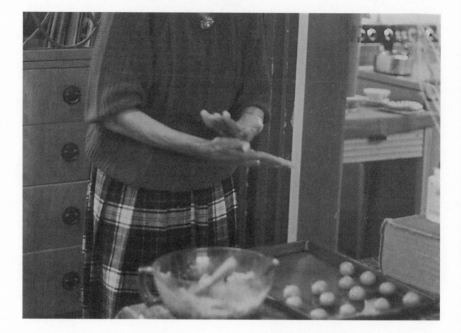

Fig. 13.2. Cookie tray preparation

section carefully before moving on to the next section. This process paralleled her organized painting style. She included detail in her dress design that reflected her love of adornment, and she added jewelry. The hair is drawn neatly, but there are some blank areas, evidence of her inability to remain attentive to detail, and she painted some lines more than once, especially in the chin area, indicating perseveration in her artwork.

As she painted this portrait, Mrs. T. revealed other meaningful facts about her self. She described a frightening time when the Ku Klux Klan surrounded the home in which she resided as a little girl and a "white woman with blonde hair" defended her presence in the community. Although this self-narration would be repeated in other types of activities, the process of making art helped Mrs. T. to organize her thoughts in a nonthreatening environment, and the release of emotion during those times was obvious even to a casual observer. Not only the paint but also her words were colorful during the creative process.

Two years later Mrs. T. completed another self-portrait (Fig. 13.4). This self-portrait has visual elements that were not evident in the previous por-

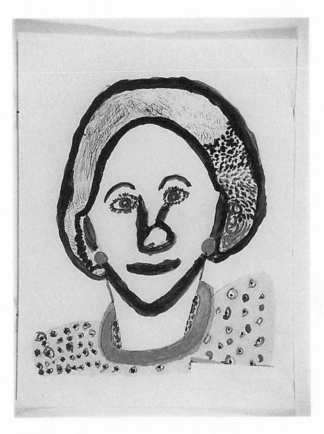

Fig. 13.3. Original self-portrait

trait. It does not contain decoration, nor was it easily drawn. It reflects some of the difficulty she was experiencing related to the progression of her disease. Compared with her earlier portrait, this portrait has no organized style, and there is minimal color. Her skin tones are painted in a medium brown. The art therapy student who assisted her with this portrait commented that "she rarely looked into the mirror before her but continued to draw ears, eyes (with lashes and eyebrows), nose, mouth, and hair." Mrs. T. referred to the subject of this portrait as "he" and said, "He's a rough guy." The features in this portrait have a crude quality that was not present in the earlier portrait (Scarpetti 1994). Mrs. T. made comments like "This doesn't look right" and "I used to do much better than this," revealing that she was aware of her inability to organize and that "things weren't right." Yet her

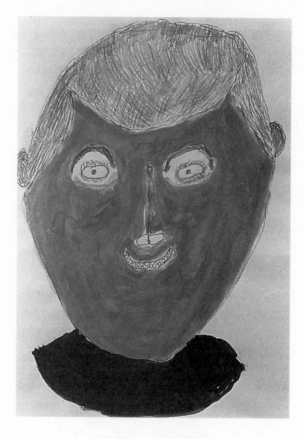

Fig. 13.4. "Rough Guy"

interactions with others at the center continued to be pleasant, and she continued her role as a helper.

Figure 13.5 shows an attempt by Mrs. T. to paint what she was feeling that day. There is no color, only black and white. The omission of color may indicate that her attitude at the time was not positive and that she was feeling uncomfortable. She usually described her paintings immediately after she completed them, but she could not explain her thoughts about this picture. This was reflected in her affect in the group, which was atypically quiet and reserved. She attempted to organize the picture by painting in the corners exclusively, leaving the center of the picture plane open. Leaving the center of the page blank may also indicate that she was having difficulty externalizing or understanding her present mood, which was also

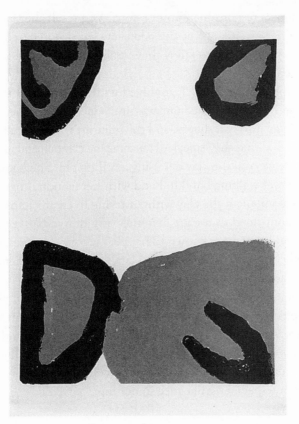

Fig. 13.5. "Feeling Miserable"

atypical for Mrs. T., who could usually verbalize her feelings to the group. At this juncture it became apparent that visual organization and using art materials had become more difficult for Mrs. T., and she eventually said that she felt "miserable." She complained that she wasn't feeling well and that she was having a bad day. The entire look of her artwork revealed a loss of detail and creative ability, and this paralleled her situation at home. In making art she could no longer pay the same attention to detail, and she spent less time completing a picture. At home, her level of physical functioning was diminishing. The family noted her inability to dress in an organized way, often layering clothes and wearing items that were not suitable for the weather. She would forget that she had eaten and insist that she receive another meal. She became increasingly argumentative toward family members responsible for her safety. As a result, her family decided to increase her attendance at the adult day care center to five times per week since she appeared to enjoy the socialization and supportive services at the center.

In an effort to keep Mrs. T. involved with art processes that still held pleasure for her, a clay medium was introduced. She cheerfully began rolling the clay into ball shapes, and the same art therapy student reported that Mrs. T. said that she "enjoy[ed] touching the clay tremendously" and that it was her idea to roll the clay out using a rolling pin. She began to recall a fond memory of walking hand in hand with her grandmother. Mrs. T. was content to manipulate the clay without trying to create a finished piece.

Mrs. T. continued to use art materials as a nonverbal vehicle for self-expression and to remain known to her peer group. However, increasingly she needed continual support and guidance from the art therapist to support her creative process. She was proud of the artwork she had compiled, totaling a minimum of twenty pieces. When she would sit down and look at several pieces at one time, she would delicately touch them with her fingertips, expressing her personal ownership of them. She would say, "I really like doing this," revealing that it was the process, not the product, that captivated her attention. Mrs. T. would selectively give her artwork to people that held some special significance in her life.

Mrs. A.

Mrs. A. had a rich imagination. Aged 89, she had been residing at a special care center for the last ten months. She had earned a B.A. degree in political science, and she had completed one year of law school before meeting her husband and beginning a family. Mrs. A. had two daughters. One daughter lived near the special care center. Mrs. A had worked in a state government office for a period of time. She had been diagnosed with "dementia with agitation," depression, anxiety, hypertension, hypothyroidism, ulcerative dermatitis, and macular degeneration. It was apparent that her level of dementia did not cause her as much difficulty on a daily basis as her physical limitations. She was slightly overweight, wore eyeglasses, and used a cane for ambulation. She had difficulty walking from one part of the special care center to another, primarily due to poor vision. However, when Mrs. A. needed an answer from the staff regarding her care or any event of the day, she would yell out loudly, insistent that she be given an immediate answer irrespective of those around her or the social situation.

Mrs. A. was referred to art therapy for two primary reasons: one, she had a casual previous interest in art, and two, she was depressed and she was becoming a daily challenge for the staff as well as the other residents. She was not easily integrated into a social situation.

When approached about the possibility of painting, Mrs. A. replied, "I can't see." However, after some coaxing and reassurance, Mrs. A. agreed to attempt a painting. The art therapist said, "If you tell me the colors you want, I will put the color on the brush." Mrs. A. proceeded to apply watercolor paint on a sheet of paper. She hesitated with her first mark, but after a few marks it appeared that she was painting a candle. The image developed into a menorah (Fig. 13.6). Mrs. A. bluntly stated that she was Jewish, and that concluded the first session. Although she could not see the total image unless it was held strategically about 3 inches in front of her,

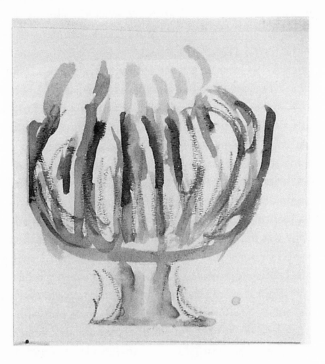

Fig. 13.6. "Holiday Time"

Mrs. A. was pleased with her accomplishment, and she agreed to try paint-ing at another time. When she did, she would usually end a session by ask-ing, "What are you going to do with the painting, put it in the trash?" She was fishing for compliments, and they were given.

After a time, Mrs. A. wanted to paint at a table with other residents. She would ask questions about the other people sitting at the table and inquire about their paintings. In the majority of social situations, however, Mrs. A.'s behavior would be considered inappropriate because her questions were loud and blunt and because at times she would ignore any responses to her questions and continue with the same inquiry. The second time Mrs. A. painted, she began with a green because she was thinking about the out-doors. Spreading the paint over the paper, she said, "I'll make some trees. . . . Now give me some brown." This time she applied the paint in a spontaneous, fluid manner, allowing the image to emerge. She asked for blue for the sky, and she asked for advice about where to put the paint on the page. Mrs. A. was freely making decisions and choices, but she allowed the art therapist to be her guide, or "third hand" (Kramer 1986). When she nearly finished with the painting, she asked, "What should I call it?" The art therapist re-sponded, "Well, what do you think?" and Mrs. A. eloquently blurted out, "The Edge of the Forest" (Fig. 13.7).

During one session Mrs. A. was struggling, and she said, "I don't feel like doing anything." The art therapist sat next to her, gently accepting her mood. Mrs. A. appeared to be depressed, withdrawn, and fatigued. After sitting silently for ten minutes, not verbalizing anything about her present state, Mrs. A. said, "Give me some paint, any color." She began a line, and it developed into a shoe. The session became a humorous dialogue about shoes, and her mood improved. The art therapist asked her if she liked shoes, to which she replied, "Not particularly." After painting two images of shoes, Mrs. A. did a painting of a pair of roller skates, which she titled "Fleeting" (Fig. 13.8). She was not able to elaborate on the meaning of the title; how-ever, it appeared that she had finally moved beyond her depressed mood. A pattern was beginning to emerge in Mrs. A.'s creative process. She pre-ferred to draw or paint more than one image each session, and usually the first or second image was not her favorite. She had to produce several im-ages before she could arrive at the one that communicated what she wanted to say. She also preferred to title her paintings, and she would consistently ask, "What should I call it?" It should be noted that Mrs. A. did not remem-

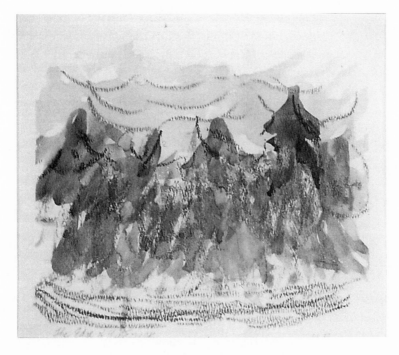

Fig. 13.7. "The Edge of the Forest"

ber her paintings or the art therapist from week to week, but she began to be more comfortable and joined each session more readily.

As her images developed over an eight-month period, Mrs. A. created several paintings that expressed freedom and movement, such as a painting of a dancer, a bird in flight, or a pair of roller skates. The images cannot be separated from the movement they portray. Having worked with Mrs. A. for an extended period to help her express herself through art, I can state with some confidence that her symbols of movement compensated for her inability to get around physically or to leave the special care center without assistance. Her imagination led her to create images that expressed some degree of freedom both literally and figuratively. Thus, through her artwork the staff came to know aspects of Mrs. A.'s personality that it would otherwise have been impossible for them to know.

As a result of her efforts in weekly art therapy sessions, her behavior in the special care center changed. When she was involved in making art, she was able to address others working at the table in a socially acceptable manner.

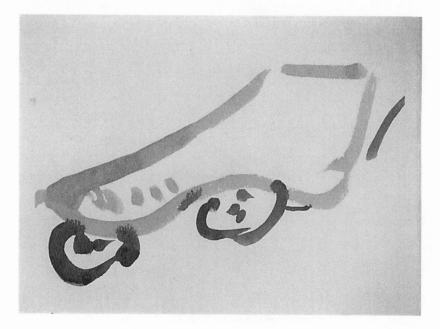

Fig. 13.8. "Fleeting"

She would ask, "What are they painting?" or "Can I see your painting?" She would often compliment them on their artwork. Sometimes members of the art therapy group would laugh at her repeated questions, which previously had been a source of annoyance, showing their acceptance of her creative personality and her new-found role as an artist. She was the most prolific artist at the special care center. She was able to paint for one to two hours at a time, showing a stamina that she did not show in any other type of activity.

At an art exhibit held for family members at the special care center Mrs. A. was asked, "What do you like about painting?" Immediately she replied, "Just doing it." After a short pause she added, "I like to feel like it's part of me."

Mrs. W.

Mrs. W.'s interest in using art materials was initially social: she wanted to be part of the group. Over the course of eight years, however, she was able to use the images she created to show what her disease process felt like and to make herself known to the staff. She was unswerving in her desire to describe what was happening to her and to understand what was to come.

Mrs. W. moved into the independent-living section of a large retirement community at age 79. Within a few months her friends and the staff noticed that she was missing luncheon and medical appointments. Over time it became apparent that her cognitive impairments were increasing and that supportive services were needed to maintain her present lifestyle within the retirement community.

She was attractive, well groomed, and in excellent physical condition. She walked at a fast pace and was known as the woman who always wore high heels. She was a widow with no children. She had been one of the first female vice presidents of a major financial institution in a large American city. She was accustomed to competitive situations and demanding time schedules. Eventually she was referred to the adult day care center of her retirement community. The staff at the day care center were told that she would view her participation at the center as a work situation. She responded well to the idea of arriving at the center early in the morning and staying until she had completed a full day's activities. She assumed the role of a worker while at the center, assisting other participants in whatever way possible with the staff's support and guidance. She identified with the staff far more than she did with the other adult day care participants.

Mrs. W.'s initial experience with art materials at the center came about casually. The staff did not expect her to enjoy an art therapy group since it would mean that she would be a participant and not a helper. However, she quickly took an interest in the art sessions as a means to socially join the group. She approached art in a manner that was consistent with her work experience: as a challenge, something new to master. Occasionally she would talk about past work experiences, such as attending meetings at which she was the only woman present and how difficult that was for her. When she made these statements, however, there was a smile on her face, indicating that she remembered those days with pleasure.

The appearance of the painting was less important to Mrs. W. than applying herself to the task. She was not discouraged by her efforts, as many others would have been, and were, in a similar situation. The involvement kept her committed. Figure 13.9 shows a sunflower that Mrs. W. painted from life. There are short, scattered lines outside the form of the flower and

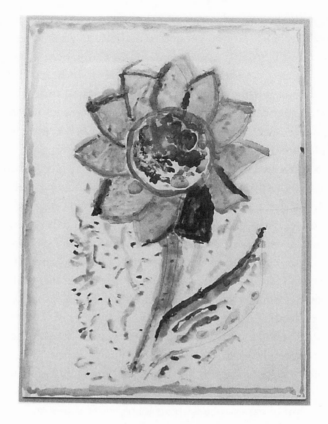

Fig. 13.9. Sunflower

a few inside the leaf form. She painted over one flower petal repeatedly (the darkest area shown), and her perseveration is evident. She painted some lines over and over, as if she did not comprehend their completion. A few months later she completed the painting shown in Figure 13.10. Mrs. W. created this heart in a group setting in which the discussion revolved around Valentine's Day and some members reminisced about past loves. She responded to the suggestion of a heart and began filling in the form with short, somewhat scattered lines and randomly placed dots, using no broad strokes to fill in an area.

During this same period of time a move from independent living to a special care center was being considered for Mrs. W. because her diagnosis of AD had been confirmed. At the adult day care center, now with limited

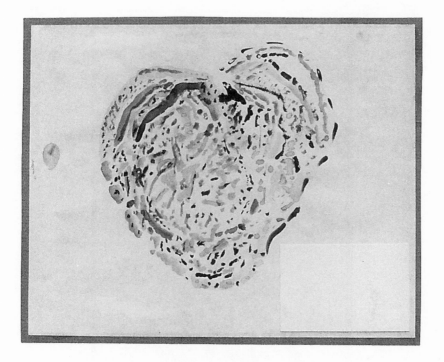

Fig. 13.10. Valentine's Day

speech capacity (forming full sentences was increasingly difficult), she would ask the staff, "Am I going?" and she would point to an area within the retirement community that was to become the new special care center. Even with increased functional losses, she persisted in trying to understand what was happening to her and where she would be residing in the future.

Figures 13.11 and 13.12 illustrate the progressive nature of her disease. These two pictures, painted within six months of each other, are characterized by a lack of form and scattered, disconnected lines. There is more space between the lines than previously. In Figure 13.12 there are fewer lines overall, and the lines are placed farther apart. The application of each line was a struggle for Mrs. W. She used a variety of colors—yellow, blue, red, and black—but she paused after applying each stroke of paint, indicating an increased struggle to make connections between the parts. She would pause and say, "Do I, do I . . . have [and she would pause again]?" That she was searching for the word *Alzheimer's* was confirmed when a staff mem-

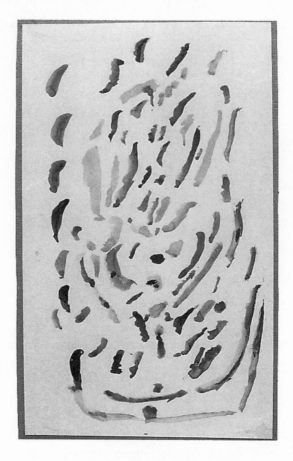

Fig. 13.11. Abstract I

ber completed her sentence and she wanted to continue with a discussion of memory loss. She was aware of her difficulty in processing her painting, just as she was aware of her difficulty in processing her thoughts. Yet she was persistent in trying to come to terms with what was happening to her. The artwork she produced seemed to graphically mimic the course of a progressive dementia. It was like an x-ray, reflecting the disconnections in her brain activity.

Almost two years later, while residing at the special care center, Mrs. W. completed the painting shown in Figure 13.13. This piece is smaller than her previous paintings, measuring 4 by 6 inches. The painting lacks color,

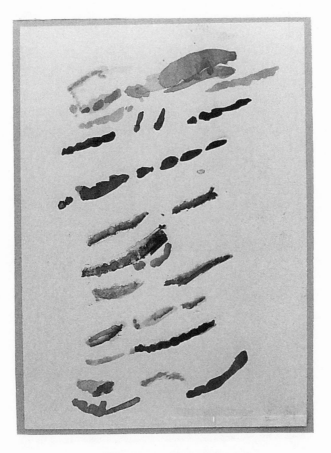

Fig. 13.12. Abstract 2

and Mrs. W. applied the paint with a scribbling motion. She occasionally made a mark in an attempt to border or frame the piece, with little success. She appeared to wander in her production of this painting. In the paintings shown in Figures 13.9 through 13.12 the paint was applied more energetically, and the placement was more deliberate. During the three years following the painting shown in Figure 13.13 there were many times when art materials were not offered to Mrs. W. out of a concern that it might create a confusing situation, yet she continued to try to take part. She would sit with the group and stare at the art materials, but she was not able to initiate any purposeful use of them. Near the end of her life, when verbal

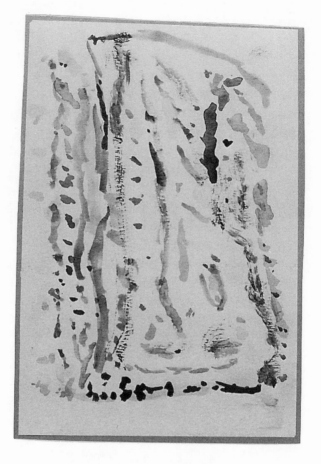

Fig. 13.13. Abstract 3

speech was not available to her, she would walk into the office of the special care center's coordinator and stand silently in front of the telephone, looking down at the phone and then glancing up at the coordinator. Each day she spent time in the coordinator's office just looking around. She seemed to be trying to connect or analyze her situation, still persistent in wanting to be heard and wanting to understand.

Eventually Mrs. W. was moved to the nursing division of the same retirement community. Her expressive abilities in art dissipated, but she would walk up to the art therapist as an equal and stare. She seemed to recognize that the two of them had worked together and were now struggling together to make sense of this final phase of her life. Three weeks after her placement in the nursing division, Mrs. W. passed away. Over the course of the disease Mrs. W. had persisted in her artwork, in her verbal inquiries about her disease, and in her nonverbal actions.

Conclusions about the Three Cases

In each of the cases discussed above, the process of creating subjective images gave the person with dementia a means to gain control over her own reality. The emphasis on affect or feeling levels rather than on normative reality provided a bridge to her remaining strengths. Mrs. T. had a need to share autobiographical information, both verbally and nonverbally. Her images distilled what was essential to her alone, in the past and in the present. Her desire to maintain a sense of aesthetics was evident in the decorative designs of her artwork and in the pride she took in her personal appearance. She wanted to show that she was proud of her accomplishments as a caterer and as a person who had had to persist in the face of prejudice. Even though her social abilities were now limited, she wanted to enter into new relationships.

Mrs. A. found a means to compensate for her limited eyesight by visualizing through her imagination. She expressed her desire for a greater degree of freedom. Her images and her titles enabled observers (the art therapist and caregivers) to glimpse her unique imagination. She was only trying to express her own reality at the time.

Mrs. W. still embraced a challenge, a new opportunity. She did not passively submit to the obstacles before her, and even with severe limitations, she tried to comprehend her current situation and what was to come. Her artwork revealed both her strengths and her deficits. The paintings illustrated broken connections, yet she was determined to complete each picture.

None of these women revealed anything new about themselves in their artwork, which would have been difficult or nearly impossible because of the severity of their disease, but they were able to make their experiences known in spite of their cognitive deficits. The images suggested the women's internal worlds. The artworks allowed the observer to glimpse the person who had created them in a way that words could not have done.

Lessons Learned

Personal Expression of Self versus Competence

Like any other artist faced with obstacles to overcome due to an illness, the three women discussed above did not let their incapacities determine the level of their personal, creative competence. Competence was not their reason for making art. The process of creating evolved into a special way to become known as a person. Each of these women began with a feeling of insecurity. However, initial resistance and insecurities gave way to making an initial mark that led to involvement and concluded with a final product. Each person, with the help and comfort of a supportive person, found a way to comfortably use art materials to become known to herself and to others. It is thus fair to assume that a caregiver (professional, family, or friend) could use art materials as an alternate form of communication. Some people with dementia who previously never would have considered communicating nonverbally through artwork might turn to this expressive medium. However, as with other artists, there are times when creating is a struggle with no obvious personal gain. At these times the caregiver needs to consider the impact making art has on the individual. The act of making art should be pleasurable, should encourage qualities in the creator such as involvement and spontaneity, and it should allow him or her a way to express feelings and perhaps a way to socialize with others. It should not create additional confusion or stress. People with dementia are able to measure their own interest in using art materials; therefore, the caregiver can sense when to discontinue art as a means of personal communication.

The Senses: Benefits of Process, Not Product

People with dementia can find ways to connect with their sensory world through art. Using art materials to exercise and experience personal choices and control in a symbolic way can be valuable for people with difficulties (Wood 1998, 5).

Simply structured art activities that have no purpose other than to experience the use of a sensory medium are worthwhile. A person can be captivated by a vibrant color such as a warm yellow or a bright orange. The feel of clay can evoke an unexpected response. The art therapist or a caregiver needs to ensure that the art materials serve to enhance sensory exploration and do not create more obstacles.

A Tangible Product

Over the course of the disease, artwork illustrates to the person with dementia and to his or her caregiver(s) some facts of the person's experience. Often a song or a melody is remembered and sung, but the song cannot be held in the hands of the person singing, nor can it be seen. For the person with dementia, there can be great comfort and value in using one's hands, especially when one's level of cognition wanes.

An image provides the viewer with a piece of the person's experience. Yet the influence of the artwork can extend beyond the individual who created it. The artwork, as mentioned, can be a gift or a piece to be viewed by staff and family members. It can be viewed by visitors and casual observers can note the efforts of the creator, thus validating the person as a productive, contributing human being.

Analysis of the Artwork

A qualitative analysis of features that are typically observed in the drawings of people with a progressive dementia suggests that there are some common elements that indicate physical changes in the brain. Such elements include short, scattered lines; perseveration, or repetition of a line, shape, or color; a small, cramped appearance; disconnections in the creative process, that is, the inability of the person to perceive the parts as fitting into a whole or abrupt interruptions in the process of creating; an impoverished appearance, with essential features often omitted from the drawings; and difficulty in comprehending or following directions. Attention deficits may also be apparent in the artwork, resulting, for example, in the failure to integrate separate features into a coherent whole (Cronin and Werblowsky 1979; Moore and Wyke 1984; Wald 1983, 1984, 1986).

Such features can help the staff and family caregivers to evaluate changes or the progression of the disease. Although it is tempting to consider the artwork on its own, it is important to remember that the artwork is never divorced from the individual who created it, that it reflects the individual's personal state.

Conclusion

Working with art materials allows persons with dementia to create and re-create their unique selves, complete with losses and gains. In the cases discussed here the gains were self-evident, one person momentarily being able to express her past, another finding an imagination that could only be revealed through art. In addition, the experience allows a social connection, an interpersonal process between the person with dementia and the art therapist. Making art minimizes verbal demands on the individual and provides an alternate outlet for negative feelings or confusion in an environment where it is safe to release them.

An image, a spoken word while creating, a refusal to participate, a title for a picture, an expressed feeling, a choice of color or medium, a desire to share a painting with another person—all are pathways to understand the creator, the originator, the person, who happens to be diagnosed with dementia.

REFERENCES

Ackerman, D. 1990. *The natural history of the senses*. New York: Vintage Books.
Cronin, S., and J. Werblowsky. 1979. Early signs of organicity in art work. *Arts Psychotherapy* 6:103–8.
Johnson, C., P. Lahey, and A. Shore. 1992. An exploration of creative arts therapeutic group on an Alzheimer's unit. *Arts in Psychotherapy* 19:269–77.
Kahn-Denis, K. 1997. Art therapy with geriatric dementia clients. *Journal of American Art Therapy Association* 14 (3): 94–99.
Kramer, E. 1986. The art therapist's third hand: Reflections on art, art therapy, and society at large. *American Journal of Art Therapy* 24:71–86.
Lowenfeld, V. 1975. *Creative and mental growth*. 6th ed. New York: Macmillan.
McNiff, Shaun. 1992. *Art as medicine: Creating a therapy of imagination*. Boston: Shambala.
Moore, V., and M. Wyke. 1984. Drawing disability in patients with senile dementia. *Psychological Medicine* 14:97–105.
Scarpetti, S. 1994. Clinical orientation II: Case study. Paper presented in clinical orientation studies course at Ursuline College, Cleveland, Ohio, April.

Wald, J. 1983. Alzheimer's disease and the role of art therapy in its treatment. *American Journal of Art Therapy* 22 (3): 57–64.

———. 1984. The graphic representation of regression in an Alzheimer's disease patient. *Arts in Psychotherapy* 2:165–75.

———. 1986. Art therapy for patients with dementing illnesses. *Clinical Gerontologist* 4 (3): 29–39.

Wood, M. 1998. What is art therapy? In *Art therapy in palliative care*, ed. M. Pratt and M. Wood, 1–11. London: Routledge.

14

"I Can't Place This Place at All"

The Nursing Home Experience

JOHN KILLICK

In a sense, all aging involves gains and losses. The longer we live, the more experience of life we accrue, and this can lead to an accumulation of what used to be called wisdom. But as we grow older, there can be a deterioration in physical capacity or failing mental powers. Dementia is not an inevitable part of this process, but since it is largely a disease of age, as we tend to live longer it affects a growing number of people in our society.

Among losses that come with age, bereavement has received the most attention. We now understand more about the natural psychological consequences of losing someone close. A range of emotions, preoccupations, and actions occur and recur during the period of mourning (Kubler-Ross 1970; Worden 1991). But death is not the only event that occasions feelings of loss. We recognize the need for grieving in response to other losses in people's lives—of relationships, of jobs, of valued possessions. In the area of health there are potentially many losses. People with dementia will be affected by these as a matter of course.

This chapter is concerned with the consequences for people whose dementia has caused a change in their circumstances requiring them to enter a nursing home. I attempt to identify some of the additional losses involved, quoting extensively the words of residents, and to make some positive observations about how individuals adapt and how stresses may be ameliorated. My material comes from more than nine years as a writer in residence for a private health care company in Great Britain.

Before I enter into this discussion, however, I need to explain exactly what my work entails and how the texts provided here came about. I work one-to-one in mental health units where everyone has a diagnosis of dementia. Mine is a listening brief, but that also involves essential relationship-building before insights are vouchsafed. The principles I follow include the following:

- *Let the resident choose you.* I let the resident choose me rather than picking individuals based on my own preference or on the recommendation of staff. This imparts a much greater naturalness to the conversations and harnesses the motivation of my subjects.
- *Do not ask questions.* I do not ask questions, and I have no agenda. I let the residents choose the topic and set the pace. My role is an enabling one.
- *Ask the individual for permission.* At a certain point in the interaction I may ask permission to write down or tape-record what the person says. I explain that this is so that I can concentrate on the individual's remarks, which seems to have an empowering effect. Any transcript made is shared with the individual on a subsequent visit. With the individual's permission, it may also be shared with relatives or staff.
- *Some texts have natural poetic qualities.* I talk to the individuals and ask permission to shape their words as poems. If permission is given, I return with a finished piece and seek the person's approval. I never add anything, only subtract material that seems irrelevant to the main subject; this process resembles that of any writer revising and refining a text. Often I am given permission to share the poem with a wider audience. Occasionally this practice is actually requested by the person with dementia.

Entering any institution necessarily involves being subjected to regimes and privations. These have been well documented by Goffman (1961). The age at which most people enter nursing homes may well exacerbate the situation: the institutional experience after a lifetime of independent living can prove traumatic for some. The variability of the quality of institutional care must also be put into the equation. The report commonly referred to as the Wagner Report (Wagner 1988) enumerated desirable characteristics, but it is by no means certain that all establishments match these or meet even acceptable standards of nursing care.

Entering a long-term-care facility can mean different things to different people. I would not wish to suggest that the experience is predominantly one of loss for everyone. For those who have lived alone for a long time the social aspects of nursing home life can prove beneficial. The constant availability of assistance and medication may bring peace of mind. The routines of an institution can prove profoundly reassuring to one whose established regime has been disrupted. Wade (1994) identified these and other positive characteristics.

Entering nursing care may also entail a series of losses. The first and most obvious of these is the loss of a home over which one had a claim of ownership or tenure and that was comfortingly familiar in its layout, its furniture, and its many smaller objects. It is likely to have constituted a highly personalized environment. The individual may have lived in these surroundings for many years. Nothing that can be supplied in the communal setting will come close to replacing it, and the fact that that personal stamp, that unique authenticity, is gone, probably forever, is difficult for many people to accept. In someone with dementia it can exacerbate already existing feelings of confusion:

> It's really scary when you're an old woman.
> I'm bereft. I hate being stranded like this,
> I want to be down in the middle of town.
> But I have no money to speak of,
> and I don't know how to get away from here.
> I can't open it! The door won't open!
>
> I shall have to grit my teeth and walk like hell.
> And it's cold out there without a coat.
> How stupid I didn't think of this before.
> I've never been in such a situation.
> I've missed buses, but this is different.
> This door won't open! And that's another!
>
> I didn't expect this predicament. Well, if I'm stuck
> I'll just have to ask them for a bed for the night.

The longing to be home is very frequently expressed by residents of nursing homes, and it is often part of a larger desire, to be in familiar surroundings, which will bring some consolation. As another woman, the woman whose words provided the title for this chapter, put it, "I can't place this place at all. . . . Isn't that terrible? . . . Can you take me home so far? I'll reward you."

Second, there is the loss of access to friends and family. Although residents of a nursing home may have visitors, they cannot drop in in quite the same way that they would in a private dwelling. There are established routines to be observed, and there is not the same opportunity to offer hospitality to guests. Depending on where the establishment is situated, those who wish to maintain links may have to travel a considerable distance. Some friends and family are likely to be about the same age as the resident, and that poses special problems. The result is an inevitable sense of loss, feelings of isolation and losing touch with one's community outside. Here is a lady trying to place me, a visitor, in relation to her family:

> *You didn't have a house in them days, you had rooms.*
> *I came to live around this part, and it's a nice part, isn't it?*
> *Now I've a house with two rooms to spare.*
>
> *Are you my uncle, then?*
>
> *The girls were nice. Not like now when they get a bit hoity toity.*
> *My girls quarrelled, it got a bit touchy at times.*
> *I think it's better if you get strangers bringing them up.*
>
> *You are gran's father, then?*
>
> *My grandmother never seemed never to make nothing hard.*
> *My dad was a very strict man. Still is.*
> *My man never comes in and grouses, nothing like that.*
>
> *Are you one of the sons, then?*
>
> *All those old 'uns'll be gone, spent their days.*
> *Old people today don't try to do what they shouldn't.*
> *If there's anything here I try to keep it on the level.*
>
> *Are you a bit of a relative, then?*

Third, there is the loss of role. We play many roles in the course of our lives, and society's attitudes toward age tend to erode these, often putting nothing in their place. People who are retired may have had to adjust to a life lacking the sense of purpose that work supplies. Now other statuses confirmatory of dignity and purpose have been taken away—housewife, handyman, manager of personal finances, car driver. One man uses the symbol of a barrow to represent his losses:

> *Have you seen my barrow?*
> *I joined the group,*
> *and now it belongs to all of us.*
> *But I don't know where it's gone.*
>
> *It seems as if*
> *I'm like a buzzing toy—*
> *it buzzes round and round*
> *but it doesn't mean much.*
>
> *Altogether you won't find*
> *much toing and froing*
> *and doing or being*
> *with me. I never carry*
> *as full as you do.*
>
> *The way this country's going*
> *men can just go round*
> *and do as they choose.*
> *They can take my bed*
> *and my barrow.*
>
> *I think I just drift about.*
> *I think that's what I do*
> *usually. I'm just a kind*
> *of quiet nobody.*

Next comes loss of privacy. Not everyone in nursing homes has a room of his or her own, though this should surely be regarded as a basic right regardless of income. And even where sharing does not occur, all the other rooms are communal. Many people end their days forced to endure a social life with people they have never met before, with whom they may have little in common, and in any case have not chosen as their companions. Here is a lady searching for a place and rejecting the people she meets on the journey:

> *Which way shall we go?*
> *We could go this way round*
> *And round and round again.*
> *Or we could go that way round*
> *And round and round again.*
>
> *You get these girls coming along,*
> *About six of them at least.*
>
> *Which and Whatsum, I say.*
> *I can't catch them up.*
> *It's all too much for me.*

There is a loss of continuity too. The person with dementia has probably not met any of the staff or residents before, and they may know little or nothing of the person's past life, so even though the present may offer little in the way of opportunities for achievement, past roles, relationships, and successes are likely to be "a closed book" to those with whom they must spend their days. This is particularly unfortunate where the staff are concerned: the person before them may seem little more than an amalgam of ailments, and relationships are bound to suffer from this two-dimensional view.

In addition, many of the habits and rituals of a lifetime may have to be abandoned when a person enters an institution. And the ability to take decisions even over small matters appears to be blocked, so that people feel powerless to affect the circumstances of their daily lives. Sometimes, as in the following text, this finds expression as a sense of impotence, even victimization:

> *I'm not to ask for any help.*
> *They've told me, I'm not to ask.*

They told me up the corridor.
So I'll do as others do:
I'll just go to sleep.

I can't have any help.
No wonder, there is none.
She came through
when they were telling me
so she knows.

Can I get undressed?
Be careful, they might hear you,
you can't be too careful.
I'm not to get washed or that—
Orders of the Management.

They don't give you a chance:
if you do this you'll get that;
if you do something else
you'll get the other.
I'm not asking any questions,
I get jumped on every time.

The speaker in the following text has only recently been admitted to the nursing home. He pours scorn on everything, from cups of tea to the construction of the building. Despite its humor, the text is an expression of frustration rather than a balanced view of his situation:

In this place all the cups of tea
end half-way up. If I get tea
in a saucer, anyone can have it.
What I want to know is:
is there any limit to when I get the top half?

The object of golf is to hit the ball
as fast as you can, direction immaterial.
I've never owned a set of clubs

and I've never owned a trolley.
The truth is I'm here on a golfing holiday
and they haven't even got a course!

This isn't a building, no way
is this a building. I'd describe it
unkindly. Somebody came along
and stuck three rooms together
and called it "A Home"!
Then 33 other people came along
and each tacked a piece on.
In short, it was thrown together
and the bits didn't meet,
and'll never be got right.

The best way to improve this place is. . . .
bigger cups! And I don't know whether
that's my view of tea or golf!

The cumulative effect of losses causes the most concern. Listlessness, boredom, and pessimism are commonplace in these institutions and may be responsible for a further decline in mental functioning that would usually be attributed to a progression of the dementia. Loss of control of their lives and of the skills necessary for exercising such control will inevitably lead to a loss of self-esteem in the short or long term. And where the will to survive and stay healthy has been sapped, it may well be that the very physical conditions that nursing care exists to treat will be exacerbated. Here is a lady reflecting vividly on the process and its effects on those around her:

I've lived here since the War finished.
It's a nice place and nice people, but it isn't home.
That man is completely up a gum tree,
but he'll be able to get down again.

That's one of the children in the playground crying.
Her parents are here looking after her.

> *That door's squeaking. It hasn't very much sense.*
> *It makes you wonder who's looking after it.*
>
> *There were people here yesterday who had the pull with us,*
> *but then they had to let their ropes go.*
>
> *There's a party coming in tomorrow*
> *which will make this place overcrowded.*
>
> *There's so much space down below*
> *that it seems ridiculous not to use it.*
>
> *I think it's a pity to have all these people together in here.*
> *They don't wear as well as they would outside.*

The last two lines throw down a challenge: how are we to attempt to counteract the negative effects of institutional life on the increasing numbers of people with dementia who are entering special units in our nursing homes? The answer is, with difficulty, particularly when large numbers of untrained staff are employed. But there are things we can do. The overall message is that the staff must be encouraged to realize that the transition from one's own home to a nursing home can often be traumatic. They need to recognize the signs of disorientation, distress, and depression, which often result from this. In some cases treatment can be offered; in others counseling must be made available. Individuals must be given the opportunity to talk through their fears and distresses.

Lessons Learned

Here is a list of other practical measures that can be taken. Although these suggestions are not new, they are often forgotten and thus can bear restatement:

- Relatives can be encouraged to surround their loved ones with familiar furniture and objects. They will not only help people to settle into their new environments but also remind them of their past lives, emphasizing a vital sense of continuity and providing topics of conversation for staff and visitors.

• There should be an open-door policy. Relatives should be able to visit at any time rather than at certain advertised hours. A flexible arrangement such as this encourages more visits and also gives more stimulation to residents.

• Ways should be found to consult residents whenever possible about their preferences with regard to routines, food, entertainment, and so on. The times for getting up in the morning and going to bed at night, as well as for taking a bath, can be varied according to individual preferences. Similarly, menus that involve real choices can be compiled, and individuals can be asked what entertainments they prefer and when they wish them to be provided.

• As long as individuals are able to carry out everyday tasks and take on responsibilities, they should be encouraged to do so. Examples might be tidying and dusting, food preparation, washing up, and gardening.

• Life-history work and the sharing of insights gleaned can help to establish residents as three-dimensional people in the eyes of staff and encourage the building of fruitful relationships. This involves consulting residents and relatives about details of residents' past lives, interests, tastes, and preferences. It also involves ensuring that all staff are aware of this information source and make use of it.

• A varied activities program that takes account of minority interests should be instituted. Not everyone enjoys bingo or wants to watch the same television program. Efforts should be made to discover people's specific enthusiasms and cater to them even though it may involve special provision for the individual.

• Links should be forged with individuals and organizations in the community so that a sense of interconnectedness is developed between those outside and those inside the walls. There are many public-spirited people who would be prepared to visit a nursing home for an hour or two a week to chat or to provide a service. Similarly, there are organizations that might be persuaded to use the premises and include residents in their meetings.

I would like to end on a positive note. An important resource that we so easily neglect within these institutions is the residents themselves. Between them they have much to offer in the way of interests and enthusiasms, and even more in terms of humor and human sympathy. We can harness these by creating opportunities for them to be exercised. It only takes imagination and a little effort. By way of example I want to introduce you to Peachey—that is her nickname for herself. I spent an hour with her, and she more than repaid my time with her irrepressible high spirits and warmth. This is the piece of writing I made from her words. She immediately sought out all the staff on the unit, gathered them together, and declaimed it to them with great enthusiasm:

> *When we got off the plane*
> *the man in the little hut*
> *was selling the photographs he took.*
> *He said "This is the lady."*
> *He didn't need any building-up of acquaintance.*
> *It was straight from the horse's mouth.*
>
> *I wasn't brill at school,*
> *but the boys called after me.*
> *The boys christened me "Peachey."*
> *They'd say "Tell Peachey."*
> *And I didn't like it.*
>
> *I didn't know it was a gift.*
> *But the teacher had a soft spot,*
> *he never said anything, of course,*
> *but it was in his eyes.*
>
> *I roar with laughing at people,*
> *and they laugh at me.*
> *But I don't know any jokes,*
> *it's all home-made humour.*
> *It fits if I say the phrase.*
> *Sparsmodic. I can laugh and like it.*
> *I used to sing for people,*
> *sing what fits the emotion at the time.*
> *When I first did it*

I thought I was going to be reprimanded
for singing out of line.
But Life is Singing.

I'll talk, but it's not my scene,
chatting somebody up.
I'm not a grabber of situations.
I come out in little phrases, that's me.
And I don't know anybody who's not cheerful.
I bet you've never been so near Nature before!

What should become obvious from the texts is that people with dementia in nursing homes do not, as was once thought, talk gibberish. Their speech is worthy of consideration by those without the condition. What we have here are serious statements that we must take seriously.

These people are individuals, clearly differentiated from one another. The idea that they can be lumped together as "the demented" is proven false by these examples. Their use of words is inventive and memorable. Here are people using the affective properties of language, not the intellectual.

What these people with dementia in nursing homes do have in common is that they are all engaged in the struggle to make sense of what the condition is doing to them and to come to terms with the change in their situation. These poems are positive achievements, expressive of feelings, and testimony to the strength of the human spirit, despite dementia.

ACKNOWLEDGMENTS

The poems are taken from J. Killick, *You are words: Dementia poems* (London: Hawker, 1997); and J. Killick and C. Cordonnier, *Openings: Dementia poems and photographs* (London: Hawker, 2000).

REFERENCES

Goffman, E. 1961. *Asylums*. New York: Doubleday.
Kubler-Ross, E. 1970. *On death and dying*. London: Tavistock.
Wade, B. 1994. *The changing face of community care*. London: Daphne Heald Research Unit.
Wagner, Lady. 1988. *Residential care: A positive choice*. London: HMSO.
Worden, J. W. 1991. *Grief counselling and therapy*. London: Tavistock and Routledge.

Index

acceptance of disease, 157–58, 159, 171
activities: awareness of symptoms and,
    208; choice and, 279; at day care cen-
    ter, 193–95; past, connection with,
    174–75
adaptation, 176. *See also* coping strategies
adult day care. *See* day care center
aging, comments on journey of, 145–46
agitation in support group setting, 239
altruism, 175, 209. *See also* volunteerism
Alzheimer, Alois, 5
Alzheimer's Family Care Center, 127–28
ambivalence about disclosure of diagno-
    sis, 123–25, 236
anger: forgetting and, 54–55; with med-
    ical experience, 36–37, 39, 41
anticipatory adaptation, 176
anxiety: in assessment experience, 16–
    20; strategic resistance and, 19–20, 21
art therapy: analysis of artwork, 267–68;
    behavior and, 256, 257–58; clay me-
    dium, 254; feelings, 252–53; Mrs. A.
    case presentation, 248, 254–58, 265;
    Mrs. T. case presentation, 248–54,
    265; Mrs. W. case presentation, 248,
    258–65; overview of, 246–47; prod-
    uct of, 267; progression of illness and,
    261–64; self-expression *vs.* compe-
    tence, 266; self- portraits, 249–52;
    senses and, 266–67; symbolism in,
    257; titling work, 256–57

assessment experience: acknowledging
    the challenge, 14–16; background of
    study of, 9–11; biographical approach
    to, 23–24; conditions necessary for,
    22–23; considering future options,
    20–22; overview of, 3–4; playing
    game, 16–20; primary health care
    and, 5–6; recommendations for, 23–
    25; seeking help, 14; social context
    and, 8–9; temporal dimensions of, 4
attributes and selfhood: Dr. M case ex-
    ample, 95–100, 102, 103–4; Mrs. D
    case example, 106, 107; overview of,
    92–93
autonomy, loss of, 120, 275–77
awareness of symptoms: activities and,
    208; burden and, 118; description of,
    xxxi–xxxii; "I'm sort of oblivious"
    theme, 66–69; need for support and,
    207; research on, 49–50. *See also*
    lived experience; losing one's way,
    worries about

befriending service, 189, 199–204
biographical approach to assessment,
    23–24
Bradford Dementia Group, xv–xvi

caregiver: concern of persons with
    Alzheimer's disease for, 116–18,
    208–9; conjoint interview with,

caregiver (*cont.*)
128–29; conversation strategies for, 89–90; dependency and, xxxii; interview in home and, 205; quality of life of person with Alzheimer's disease and, 83; research on, xv; spirituality and, 160–61; stress and coping model and, 165–66; support group and, 230–32, 240; view of person with Alzheimer's disease of, 106, 107–8, 109, 110. *See also* family; spouse
"caring congregation," 156–57
choice, 208, 279
Cleveland community dialogue, 155–60
cognitive restructuring, 37, 38, 167
communication: affective *vs.* intellectual, 281; "barriers to communication" theme, 115; changes in, 129–30; difficulty expressing self, 63–64; in group process, 229–30, 231–32, 239; intervention strategies for, 71, 89–90, 147–48; with physician, 39–42. *See also* art therapy; conversation strategies; meaningful communication
community services: befriending service, 189, 199–204; evaluation of, 188–90, 207–9; interview approach to evaluation of, 204–7; overview of, 187–88. *See also* day care center; support groups; volunteerism
compassion and empathy, 141–42, 279–81
competence: art therapy and, 266; volunteerism and, 213, 223. *See also* attributes and selfhood
conceptual framework, xvii–xix. *See also* person-centered care
confusion, feelings of, 60–62
conjoint groups, 230–32
consent issue, 204
conversation strategies, 71, 89–90. *See also* expressing self; "indirect repair";

participation in conversation; symptoms
coping strategies, 166–67; acceptance and ownership, 171; altruism, 175; anticipatory adaptation, 176; assessment process, 19–20; after diagnosis, 36, 37–38; disclosure, 171–72; fluidity, 174; holistic practices, 176; innovative techniques and technology, 173–74; interventions for caregivers, 177, 178–79, 180–82; past activities, connection with, 174–75; positive attitude and self-acceptance, 172; proactive stance, 175–76; religion and spirituality as, 155; role relinquishment and replacement, 172–73; spirituality, 176–77; stress and coping model, 165–66
counseling, xxxiv–xxxv. *See also* intervention strategies
cultural considerations for support group, 237–38

Davis, Robert, 154, 161
day care center: activity evaluation, 193–95; art therapy at, 248–54, 258–61; benefits of attending, 195–96; choice and, 208; data on communication gathered at, 137–39; Dementia Care Mapping findings and, 196–97; family view of, 192–93; greetings at, 147; interviews at, 190–91; Leith area of Scotland, 189–90; member recommendations for, 197–99; personal identity, social selves, and, 105–7; reasons for attending, 191–92; social relationships and, 208; Stirling area of Scotland, 188–89. *See also* volunteerism
"Decade of the Brain," xv
demented, meaning of, xxxvi–xxxvii
dementia, description and causes of, xiv
Dementia Care Mapping (DCM) tool, 196–97, 205

denial, 37, 238

dependency, xxxii

depression: dependency and, xxxii; diagnosis and, xxvi, 30, 34–36, 42; in family, 36; journaling and, xxxiv; quality of life and, 83; support group and, 236–37

diagnosis: acceptance of, 157–58, 159, 171; accuracy of, xiii, 5; coping strategies after, 36, 37–38; depression, after, xxvi, 30, 34–36, 42; disclosure of, 23, 123–25, 171–72, 236; neuropsychological assessment, 6–7; primary health care and, 5–6; reacting to, 33–34, 43

direct questioning of person with Alzheimer's disease, 43, 44

disclosure of diagnosis, 23, 123–25, 171–72, 236

drug research, xxxii–xxxiii, 214

"excess disability," 89–90, 109

expressing self, difficulty with, 63–64. See also conversation strategies; symptoms

facilitator for support group, 237, 238–39, 240, 242

family: day care center evaluation by, 192–93; depression in, 36; fear or recognition of being burden for, 116–18; intervention strategies for, 177, 178–79; loss of autonomy and, 120; medical care, role in, 39–40; mutual adjustments in, 121–22; participation in research by, 10–11; receiving and reacting to diagnosis, 34; role changes, 4, 17–18, 119–20; strategic resistance and, 21; support group and, 230–32, 240; as survival, 122–23. See also caregiver

Fazio, Sam, xvii

fear: of being a burden, 116–18, 211–12;

of losing one's way, 55–58, 70–71, 219; memory failure and, 55

forgetting, 52–55. See also memory; memory clinics; symptoms

friendly visitor, 189, 199–204

frustration: with medical experience, 38–41, 42–43; with memory, 54–55; prayer and, 157, 159

general practitioner (GP). See primary health care

gene therapy, 42

Goldsmith, Malcolm, xvi–xvii

grief, 241–42, 270

grounded theory, 14. See also qualitative research

health care provider: intervention strategies for, 177, 180–82. See also primary health care

help: receiving, 71–72; seeking, 14–22

Henderson, Cary, 112, 116, 117, 122, 126, 127

holistic practices, 176

hope: diagnosis, prognosis, and, 42; instillation of, xxv, 24; spirituality and, 154–55, 160–61

humor, comments on, 146, 236–37

identity. See personal identity; selfhood

immediacy in interview, 205

Index for Managing Memory Loss, 166–67

"indirect repair," 90

information seeking, 37–38

insight. See awareness of symptoms

intervention strategies: art materials, 266; communication, 71, 89–90, 147–48; family, 177, 178–79; health care provider, 177, 180–82; life-story work, 209–79; lived experience and, 70–72; nursing home, 278–81; quality of life, 83; spirituality and religion,

intervention strategies (*cont.*)
    maintaining connections to, 162–63;
    support services, 126–28, 129
interview approach: direct questioning,
    43, 44; ethical and practical consider-
    ations and, 204–7; researcher bias
    and, 169–70; semistructured, 190–
    91; unstructured, 11. *See also* qualita-
    tive research
isolation and withdrawal, 125–28, 192,
    215

journey metaphor, xiv

King's Fund Centre, 22–23
Kitwood, Tom: Bradford Dementia
    Group and, xv–xvi; Dementia Care
    Mapping (DCM) tool, 196–97, 205;
    paradigm shift and, xvi, xviii; person-
    centered care and, xviii, 113, 153;
    qualitative methods and, xix; on
    well-being, 130, 214, 223
Korsakoff's syndrome, 89
Kuhn, Daniel, xvii

language. *See* communication; conversa-
    tion strategies
lessons learned, overview of: clinical im-
    plications, xxv–xxvi; general insights,
    xxv; research recommendations,
    xxvi–xxvii
level of care, transition to different, 220,
    225–26, 240–42, 278
life-story work, 209, 279
"listening with the third ear" (atten-
    tively), 147–48
lived experience: Bradford Dementia
    Group and, xv–xvi; "Conversations
    don't always fall into place" theme,
    62–66; "Everything is more difficult"
    theme, 58–62; expressed in poetry,
    272, 273, 274, 275–78; fog in head,
    xxxi–xxxii; "I can't remember"

theme, 52–55; "I'm sort of oblivious"
    theme, 66–69; insights about, 143–
    45; intervention strategies and, 70–
    72; "I worry about getting lost"
    theme, 55–58; overview of, xiv;
    symptoms, xxxi–xxxii, 49–50; unre-
    ality, sense of, xxxi–xxxii. *See also* art
    therapy; coping strategies; meaningful
    communication; relationships; spiri-
    tuality and religion
losing one's way, worries about, 55–58,
    70–71, 219
loss: of access to friends and family, 273;
    with age, 270; of autonomy, 120,
    275–77; cumulative effects of, 277–
    78; of place, 272–73; of privacy, 274–
    75; of role, 274, 275; of things, 59–
    60; viewing persons with Alzheimer's
    disease in terms of, 165, 217–18, 225
love, 130–31

"malignant social psychology," 89
marriage, effects on, 113–14, 121
meaning: of disabling illness, 33; search
    for, 212–13, 214; volunteerism and,
    222–23. *See also* spirituality and reli-
    gion
meaningful communication: on building
    sense of community, 147; on compas-
    sion and empathy, 141–42; data on,
    137–39; definition of, 134; examples
    of, 139–40; on humor, 146; on jour-
    ney of aging, 145–46; on living with
    Alzheimer's disease, 143–45; sources
    of information on, 135–37; on spiri-
    tuality, religion, and humanity, 140–
    41
medical experience: depression, anger,
    and coping, 34–38; identification of
    issues and concerns, 30–32; overview
    of, 29–30; receiving and reacting to
    diagnosis, 33–34; as unsatisfactory or
    frustrating, 38–41, 42–43

medical model: assessment and, 8, 135–36; holistic model compared to, 148; as paradigm, xv

memory: forgetting and, 52–55; senses and, 153–54; support group participation and, 238–39. *See also* symptoms

memory clinics, 6–8, 9–10, 23

mental health needs: "listening with the third ear" (attentively), 147–48; well-being, 97, 214, 223–24. *See also* coping strategies; depression; support groups

methodology, xvii–xix. *See also* qualitative research; research

Mini-Mental State Examination (MMSE), 6, 78

mood state instrument, 31–32

musical expression, 38, 153, 157

mutual adjustments, 121–22

National Institute on Aging, research funded by, xv

neuropsychological assessment: best practice for, 6–7; examples of, 95, 105–6; individual variability and, 103–4, 108–9; overview of, 135–36; room design for, 17. *See also* assessment experience

nursing home: interacting with residents of, 271; intervention strategies for, 278–81; loss and, 270, 272–78; move to, 271–72

paradigm shift, xvi, xviii. *See also* Kitwood, Tom

participant-observer approach, 138

participation in conversation, difficulty with, 64–66. *See also* conversation strategies

personal empowerment, 22–23

personal identity, 91–92, 95–100, 102, 107

person-centered care: assessment and, 8–9; attachments and, 113; communication and, 148–49; coping strategies and, 177, 179, 182; programs and, 225; spiritual care and, 153

person's perspective. *See* assessment experience; lived experience; medical experience

pet, relationship with, 116

physician-person dyad, xxv, 39–40, 42

positive attitude, 172

prayer, 157, 159

primary health care: diagnosis and, 5–6; first contact with, 14–15; referral to memory clinic, 15–16, 17–18; as unsatisfactory or frustrating, 38–41, 42–43

proactive stance, taking, 175–76

prosopagnosia, 121–22

proxy view, 207

psychometric assessment, 135–36

qualitative research: descriptive study, 167–70; limitations of, 168; purpose of, xix; thematic analysis, 32. *See also* methodology; research

Quality of Life–Alzheimer's disease (QOL–Alzheimer's disease), 77–81

quality of life (QOL): Alzheimer's disease and, 76–77; assessment of, xviii, 77–81; case examples, 81–82; intervention strategies for improving, 83; overview of, 75; volunteerism and, 213

quantitative research, xviii

Reagan, Ronald, 117, 211

relationships: barriers to communication theme, 115; devaluation theme, 115–16; disclosure and, 23, 123–25, 171–72, 236; environment and, 129–30; establishing connections, 126–28; family as survival, 122–23; fear or

relationships (*cont.*)
  recognition of being burden, 116–18;
    inquiry about, 128–29; loss of auton-
    omy, 120; love and, 130–31; mutual
    adjustment in, 121–22; overview of,
    112–14; primacy of, 112–14; re-
    sponses from others, 124–25; role
    changes, 119–20; withdrawal and iso-
    lation, 125–28, 192, 215
"relative well-being," 97
religion. *See* spirituality and religion
research: focus group interviews, 30–31;
    participation in, xxxii–xxxiii, xxxv,
    214; qualitative, xix, 132, 167–70;
    quantitative, xviii; recommendations
    for, xxvi–xxvii; in United Kingdom,
    xv–xvi; in United States, xv. *See also*
    methodology; qualitative research
resilience. *See* coping strategies
role changes, 119–20, 172–73, 274, 275
routine, establishing, xxxv–xxxvi, xxxvii

Sabat, Steven, xvii
seeking help: acknowledging challenge,
    14–16; considering future options,
    20–22; playing game, 16–20
self-acceptance, 172
selfhood: Alzheimer's disease and, 90–
    91; art therapy and, 246–47; case ex-
    amples, 94–95; Dr. M case example,
    95–105; memory and, 89; Mrs. D
    case example, 105–9. *See also* per-
    sonal identity; Social Constructionist
    approach to selfhood
self-portraits, 249–52
Seman, Dorothy, xvii
senses: art therapy and, 266–67; memory
    and, 153–54
Snyder, Lisa, xvi–xvii
Social Constructionist approach to self-
    hood: overview of, 91, 104, 109; self
    of mental and physical attributes, 92–
    93, 95–100, 102, 103–4, 106, 107;

self of personal identity, 91–92, 95–
    100, 102, 107; social selves, 93–94,
    99–104, 105–9
social relationships: art therapy and, 247;
    community services and, 207–8; at
    day care center, 194; disclosure and,
    123–25, 171–72; establishing con-
    nections, 126–28; responses from
    others, 124–25; role changes, 172–
    73; spirituality and, 159; support
    group and, 236–37; withdrawal and
    isolation, 125–28. *See also* befriend-
    ing service; volunteerism
special care unit, art therapy at, 254–58
spirituality and religion: Alzheimer's dis-
    ease and, 150–51; Cleveland com-
    munity dialogue, 155–60; comments
    about, 140–41; as coping strategies,
    176–77; definitions of, 151; guide-
    lines for maintaining connections,
    162–63; hope and, 160–61; spiritual
    care, 153–54; subjective voice, 154–
    60; theology of Alzheimer's disease,
    151–52
spouse: definition of person with
    Alzheimer's disease by, 106, 107–8;
    effects of Alzheimer's disease on mar-
    riage, 113–14, 121; as support-giver,
    xxxi, xxxii, xxxiii–xxxiv, xxxv,
    xxxvi. *See also* caregiver; family
Stansell, Jane, xvii
stereotype of average or typical person
    with Alzheimer's disease, 104–5,
    108–9
stigma: enacted, 124–25; felt, 123–24
strategic resistance, 19–20, 21
strengths, focus on, and quality of life,
    82. *See also* coping strategies; volun-
    teerism
stress and coping model, 165–66
subjective experience, research on, 166.
    See also assessment experience; lived
    experience; medical experience

suffering, bearing witness to, 72–73

supporter. *See* caregiver

support groups: agitation and, 239; criteria for participation in, 233–34, 241; cultural considerations for, 237–38; denial and, 238; evolution of, 228–29; facilitator for, 237, 238–39, 240, 242; family involvement and, 230–32; future of, 242–43; memory impairment and, 238–39; models for, 232–33; moving on from, 240–42; participation in, xxxiv, 229–30; perception of, 100–103, 236–37; themes and interactions, 234–36; volunteerism and, 224

support groups, "curative" factors of, 229

support services, 126–28, 129

symptoms: "Conversations don't always fall into place" theme, 62–66; "Everything is more difficult" theme, 58–62; "I can't remember" theme, 52–55; "I'm sort of oblivious" theme, 66–69; "I worry about getting lost" theme, 55–58; living with, 69–70; overview of, 75, 88–89; perception of, 49–50. *See also* awareness of symptoms; conversation strategies; memory

technology, use of, 173–74

thematic analysis, 32, 52, 170–71

theology of Alzheimer's disease, 151–52

therapy, xxxiv–xxxv. *See also* intervention strategies

transition to different level of care, 220, 225–26, 240–42, 278

volunteerism: "being who I am" theme, 221–22; as coping strategy, 174–75; description of program, 216–19; feeling competent theme, 223; helping others theme, 222; importance of, 212; limitations to participation, 219–20; meaning and purpose theme, 222–23; older adults and, 212–13; personal support system for, 218–19; person with Alzheimer's disease and, 214–15; philosophy of program, 215–16; recommendations for, 224–26; responses of participants, 220–21; staff for program, 226; well-being and, 214, 223–24. *See also* altruism

well-being, 97, 214, 223–24

withdrawal and isolation, 125–28, 192, 215

Yale, Robyn, xvi–xvii